Natural Strategies for Cancer Patients

NATURAL STRATEGIES FOR CANCER PATIENTS

RUSSELL L. BLAYLOCK, M.D.

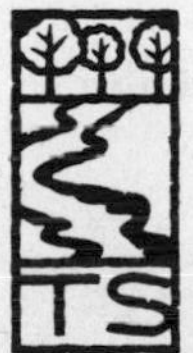

TWIN STREAMS
Kensington Publishing Corp.
http://www.kensingtonbooks.com

This book presents information based upon the research and personal experiences of the author. It is not intended to be a substitute for a professional consultation with a physician or other healthcare provider. Neither the publisher nor the author can be held responsible for any adverse effects or consequences resulting from the use of any of the information in this book. They also cannot be held responsible for any errors or omissions in the book. If you have a condition that requires medical advice, the publisher and author urge you to consult a competent healthcare professional.

TWIN STREAMS BOOKS are published by

Kensington Publishing Corp.
850 Third Avenue
New York, NY 10022

All Kensington titles, imprints and distributed lines are available at special quantity discounts for bulk purchases for sales promotion, premiums, fund-raising, educational or institutional use.

Special book excerpts or customized printings can also be created to fit specific needs. For details, write or phone the office of the Kensington Special Sales Manager: Kensington Publishing Corp., 850 Third Avenue, New York, NY 10022. Attn. Special Sales Department. Phone: 1-800-221-2647.

ISBN 0-7582-0221-0

First Trade Printing: October 2003
10 9

Printed in the United States of America

I dedicate this book to the memory of the brave people who fought this terrible disease and lost, and to their families. I also dedicate it to the memory of my mother and father, who taught me the value of wisdom.

Contents

Preface

This book is the result of more than twenty years of nutritional research directed toward improving the results of conventional cancer treatments and of the treatment of cancer by nutrition alone. I became interested in cancer treatment while in medical school, during which time I explored one of the newer methods of treatment using the body's own immune system. It was during this study that I discovered the critical importance of nutrition in immune function.

My goal has been to supply cancer patients, and their families, with the latest in the nutritional methods to boost the immune system and fight cancer. In addition, I offer important nutritional ways to prevent many of the complications associated with the conventional treatments. Most cancer patients are aware that these complications, such as nausea, loss of appetite, and fatigue, can lead to severe depression and a sense of hopelessness. Recent research emphasizes the importance of the cancer patient's mood in overcoming the disease.

Chapter 1 presents an overview of nutrition and how simple things such as food preparation can make a critical difference in the ability to overcome this dreaded disease. It also discusses the importance of choosing quality nutritional supplements, the special cancer killers contained in fruits and vegetables, and how nutrients interact to strengthen or reduce the cancer-controlling properties of foods and supplements.

Chapter 2 reviews what we now know about how cells become cancers and how cancer cells differ from normal cells. Armed with this knowledge, the reader is better able to understand the vital role played by nutrition in controlling and even eliminating cancer. To many, the idea that nutrition could play such a powerful role in cancer control seems simplistic. This chapter will demonstrate how complex the process really is and how nutrition, by controlling the wayward biochemistry of cancer cells, can often halt the cancer process.

Chapters 3 and 4 review two of the mainstays of conventional cancer treatment—chemotherapy and radiation therapy—and discuss how they can either benefit or, in many cases, actually do great harm. Included are ways to reduce the harm, while at the same time increasing the effectiveness of both treatments. Specific recommendations are offered for each of the complications caused by the treatments.

Of critical importance to anyone facing cancer is the issue of nutrition possibly interfering with conventional treatments. Many oncologists warn their patients not to take antioxidant vitamins due to an unfounded fear that these vitamins will interfere with the treatments. This fear is based on the idea that chemotherapy and radiation treatments both kill cancer cells by generating large numbers of destructive free radicals. In Chapter 5, I demonstrate the fallacy in this thinking and show that, in fact, just the opposite is true—that specific nutritional treatments actually make conventional treatments much more effective.

The remaining three chapters go into detail concerning how what you eat can make the difference between treatment failure and success. This includes a discussion of the effects of certain types of fats and proteins on cancer growth and how many of these cancer-promoting foods are being recommended by oncologists and oncology dietitians. In Chapter 6, I explain exactly how special nutrients act to inhibit cancer growth and can turn off the genes responsible for cancer spread and invasion.

The special role played by the immune system in controlling cancer was first recognized more than forty years ago. Recent studies have not only confirmed these early observations but have fine-tuned the treatment so that it is much more effective. We have also learned that nutrition plays a major role in immune function, especially in that part of the immune system that combats cancer. In fact, even single-nutrient deficiencies can cause profound immune malfunction. In Chapter 7, I discuss some of the more powerful ways to enhance the cancer-fighting portions of the immune system.

Finally, in Chapter 8, I tie all of this information together. I also discuss how exposure to commonly found additives can sabotage treatment. For example, we know that fluoride can increase tumor growth by 25 percent, yet few oncologists warn their patients to avoid fluoride. Mercury, monosodium glutamate (MSG), aspartame, and other toxic substances can also increase cancer incidence, interfere with cancer treatments, and lead to treatment failures.

At the end of the book, I provide a list of recommended suppliers of quality supplements as well as of diagnostic laboratories capable of performing the tests recommended in the book. I also supply a recommended reading list that offers some of the more helpful material for cancer patients.

While I have tried to include most of the information needed by cancer patients, I have had to limit some topics because of space. In addition, I never intended to supply information concerning specific chemotherapy drugs or drug protocols in this book. The book will provide readers with all of the critical information needed to maximize treatment effectiveness, reduce or prevent the complications associated with conventional treatments, and make a successful outcome more likely. The vast majority of patients following these recommendations will feel better and will be more energetic as well.

Acknowledgments

I would like to thank my beautiful wife, Diane, for her tireless work in making this book possible. Without her support, careful reading of the text, and suggestions for important changes, it would not have been possible. I also thank my grandson, Gabriel, for keeping me entertained during the long hours of research and writing.

Special thanks go to Mr. Lee Heiman for his valuable input both as a person who understands the concerns of cancer patients searching for information and as a person looking for ways to enhance the effectiveness of their treatments. I also thank Mrs. Elaine Will Sparber, senior editor at Kensington Publishing, for her valuable assistance in preparing the manuscript for this book.

Finally, I would like to thank the staff of the American Nutraceutical Association for providing me with access to many valuable studies used in writing this book.

Introduction

Cancer is probably one of the most horrifying words in the English language. We have been conditioned to associate it with a slow, gruesome death. When I was a medical student many years ago, my professors emphasized that we should not use the word *cancer* in front of patients. It would be too frightening. Instead, they said, we were to use the terms *neoplasm* or *growth*.

During the past thirty years of treating cancer patients, I have observed that often the treatment is worse than the cancer. This is especially so with childhood cancers involving the brain because the few children who survive their cancers are left severely impaired neurologically and cognitively. This loss of intellectual function is a direct result of the treatment.

When I point this out to my radiotherapist and oncology colleagues, they retort, "Sure, but it's better than being dead." The problem with this way of thinking is the assumption that there is no third way. This book describes that third way.

Today, more and more patients are asking their doctors tough questions and demanding straight answers. They expect their doctors to be well informed about all of the newer techniques and treatments, including the alternative medical treatments. Many doctors resent these intrusions into their world and react angrily, or even refuse to treat such bold patients.

Personally, I think this change is good for medicine. Patients should be involved in their own care. I have always enjoyed knowledgeable patients and families, since it makes it much easier to discuss the disease with them and explain the treatment options. Despite this change in attitudes, however, a minority of patients remain passive and just follow everything the doctor suggests without question. These are the people in the greatest danger, since they are attempting to weave their way though a very dangerous minefield.

This book is about a revolution in our understanding of cancer prevention and especially its treatment. The field of cancer treatment is shrouded in a series of myths that are unquestionably harmful to the cancer patient. For example, we have known since 1932 that the most common cause of death among cancer patients is starvation. When I first learned this fact, I was shocked and puzzled. If starvation is the leading cause of death among cancer patients, why don't we just feed them? After all, we have at our disposal numerous ways to supply nutrients to cancer patients, even to those who cannot swallow. Tube feedings and intravenous infusions of high-powered nutrition are commonly used in other conditions.

When I was still a green medical student, I posed this question to one of our prominent oncologists. His terse and condescending reply was, "You cannot give cancer patients enhanced nutritional feedings; it will make their cancer grow faster." At first this made sense. The tumor, after all, uses the same fuel as the rest of the body. Yet, rather than accept the good professor's word for it, I explored the medical literature in a vain attempt to find scientific proof that this did indeed occur. I have continued my search for answers concerning cancer and nutrition over the past thirty years. This book is the result of that search.

What I discovered was that, even today, little evidence exists that feeding cancer patients increases the growth rate of their tumors. Recently, I reviewed this topic in an article appearing in the *Journal of the American Nutraceutical Association*. This up-to-date review of the scientific literature confirmed my earlier findings. In fact, there is considerable evidence that well-nourished cancer patients actually live longer than undernourished ones.

The second myth circulating among oncologists is that the cancer patient must avoid taking antioxidants because these nutrients might interfere with the conventional treatment. This fear is based purely on hypothetical grounds and not science. Oncologists base this belief on the idea that their treatments—chemotherapy and radiation therapy—kill cancers by inducing large amounts of free radicals within the cancer cells. Antioxidants, logically, would block the killing power of the treatments. Often, what seems to be logic fails in biology. This is because our knowledge of cancer is still incomplete and logic depends on known variables.

I have been treating cancer patients with nutritional supplementation for the past thirty years and have never seen a single case of tumor-growth acceleration or interference with conventional treatments. Yet, there are a growing number of scientific studies demonstrating that antioxidants can actually increase the killing of cancer cells.

In this book you will learn about startling findings concerning the use of plant extracts, minerals, and vitamins against cancer. The war on cancer, while not yielding a cure for this horrible malady, has opened up a whole new world of understanding concerning how normal cells function and how cancer cells differ. For the first time we are beginning to understand what we were told in the Old Testament more than 2,000 years ago—that is, that fruits and vegetables bring us good health.

Numerous epidemiological studies have shown that people who eat a lot of fruits and vegetables have much lower cancer rates than those who eat few or none. Until now, we really didn't understand why this is so. Using sophisticated instruments that can peer deep into the interior of cells, scientists have now learned that various components of plants, including vitamins and minerals, can affect cancer cells in such a way as to cause them to stop growing or even die. What is even more exciting is that these same nutrients not only fail to harm normal cells, but protect them against the harmful effects of chemotherapy and radiation. This has given us something for which the cancer specialists have always been searching: a treatment that can differentiate between normal cells and cancer cells.

The story gets even more exciting. We now know that not only will antioxidants and special plant-derived chemicals not interfere with cancer treatments, but they may actually enhance the effectiveness of these treatments against cancer. For example, a recent study using seven different chemotherapy agents found that when two vitamins were added to the mixtures of chemotherapy agents, the agents' effectiveness against tumors was greatly enhanced. Other studies have shown that certain plant chemicals called flavonoids, especially when combined with vitamins, not only enhance a chemotherapy agent's killing power against cancer, but also prevent the most serious side effects associated with such treatments.

One chemotherapy agent, cisplatin, is associated with serious side effects to the kidneys and nervous system. Quercetin, a common flavonoid found in apples, onions, and teas, dramatically reduces cisplatin's complications while enhancing its effectiveness against cancer. Even alone, quercetin has been shown to enhance the spontaneous death of malignant cells in certain types of cancer.

We now know that cancer cells hijack many of the normal cell's biochemical mechanisms so that the new cancer cell can grow and spread. Once the cancer cell is cut free of its restraints, its genes can turn on numerous enzymes and growth factors that enable it to expand, invade surrounding tissues, and eventually spread throughout the body. Chemotherapy agents, in general, are directed against only a few of the cancer cell's mechanisms. Plant chemicals and other phytonutrients, on the other hand, are directed against virtually all of these critical cellular mechanisms.

Many flavonoids, and some vitamins, can also inhibit enzymes that play a vital role in the tumor invasion of surrounding tissues. Still other plant chemicals and certain vitamins can significantly boost the immune system, especially the cells that normally attack cancers.

All of the flavonoids found to suppress or even destroy cancer cells can be found in commonly eaten fruits and vegetables. They are especially abundant in certain vegetables often referred to as cruciferous vegetables, such as cauliflower, Brussels sprouts, and broccoli.

It is now evident that these plant chemicals, vitamins, and minerals can attack cancer cells at all levels, but at the same time have no harmful effect on normal cells. In fact, they powerfully protect normal cells from becoming cancer cells. This not only is important in preventing cancer from forming in the first place, but is especially important in preventing secondary cancers from being created by the chemotherapy and radiation treatments themselves. Many people are not aware that both chemotherapy and radiation therapy are highly carcinogenic in their own right.

Estimates indicate that 350,000 people a year undergo in-hospital chemotherapy treatments. Of these, 2 to 5 percent die as a direct result of the toxicity of the treatment itself. This means that between 7,000 and 17,500 cancer patients die from their treatments alone and not from the cancer itself. One study found that 21 percent of patients receiving very high-dose chemotherapy die as a complication of the treatment.

One thing rarely discussed with patients is that mortality from these conventional treatments depends on the nutritional status of the patient at the time the treatment begins. For instance, in one experiment, 30 percent of animals given comparable doses of the commonly used chemotherapy agent cyclophosphamide died as a direct result of the toxicity of the drug. When the animals were given either vitamin A or beta-carotene supplementation, none died. It is obvious that many cancer patients are too weak from chronic malnutrition to withstand such toxic treatments, yet nothing is done to strengthen their bodies nutritionally because of the unfounded fear held by oncologists.

In this book, I not only explain the mechanism of this protection of normal cells and the enhanced killing of cancer cells, but also outline practical ways to apply this knowledge to individual patients. This includes a discussion of the factors that increase the likelihood of a good outcome versus a poor outcome, such as diet and a specially designed supplementation program.

Many patients undergoing chemotherapy or radiation treatments experience significant complications. The specific complications vary with the type of drug used or the dose and site of the radiation treatment, but can be quite severe and incapacitating. Radiation of the head and neck, for example, can result in dry mouth, ulcerations, and difficulty swallowing. Radiation of the abdominal region can cause diarrhea and poor absorption of foods, while exposure to the pelvis can result in bladder irritation, bleeding, and rectal problems. Chemotherapy can cause fatigue, mouth sores, poor absorption of food, diarrhea, suppression of bone marrow, increased infections, and liver injury. Virtually all of these complications can be either eliminated or reduced by the use of special nutritional supplements and dietary changes.

Treatment-induced malabsorption is fairly common following chemotherapy and radiation, and can result in severe malnutrition. Malnutrition in the cancer patient, especially while the patient is undergoing chemotherapy or radiation therapy, greatly increases the risk of complications and death.

We now have overwhelming evidence that nutrition, when carefully designed by someone versed in the nutritional sciences, can eliminate most of the toxic side effects of the conventional treatments, can enhance their effectiveness, and can protect the rest of the body from serious damage by the treatments. For people wishing to avoid chemotherapy and radiation treatments altogether, I explain specific programs for enhancing the body's natural defense mechanisms and ways to inhibit cancer growth using nutraceuticals.

1

Fighting Cancer with Nutrition

We have known for more than a century that people who eat a diet consisting mostly of fruits and vegetables have a cancer rate much lower than those consuming few of these healthy foods. Only recently have we begun to understand the scientific basis of this protection, however. New techniques for measuring biochemical events on a molecular level have allowed us to map out the many ways the components of fruits and vegetables inhibit cancer formation.

Even more exciting is the discovery that many of the chemicals found in edible plants can turn cancer cells into normal cells, meaning that food components may indeed be used to reverse cancer itself. In addition, these same plant chemicals can reduce the complications associated with the conventional cancer treatments and enhance, sometimes dramatically, the effectiveness of these treatments.

NUTRITION IN CANCER PREVENTION AND TREATMENT

The ability of nutrition to prevent the occurrence of cancer is now beyond dispute. In a paper appearing in the *Journal of the American Dietetic Association*, Dr. K. A. Steinmetz and his coworkers found by reviewing 206 of the best human cancer surveys and 22 animal studies that of all the dietary factors considered in relation to reducing cancer development, at all of its stages, the most important was the intake of fruits and vegetables.[1]

In fact, over all, the cancer rates were reduced 50 percent in the people who ate the most fruits and vegetables, with the greatest reduction being in cancers of the esophagus, oral cavity, larynx, pancreas, stomach, colon, rectum, bladder, cervix, ovary, endometrium, and breast. Even better protection was seen with some types of cancer.

The greatest fall in cancer rates in humans has been with cancer of the stomach, attributed almost solely to a higher intake of vitamin C–containing foods. To better appreciate the power of phytochemicals in foods in preventing cancer, let us look at a study done in Japan. It was found that people eating the most yellow-green vegetables had a stomach cancer incidence 65 percent lower than those eating significantly fewer of these vegetables. If that is not impressive enough, another study found that persons eating citrus fruits just twice a month or less had a sixteen-times higher risk of developing stomach cancer than those eating fruits at least once a week or more.

Today we hear a lot about cancer of the pancreas. It took the lives of President Jimmy Carter's sister and actor Michael Landon, as well as of 28,200 people in the year 2000 alone. It has a mortality rate of more than 90 percent. Yet, its occurrence appears to be strongly related to our diet. In one study, it was found that people who ate no vegetables had a fourfold higher risk of developing pancreatic cancer than those who ate five or more servings of vegetables. Reducing the pancreatic cancer risk depended mostly on eating vegetables and fruits high in beta-carotene and especially lycopene, the red pigment in tomatoes, pink grapefruit, and watermelon.[2]

This same red pigment appears to play a leading role in preventing prostate cancer, with the risk being lowered 35 to 45 percent in those eating a lot of such fruits and vegetables.[3] Vitamin E, especially when combined with selenium, also dramatically reduces the risk of this cancer.

While we are learning more about how these nutrients inhibit cancer, something even more exciting is occurring in the world of science. We are now finding that the very same nutrients can be used to inhibit the growth, invasion, and metastasis of cancers that already exist, and that when we combine these nutrients with conventional cancer treatments, such as radiation therapy or chemotherapy, the conventional therapies work significantly better. If that were not enough, an increasing number of studies have demonstrated that vitamins, minerals, and other phytonutrients can protect patients from the harmful side effects of these conventional treatments.

Numerous anticancer components are found in foods. A partial list includes:

- Allicin
- Antiestrogens and antiprogestins
- Carotenoids, folate, niacinamide, and vitamins A, D, K, and B_{12}
- Coenzyme Q_{10}
- Ellagic acid
- Fiber
- Flavonoids (some 5,000 have now been identified)
- Glucosinolates
- Glutathione
- Glycolipids and glycoproteins
- Immune-enhancing polysaccharides
- Indole 3 carbinol
- Isothiocyanates
- Magnesium
- Phytates
- Protease inhibitors
- Saponins
- Selenium (principally in an organic form)
- Sterols and sterolins (plant steroids)
- Sulphoraphanes
- Zinc

Most patients dread the effects of chemotherapy and radiation treatments as much as, and sometimes more than, their cancer. This is especially so for patients who already have had to go through several rounds of chemotherapy treatments. Today, it is not uncommon for cancer patients to undergo such treatments for as long as a year. Overwhelming fatigue, nausea and/or vomiting, diarrhea, loss of appetite, and severe bone marrow depression can make life seem hopeless and, for many, hardly worth living.

To be physically ill every day for months is very difficult. Yet my experience, confirmed now by many studies, has shown that patients do not have to suffer to receive benefit from the conventional treatments. The vast majority of the complications and side effects of the conventional treatments can be avoided by using simple nutritional methods.

While I do recommend many special supplements, the central and most important part of the treatment program is diet. As you shall see throughout this book, diet can mean the difference between success and failure. Many of the phytonutrients I will discuss are not available as separate nutrients, but are obtained by eating selected fruits and vegetables. By combining the two—special supplements and diet—you can supply your body with a very powerful brew of cancer-fighting nutrients.

I always tell my patients that if they try to depend on supplements alone and not change their diet, they will ultimately fail. It is estimated that as many as 70 percent of all cancers are related to the diet. To continue eating the same foods that led to your cancer in the first place is to travel down the road to disaster because, as you shall see, foods often contain extremely powerful cancer-causing and -promoting substances as well. The typical Western diet—high in red meats, bad fats, food additives, and carbohydrates—is a perfect cancer brew. Below we can see the effects that different dietary excesses can have on prostate cancer:

- High red-meat intake—200 percent increased risk
- High caloric intake—190 percent increased risk
- High dessert intake—180 percent increased risk

This brew not only causes cancer, but can promote the growth of existing cancers as well. This is especially true of fats. Certain fats, called omega-6 fatty acids, not only stimulate cancer growth, but also powerfully suppress the immune system at the same time. I tell my patients that eating these fats is like adding fertilizer to crab grass. Throughout the book I will describe other cancer fertilizers.

Another problem I see when discussing diet changes with my patients is what most people consider eating lots of fruits and vegetables to be. To many, it means eating their favorite vegetable or fruit. If they like green beans and bananas and eat them several times a day, they consider this to be eating a lot of fruits and vegetables. The beans often come from a can and have very little nutrition left plus have high levels of toxic metals. And the bananas, while having some important nutrients, are very high in sugar, a cancer growth–promoting nutrient. We see that regular consumption of these foods and a high total caloric intake dramatically increases men's risk of prostate cancer. Additional risk factors include milk consumption and a low intake of the omega-3 oils combined with a high intake of the omega-6 oils.

When I analyze most of my patients' diets, I find that the majority do not eat even two servings of fruits and vegetables a day. Most studies confirm this observation. For example, one survey found that Americans eat five or more servings of fruits and vegetables less than 25 percent of the time. The statistics are even worse for children.

In terms of health benefits (mainly in terms of antioxidants), eating fewer than five servings of fruits and vegetables a day does very little good. The health benefits begin at five servings, and for people below the age of fifty, they reach a maximum at ten servings. For those over the age of fifty, adding two additional servings—that is, consuming a total of twelve servings a day—provides the maximum health benefits. So, up to a limit, we gain greater benefit by eating more fruits and vegetables.

Several studies have shown that eating large amounts of fruits and vegetables, especially vegetables, not only retards the growth of cancers, but can convert very aggressive cancers into much more benign tumors.[4] This is a remarkable finding. In the past, we thought that once a cancer formed, its prognosis was always in one direction: Aggressive cancers stayed aggressive and less aggressive cancers could become more aggressive, but never the reverse. Newer studies are even showing, at least experimentally, that some cancer cells can be changed into normal cells using specific nutrients. So, instead of directing all our efforts into figuring out how to kill cancer cells without harming normal cells, we can simply change cancer cells back to normal cells.

THE IMPORTANCE OF UNDERSTANDING THE CANCER PROCESS

In the past, before we understood why nutrition works, most of our information was based on anecdotal stories (case histories), studies of large populations of people (epidemiological studies), and word of mouth from those utilizing nutritional treatments outside the medial establishment. This presented two major problems. First, physicians hesitated to use nutrition because little proof or explanation existed for its mechanism of action. Second, cancer patients were often afraid to rely on a treatment method that was not endorsed by the scientific community.

Despite the tens of billions of dollars spent on the war on cancer, we have not found a cure for the disease, but we have learned a lot about the cancer process and how cancer cells differ from normal cells. It is this basic knowledge that elucidated for us what many early practioners of alternative medicine knew all along: something in plants, both as foods and as herbs, has a beneficial effect in suppressing cancer growth.

Chapter 2 of this book goes into more detail about how cells become cancers, what causes this transformation, and why some people are more at risk than others. I would suggest that you read the chapter for its content and not try to memorize all of the technical terms, since they are not important to your understanding. If you find the chapter too technical, I suggest you skip over it and move deeper into the book. I include the chapter because many cancer patients spend an inordinate amount of time exploring all the aspects of their disease and develop a sophistication that allows them to better understand the intricacies of the science.

It should also be appreciated that much of the scientific work was done in an experimental setting. While thousands of cancer patients have been treated successfully with nutritional treatments, few carefully controlled studies of these large populations of patients have been properly done. This is because such studies are very expensive and no one, until recently, has taken an interest in funding them. Recently, the National Institutes of Health (NIH) has begun several studies of the nutritional treatment of cancers in large numbers of people. It will be several more years before the final results of these studies appear.

For the cancer patient, waiting for the results of academic studies is not an option. I have used nutritional methods for at least twenty-four years, more so in the last five years, and I have seen undeniable benefits—and no harm—in my patients. There is no question that the patients using these methods tolerate their treatments better and have far fewer complications. They also respond much better to their conventional treatments.

As I will show in the following chapters, selected nutritional supplements affect the cancer cell at multiple steps in its metabolism in such a way as to significantly interfere with its ability to survive. They do this without interfering with the effectiveness of chemotherapy or radiation therapy. By using different ways to kill and suppress cancer cells, nutrition, in fact, enhances the effectiveness of the conventional treatments.

To kill cancer cells, or to at least force them into a dormant state, every mechanism on which the cancer cell depends must be interfered with. Nutritional supplements do this more effectively than either chemotherapy or radiation treatments, and with little or no effect on normal cells, except to make them stronger.

Changing your diet is a very difficult thing to do, especially if the changes are drastic. Most of us are so accustomed to eating foods that are full of artificial flavors, very sweet, or creamy in texture that eating foods without these qualities becomes a chore. Dietary compliance is the most difficult problem I face in treating cancer patients. This is especially so for the patients having the worst diets. For example, a person who lives for his barbecued ribs, french fries, and soft drinks will have great difficulty switching to a plate full of fresh raw vegetables, fruits, and pure water.

If understanding why nutrition is so important does nothing else, it at least helps cancer patients to stick to the new diet. The more you understand the mechanisms by which phytochemicals inhibit cancer growth and spread, the more you will appreciate why even minor variations in your diet can have significant effects on your cancer. There is serious question as to whether cancers are ever completely eradicated. If they are not, then sticking to the diet becomes even more important, since the dormant cancer can be reactivated by a bad diet.

The longer you adhere to the diet, the easier it will be for you to follow. Tastes change with time. People on low-salt diets find normally salted foods far too salty. The same is true for low-sugar diets: people on low-sugar diets soon find foods and drinks containing sugar to taste too sweet. This readjustment process of the taste buds allows us to conform to a diet we previously thought would be unbearable. It's all what we get used to.

Supplements Versus Foods

Many health practitioners who treat cancer with alternative methods insist that no supplements are needed, only pure, healthy foods, while others disagree and promote the use of supplements. Personally, I see a third way: a program based principally on dietary changes and whole foods plus the use of specially selected supplements that have shown particular activity against cancer.

My selection of supplements is based on hard science and numerous clinical studies, as well as in my own personal experience. For example, we now know that the anticancer activity of the different forms of vitamin E varies considerably. Some forms of vitamin E, such as d- or dl-alpha-tocopheryl acetate, have very little anticancer activity, are poorly absorbed, and may interfere with other nutrients, while the d-alpha-tocopheryl succinate form of vitamin E has powerful anticancer activity, is well absorbed, and has the greatest antioxidant activity. The same can also be said for synthetic beta-carotene compared to natural forms.

We should also appreciate that we still do not know all the components in edible plants, nor do we understand many of the functions of the food components that have been isolated. By using only extracts of these plants, we may be missing an as-yet-unidentified anticancer nutrient. In addition, the process of extracting the known nutrients could destroy some of the mysterious components.

One of the big mysteries of nutritional cancer treatments is why it takes so many fruits and vegetables in the diet to have any anticancer effect. Ten servings of fruits and vegetables add up to a lot of produce. Closely connected to this mystery is the difference between the cells of animals and the cells of plants. Most of the nutritious components of plants are confined within their cells, which differ from animal cells in that they have tough cell walls surrounding their membranes. Unfortunately, humans do not have enzymes in their digestive tracts to dissolve these cell walls. As a result, we cannot absorb most of the nutrients in plants.

This leaves us with three ways to extract these locked-in nutrients. First, we can mechanically break the cell walls by chewing all our fruits and vegetables until they are fine mush. Unfortunately, most of us chew our fruits and vegetables just a few times and then swallow. Second, we can cook our fruits and vegetables, since the heating process breaks the cell wall down. The disadvantage of this method is that you also destroy some of the nutrients and wash others away. In addition, you neutralize many of the plant enzymes, which have been shown to play a part in the anticancer effects of plants. Finally, we can mechanically break down the cell walls by either juicing our fruits and vegetables or liquefying them in a blender.

I have been impressed by the number of people with advanced, near-terminal cancer who have survived after changing their diet to include blenderized or juiced fruits and vegetables. With what we know now concerning the science behind plant phytochemicals and cancer, it makes a lot of sense. People who juice or blenderize their fruits and vegetables get a much higher concentration of the anticancer chemicals than those who just eat fruits and vegetables. In addition, most of the people who go to this trouble choose fruits and vegetables that are high on the list of the most powerful edible anticancer plants.

As we shall see throughout this book, many phytochemicals have a differential effect in that they protect normal cells from the harmful effects of chemotherapy and radiation treatments while greatly enhancing the effectiveness of the conventional treatments against the cancer.

THE COMPLEXITY OF NUTRITION

Most people outside science think that nutrition is simply a matter of what you eat and that what is important is that you get enough in the way of the basic food groups and calories. In fact, nutrition is much more complex than that. First, we have to understand the purpose of eating. It is not to satisfy our taste buds or to keep our stomachs from growling from hunger, even though many in the industrialized world think this way. Second, we have to understand that the body is a collection of immensely complex chemical reactions—tens of thousands of them.

Our cells and tissues are not simple cellular organisms living together in harmony. They are extremely complex biochemical laboratories engaging in tens of thousands of biochemical reactions every second of our lives. These chemical reactions require special types of substances that must be supplied to our cells for them to function normally. Fortunately, our bodies can adapt to many deficiencies in these chemicals and can even make substitutions. Yet, these deficiencies can cause the cells to work less efficiently, making them highly susceptible to diseases, including cancer.

The nutritional requirements for cells also vary widely, with some cells requiring more of a particular nutrient than other cells. This is because the cells have different functions. For example, the thyroid gland needs a different set of chemicals than does breast tissue.

We have also learned that the distribution of vitamins and their breakdown products varies considerably from tissue to tissue. For example, the female cervix concentrates more vitamin C and folate than does the gallbladder. This should mean that a deficiency in vitamin C and folate will increase a woman's risk of cervical cancer, and that is exactly what we see. Women with very low vitamin C intake can have a cervical cancer risk ten times higher than women who consume more dietary vitamin C.[5]

In some instances, a tissue may require a lot more of a particular nutrient than normal, as for instance in the case of cervical cancer where even normal blood levels of folate are insufficient to prevent the disease. It takes higher intakes of folate to prevent cervical cancer in women at high risk. This is one of the reasons why the recommendations for the vitamins and minerals are constantly being revised upward.

Sometimes a person can be eating a perfectly healthy diet, with lots of fruits and vegetables, low amounts of harmful fats, and little sugar, and still have a high risk of cancer. One reason for this is that unless the nutrients can enter the bloodstream, they do little good. We call this inability to enter the bloodstream malabsorption. Occasionally, malabsorption involves only a single type of nutrient or even a single vitamin or mineral.

So how can we know if we are absorbing our nutrients properly? One way is to have our blood levels of the nutrients measured directly. Several laboratories measure vitamin and mineral blood levels. Yet, even then we may be fooled. Many vitamins are converted from the form found in food into an especially active form required by the cells in the body. For example, the riboflavin from food is converted into riboflavin-5-phosphate in the body, and the pyridoxine (vitamin B_6) from food is converted into pyrodoxal-5-phosphate in the body. The conversion processes for these vitamins require special enzymes, which are often impaired in the elderly, in people undergoing cancer treatments, and in people suffering from a chronic disease.

The Quality of Supplement Products

One question I am frequently asked concerns whether synthetic vitamins or natural vitamins are better. In most cases, the natural vitamin is better, yet some synthetic vitamins are converted into numerous metabolic breakdown products when absorbed and these products can have powerful anticancer effects of their own. This has been shown to be the case with synthetic beta-carotene, which can be converted into numerous other compounds.

A recent study of commonly available forms of synthetic beta-carotene supplements found that many often contain no beta-carotene at all, only the breakdown products of beta-carotene.[6] This doesn't mean that these supplements are ineffective against cancer, since in animal tests these breakdown products were also effective against cancer.

In some instances, vitamins compete for absorption from the gastrointestinal tract. For example, synthetic beta-carotene interferes with the absorption of another very important carotenoid called lutein.[7] Similarly, synthetic vitamin E in high doses can lower the blood levels of beta-carotene. This competition for absorption can have major consequences for the person with cancer. Lutein, for example, is more important in preventing lung cancer and possibly breast cancer than is beta-carotene. In addition, taking beta-carotene from natural sources, such as from the algae *Dunaliella bardawil* or *salina*, results in much higher levels of the carotenoids than does taking synthetic forms of the vitamin.

Another problem with taking synthetic vitamins is that many natural vitamins consist of a number of components, whereas the synthetic forms have only one form. For example, vitamin E is actually composed of eight different fractions (alpha, beta, gamma, and delta tocopherols, and four tocotrienols), with some having more anticancer activity than others. The same is true for the carotenoids. While most people are familiar with beta-carotene, some of the other forms of the carotenoids are significantly more potent against specific cancers. Alpha-carotene, for instance, has been shown to play a more important role in preventing breast cancer, and lutein, beta-cryptoxanthin, and lycopene may be more important in preventing ovarian, prostate, and lung cancers.[8] Astaxanthin, another carotenoid, has been found to strongly inhibit bladder cancer. If you take only synthetic beta-carotene, you will miss all of these powerful anticancer carotenoids.

Even when taking synthetic vitamins, you should always try to use the form that most closely resembles the one found in nature or that has been shown to have a special anticancer effect, such as vitamin E succinate. Following are some guidelines.

Use the ascorbate form of vitamin C and not ascorbic acid. The acid form is more likely to upset your stomach, is poorly absorbed, and must be converted in your body to be used. Taking higher doses of ascorbic acid can cause acid buildup (acidosis) and can increase your risk of osteoporosis. The best forms are magnesium ascorbate and calcium ascorbate. I prefer the former.

Never use vitamin E acetate (which is also called d- or dl-alpha-tocopheryl acetate). This form of vitamin E is poorly absorbed, can cause a loss of carotenes in the liver, does not enter the brain, and has very little, if any, anticancer effect. The most powerful form of vitamin E is vitamin E succinate, which is also known as d-alpha-tocopheryl succinate or dry E. It comes as a white powder in a capsule. As we shall see, this form of vitamin E has the most powerful effect against cancer.

The second-best form of vitamin E for the cancer patient is the natural form, which is also called mixed tocopherols. In most cases, the supplement contains four types of tocopherols: alpha, beta, gamma, and delta. Technically, vitamin E also includes four other types of components, called tocotrienols, which include alpha, beta, gamma, and delta forms. Recent research has shown that the tocotrienols have powerful cancer-inhibiting effects, especially when combined with certain anticancer drugs, such as tamoxifen.

Many vitamin E supplements come in a gelatin capsule mixed with oil. In most cases, this oil is one of the tumor growth–promoting oils, usually soybean oil. This is another reason to take only vitamin E succinate, a dry powder. Unfortunately, no one has produced a vitamin E supplement dissolved in extra virgin olive oil.

Multiple vitamins should be taken only as a powder in a capsule and not as a hard tablet. Many tablets have been shown to contain binders that can prevent the absorption of the vitamins. Binders are like glue, used by manufacturers to keep the tablets from breaking during shipping. The ease with which a tablet can be broken down is of special concern for people who have undergone chemotherapy or radiation, since many have poor digestive abilities.

In general, avoid supplements that contain aspartate, glycine, or amino acid chelates—the so-called chelated vitamins or minerals. While they claim to improve absorption, and many do, these amino acids are excitotoxins. Excitotoxins not only can damage the brain, but some individuals have an extreme sensitivity to them. Granted, they are present in small doses, but for a person with a brain tumor, they might stimulate the tumor to grow faster.

You should also avoid gelatin capsules as much as possible, since gelatin is very high in glutamate, a powerful excitotoxin. In addition, gelatin is a bovine product and therefore carries a risk of mad cow disease.

Beware when buying plant extracts—that is, supplements containing extracts of fruits or vegetables. Many of these supplements contain such low amounts of the extract that you gain little nutritional benefit. This is a problem with vitamin C brands that claim rose hips as an ingredient. In truth, most of these brands have only a trace of rose hips, nowhere near enough to have any benefit, but enough to jack up the price.

Buy only fruit or vegetable extracts that come either as a loose powder or as a powder in a capsule. The label should list the amount of each ingredient. Note that these products require freeze drying or low-temperature drying to preserve the phytochemicals. None of the brands I have examined are complete, and none should be used in place of a multivitamin-and-mineral supplement. Most are also low in magnesium. Do not buy a vegetable supplement that comes as a hard tablet with little flecks of green or red, since most such products are worthless.

Another common problem is supplements that come as a dry powder or tablet, but that are, in fact, absorbed only when dissolved in oil. Unfortunately, the label never tells you this. For instance, coenzyme Q_{10} (CoQ_{10}), a very important anticancer nutrient, is absorbed poorly as a dry powder. It is fat-soluble and best absorbed when dissolved in an oil. One solution is to dissolve the powder in extra virgin olive oil. Just empty the capsule in a tablespoon of oil and take it as you would medicine. It has very little taste.

I have found several supplements in this category. Many of the flavonoids, such as curcumin, quercetin, and hesperidin, are better absorbed in an oil base as well. (At least one manufacturer makes water-soluble forms of quercetin and hesperidin that do not need to be dissolved in oil.) Often, failure to address the solubility issue explains why supplements do not seem to work for some people.

Finally, we must deal with the issues of quality and price. Many people shop for supplements the way they shop for toilet tissue, choosing whichever is the cheapest brand. This is like buying spoiled food to save money. In many cases, the brands with the highest quality cost more, sometimes significantly more. This does not always hold true, however, because occasionally some worthless brands have high prices.

The only way to tell is to take a close look at the manufacturer. Some will hold a pharmaceutical manufacturer's license, which requires the company to pass rigorous standards and meticulous examinations of its manufacturing methods. Others sell their products to university laboratories and therefore must meet certain standards of quality and purity.

While the length of time a company has been in business and its size are major considerations, some smaller, younger companies make very high quality products. Most supplement companies keep records showing the analysis profiles of their supplements. These are available to health food stores and pharmacies. You should ask to look at the analysis of any supplement in question.

Quality is especially important in patients undergoing chemotherapy or radiation treatments because often they have difficulty absorbing nutrients. How a supplement is manufactured makes a great deal of difference. For example, most supplement manufacturers add what is called an excipient to their products. One of the most commonly used is magnesium stearate, which has been shown to reduce nutrient absorption by more than 60 percent, even when used in a capsule. Other excipients are ascorbyl palmitate and stearic acid, both of which cause the same absorption problem.

Supplements can also be coated with a substance to make them easier to swallow. This coating is, in fact, nothing more than shellac, just like the kind used on furniture. Some companies use none of these additives and instead utilize a process that preserves the quality and purity of the product, maximizing absorption.

Herbs are in a special category all their own. Unlike most plants, herbs contain powerful chemicals that have pharmaceutical effects. The amounts of these chemicals in an herb depends on the soil the herb was grown in, the climate of the area, the moisture of the soil, and even the time of day the plant was harvested. When making large batches of herbal supplements, manufacturers must use exacting methods to make sure each capsule has the same amount of active ingredient.

To be sure your herbal supplement has the right amount of the active ingredient, check the label for standardization information. For example, a ginkgo biloba label should say the product is standardized to 24 percent heterosides and 6 percent terpenes. This guarantees that each capsule contains at least these amounts of active ingredients. The best protection is to only buy herbal products that have "Guaranteed Potency Herb" written on the label. This assures you of a very high standard herb. Never buy cheap herbs.

NUTRIENT INTERACTION

This brings us to another important topic: nutrient interaction. Medical science has, for far too long, treated nutrients as just more objects to explore. In their way of thinking, which is very archaic, if you want to know why something works—for example, why fruits and vegetables can reduce the risk of cancer—you simply extract the components found in the highest concentrations and test them. Citrus fruits have a lot of vitamin C, so to the popular way of thinking, you just give test animals and people lots of vitamin C and see if it works. Sometimes it does, sometimes it has no effect, and on rare occasions, it actually increases the growth of cancer.

The problem with this way of thinking is that nutrients do not normally work alone, especially in as complex a biological system as exists in people. To a large part, this is because of the interactions of the biochemical systems, where altering one part of the system may affect a dozen or more other parts of the system. Another important consideration is that the nutrients themselves interact. This is especially true when dealing with anticancer effects.

One of the more powerful interactions between nutrients and anticancer effects is seen with vitamin E and selenium. Several animal studies as well as studies of large populations of women have shown that vitamin E reduces the risk of breast cancer, especially in women at very high risk of the disease. But when you add selenium to the vitamin E, an even greater lowering of the risk is seen.

If we look at whole fruits and vegetables, we notice that vitamins never occur alone. This is very important, since vitamins keep each other from oxidizing. Vitamin C protects vitamin E, beta-carotene protects vitamin C, and so on. Recent studies emphasize the importance of mixing these nutrients in our diet and as supplements.

To emphasize the importance of nutrient interaction, let us look at the Physicians' Health Study, which involved 22,071 doctors, making it one of the largest nutritional studies ever done. The researchers isolated 578 men with prostate cancer in the study group and compared their diets to those of 1,294 controls. They found that the men with the highest blood levels of lycopene, the red pigment in tomatoes, had a dramatically lower incidence of prostate cancer, especially of the very aggressive type; some had as much as a 60 percent lower incidence. Yet, beta-carotene had no effect on the risk of the disease—at least, not in the men with normal levels of lycopene. To the researchers' surprise, beta-carotene did have a major effect on reducing the prostate cancer risk if a man's lycopene level was low. This, once again, emphasizes the interrelationship between nutrients and anticancer effects.

Special Cancer Killers in Plants

While most people think of vitamins as antioxidants and as the major nutritional weapons against cancer, other plant chemicals are, in fact, infinitely more powerful. Of major interest to cancer researchers are the flavonoids, a group of 5,000 very complex chemicals. Like vitamins, they also work best when together. A single vegetable or fruit can contain hundreds of these chemicals. In addition, their anticancer activity is further enhanced by the presence of vitamins.

There is growing evidence that the effectiveness of nutrients when combined is not only additive, but synergistic. An additive effect is two plus two equals four, whereas a synergistic effect is two plus two equals twelve or twenty.

Not only do certain nutrients enhance each other's anticancer activity, they also dramatically enhance the ability of anticancer drugs and radiation to kill cancer cells, as we shall see later.

Not All Foods Are Created the Same

One factor that is rarely considered is the nutritional variation among foods. For example, we often hear that apples are a good food for preventing cancer. Yet, all apples are not the same in terms of cancer-preventing abilities. One of the known anticancer constituents in apples is a chemical called chlorogenic acid, yet the content of chlorogenic acid varies considerably among the different species of apples, with the McIntosh containing a very high level and the Golden Delicious a very low level.

Whether a fruit or vegetable is vine ripened also makes a difference. Many fruits and vegetables found in our local market were shipped across the country. To keep produce from spoiling during shipping, the produce companies pick the plants before they ripen, which means that these fruits and vegetables have lower concentrations of nutrients. Sometimes young sprouts have a greater concentration of a particular beneficial nutrient than the fully matured vegetable. For example, broccoli sprouts have been shown to have as much as 100 times more indole-3-carbinol, a powerful inhibitor of breast cancer, than mature broccoli.[9] Several nutritional companies have taken advantage of this observation by offering numerous types of plant sprouts, such as wheat, rye, and barley.

Not all vegetables and fruits have the same cancer-fighting power. The produce with the greatest anticancer effect are the cruciferous vegetables, which include kale, broccoli, Brussels sprouts, cauliflower, and cabbage.

This is not to say that other vegetables are of no help because beets, parsley, spinach, carrots, and tomatoes have all been shown to have equally powerful anticancer effects. In general, fruits and vegetables with deep colors have the greatest anticancer effectiveness.

Most people are aware that our soil—the sole source of nutrients for plants—is terribly depleted of nutrients. For example, the soil in many areas of the United States is severely depleted of the mineral selenium. People eating vegetables grown in selenium-depleted soil can develop severe selenium deficiencies, thereby greatly increasing their risk for certain cancers, including breast and prostate cancers. Selenium plays a major role in immune system function as well, especially in the immune cells that attack cancer.

Things That Deplete Nutrition

In addition to a poor diet, there are many things we do, such as smoking and taking medications, that can severely affect our nutrition. Smoking has been shown to dramatically lower the level of vitamin C in the tissues. Even secondhand smoke can have this effect. For some as-yet-unexplained reason, smokers cannot improve their vitamin C levels unless they take very high doses of the vitamin every day. To reach normal tissue levels of vitamin C, they need to take a minimum of 500 milligrams daily. In addition, smokers have significantly lowered beta-carotene levels. One study found that flavonoid intake, a reflection of fruit and vegetable consumption, was 21 percent lower in smokers than in nonsmokers. Taken together, these facts may explain why smokers have a much higher incidence of lung cancer (from among all cancers) than nonsmokers. It also means that when smokers begin treatment for cancer, they are less likely to respond well and are more likely to suffer serious complications.

One of the biggest culprits in depleting nutrition is taking a medication over a long period of time. Numerous medications can severely lower the body levels of critical vitamins and minerals. For example, oral contraceptives lower the levels of vitamin C, folate, riboflavin, vitamin B_6, vitamin B_{12}, magnesium, selenium, and the amino acid tyrosine (which is critical to brain function). As we have seen, low vitamin C levels in women can increase their risk of cervical cancer by tenfold. One study found that vitamin C levels may be lowered by as much as 30 percent in women taking birth control pills.

Chronically low levels of folate have been shown to increase the risk of numerous cancers, especially cancer of the cervix, breast, and colon.[10] Antiseizure medications, blood pressure medications, and antiulcer medications can also dramatically lower folate levels. One type of antidiabetic medication, the biguanides, can significantly deplete folate as well. Millions of people have been taking these medications every day for decades.

We now know that chronically ill people are much more likely to develop cancer than healthier people and that one of the reasons for this may be the prolonged nutritional depletion caused by both their illness and their medication.

Many medications, even when taken alone, can cause depletion of numerous nutrients. As already stated, oral contraceptives deplete a number of essential nutrients. Another group of notorious culprits is the antihypertensive medications used to control blood pressure. These medications have been shown to cause deficiencies in vitamin B_6, calcium, zinc, magnesium, CoQ_{10}, ascorbate, thiamine, and vitamin K.

Of special concern to cancer patients is the effect of medications on lowering the body's supply of CoQ_{10}, a powerful antioxidant, supplier of cellular energy, and cancer preventative. It has been shown that virtually all cancer patients have low CoQ_{10} levels and that raising these levels significantly improves these patients' chances of survival.[11] Of the medications known to deplete CoQ_{10} levels in the body, the most commonly used include:

- Most cholestrol-lowering drugs, referred to as statins
- Blood pressure medications, such as the hydralazines, thiazides, beta-blockers, clonidine, and methyldopa
- Antidiabetic drugs, such as the sulfanylureas and biguanides
- Phenothiazines and tricyclics, which are antinausea medications and types of antidepressants

The drugs used to lower cholesterol, the so-called statin drugs, have been known for some time to cause dramatic deficiencies in CoQ_{10} levels. Tens of millions of people who take these drugs, usually for life, are never told of this very serious side effect. These drugs also deplete other nutrients, such as beta-carotene, folate, and vitamins A, B_{12}, D, E, and K, as well as calcium, magnesium, zinc, and phosphate.

Magnesium depletion is a special problem with certain chemotherapy drugs, such as cisplatin. In fact, magnesium levels can fall to dangerously low levels, leading to cardiac and brain damage. Many commonly used prescription drugs deplete magnesium as well. Women who have taken birth control pills for decades often have severely low tissue magnesium stores. When they develop cancer, their chemotherapy treatments are much more hazardous and likely to produce complications than those of women with normal magnesium tissue levels. This problem is rarely considered by oncologists.

It has been shown that patients going into chemotherapy and radiation treatments with good nutrition are far less likely to suffer complications, respond better to the treatments, and have a lower risk of dying during the treatment than do people with a poor nutritional status. This has been confirmed in experimental settings.

In one experiment, it was found that when rats were given cyclophosphamide alone and were operated on alone, they rarely died, but when they were given the two treatments combined, more than 75 percent died. When the rats were treated with vitamin A or beta-carotene before surgery, the mortality rate was reduced to zero—that is, none of the rats died.

So, it is fairly obvious that there are a number of things you can do immediately to boost the effectiveness of your cancer treatments. First, do not smoke and avoid being in enclosed areas where others are smoking. Not only does tobacco contain numerous carcinogens, but the nicotine in tobacco—even in the form of the nicotine patches used to stop smoking—is a rather powerful inhibitor of the immune system. The last thing you want to do is further suppress your immune system.

Second, if you have been taking medications known to lower the levels of vitamins, minerals, or CoQ_{10}, take supplements to correct the deficiencies in order to remain on the medications. Check with your doctor to see which medications you can discontinue. In many cases, doctors are either not aware that their patients are still on inappropriate medications or they have forgotten they prescribed the medications. It is your responsibility to review your medications with your doctor on a regular basis.

Finally, take a magnesium supplement. This is one supplement rarely suggested by conventional doctors. It is particularly important to supplement with this mineral since deficiencies are so common, even in healthy people. For example, one survey of more than 30,000 people found that 75 percent were deficient in magnesium intake, with two-thirds of these people drastically deficient. People taking diuretic medications are at special risk, since these medications not only wash out potassium, but also remove magnesium. Fortunately, vegetables are high in magnesium.

FOOD PREPARATION TECHNIQUES AND CANCER

Many people have heard that searing meats—that is, cooking meats over an open flame or allowing them to burn—increases the risk of cancer. The presence of powerfully carcinogenic compounds in seared meat was first discovered in 1977 when material was extracted from the charred surfaces of fish and beef and tested for its ability to mutate genes. The mutagenic compounds are called heterocyclic amines.

When analyzed, these carcinogenic compounds were found to be formed from several chemicals in meat (creatine, certain amino acids, and sugar).[12] When exposed to high temperatures, these chemicals can form a series of compounds that can damage the DNA, eventually resulting in cancer.

In general, grilling and panfrying (but not broiling) at high temperatures can produce significant amounts of heterocyclic amines in meats and fish.[13] Deep-frying, baking, and roasting meats and fish also produce carcinogens, but in general the amounts are low. Barbecuing produces among the highest levels of heterocyclic amines, especially when done over a grill. Exactly how many of these dangerous compounds are produced depends on the degree of the heat, the cooking time, and if the cooking is done over wood, the type of wood used. The worst type of wood to use is mesquite, which produces large amounts of these carcinogens during cooking. Hardwoods burn cleaner and are less likely to cause a problem.

Heterocyclic amines have been shown to cause cancer in a large number of animal species. While most of the cancers they cause involve the gastrointestinal tract and liver, they can also increase the incidence of tumors in the lungs, breast, and blood vessels, and can produce lymphomas as well. One particularly frightening finding was that even the children of mothers who eat diets containing high levels of these compounds during pregnancy suffer a high risk of cancer later in life.[14]

In one study, researchers found a strong association between a mother's prenatal vitamin C intake and a lower risk of brain tumors in the child.[15] In addition, they found that the women in the study who took high doses of folate, multivitamins, and vitamin C and ate the most fruits and vegetables, especially during the first six weeks of pregnancy, had the lowest incidence of brain cancers in their children. Especially frightening was the finding that the children who did not eat any fruit in the first year of life had a 430 percent increased risk of developing a brain cancer, especially of the neuroectodermal type, such as the horrifying medulloblastoma.

There is also evidence that searing the fats in vegetables, such as when panfrying, can increase the production of these cancer-causing chemicals. Fortunately, vegetables contain many compounds that block these carcinogens. For example, green tea, consumed as either a tea or a supplement, has been shown to dramatically reduce the cancer-causing ability of heterocyclic amines.

Another set of compounds found in foods that can increase cancer risk are the nitrite food additives, used as food preservatives. When ingested, they are converted into nitrosamine compounds, which have been shown to produce cancer in animals and are suspected to do so in humans as well. A diet high in foods containing these preservatives has been recognized as a major risk of stomach cancer and possibly also of other cancers, including brain tumors. The artificial sweetener aspartame is also converted into a mutagen in the stomach by this process.[16]

So, what can you do to reduce the danger from seared meats and fish? Most important is to give up eating meats and fish prepared over an open flame, grilled, or panfried. People from the Deep South may find it difficult to completely give up barbecue. For those times when you may be tempted to break ranks and sneak a little seared meat or fish, there are a few things you can do to greatly reduce your risk.

Edible plants contain complex chemicals called flavonoids that have been shown to be very efficient at blocking these cancer-promoting chemicals. In fact, one way to reduce your risk from nitrites is to take vitamin C with the seared food. The vitamin C will prevent their conversion to nitrosamines.[17] Unfortunately, as we shall see, vitamin C also greatly increases iron absorption, something we do not want in the face of cancer.

Fortunately, there is an alternative. Two flavonoids commonly found in vegetables, caffeic acid and ferulic acid, have been shown to powerfully block nitrosamine formation. Caffeic acid is found in plums, apples, and blueberries, while ferulic acid is commonly found in all fruits. Ellagic acid, another flavonoid, is even more powerful—in fact, it is some 80 to 300 times more potent than vitamin C. Ellagic acid is commonly found in strawberries, raspberries, and blackberries.

Sometimes, we like to break the boredom of eating all our meats broiled. Frying can be made much safer through the use of extra virgin olive oil, which contains some powerful antioxidant, anticancer flavonoids. To boost your protection even more, add turmeric to the oil. Several pinches will go a long way toward making your meal less of a cancer risk. Many spices, such as sage and rosemary, have antibacterial, anti-inflammatory, and anticancer effects.

PREPARING YOUR FOOD

Another problem faced by cancer patients is how to prepare their fruits and vegetables. Some authorities insist that all fruits and vegetables be eaten raw, mainly to preserve the enzymes and prevent a loss of nutrients by heating. While there is some validity to this, I am not an absolutist. Instead, I think you should mix raw and cooked vegetables in your diet.

As I have stated previously, eating raw vegetables limits the amount of the nutritional components you can absorb. This is because they are locked within the cells of the plant by tough cell walls that we can't digest. To unlock the nutrients, you need to chew your vegetables until they are mush, cook them, or liquefy them in a blender.

The problem with the first option—chewing to a fine mush—is that most people are not that patient. Most people chew a few times and then swallow. Furthermore, some studies have shown that chewing vegetables allows only 30 percent of the nutrients to be absorbed. This means you have to eat a lot more vegetables to get the full amount of the nutrients. Using a blender or juicer releases about 90 percent of the nutrients. The other advantage is that you are consuming raw fruits and vegetables.

So, what about cooking? Will it destroy all the nutrients? Careful studies have shown that it varies with the food type. A considerable loss of anticancer (antimutagenic) activity was seen when the following foods were heated: apples, apricots, kiwi, pineapple, beets, cabbage, cauliflower, leafy lettuce, cucumber, onions, radishes, and rubarb.

Foods that maintained their anticancer power when cooked included blackberries, blueberries, sweet and sour cherries, honeydew melons, plums, strawberries, Brussels sprouts, chicory greens, eggplant, garden cress, pumpkin, and spinach.

Cooking vegetables in tap water has two disadvantages. First, most of a vegetable's water-soluble nutrients—such as its minerals, B vitamins, and ascorbate—are lost in water. Second, if the water is fluoridated, the amount of fluoride in the water becomes more and more concentrated as the water evaporates until a very concentrated solution of fluoride remains. The fluoride, being a very reactive chemical, will then bind with the vegetable and cannot be washed off. Fluoride is a carcinogenic compound. (For a discussion about the dangers of fluoride for cancer patients, see Chapter 8.)

When cooking vegetables, either steam them or cook them in extra virgin olive oil. I say cook, but actually you should just heat them in a pan for a few minutes. This will break down some of the plant cells, but not as thoroughly as when you fully cook the vegetable. If you use distilled water to cook your vegetables, you can drink the juices, since they will contain a high concentration of nutrients. Southerners call this pot liquor.

When it comes to fruits and vegetables, keep the following important points in mind:

- Eat a mixture of raw and cooked vegetables based on the above heat stability information.
- Always eat vegetables when you eat meat. The flavonoids in the vegetables will neutralize the carcinogens in the meat, especially in seared meats. They will also reduce the absorption of iron, so that you absorb only enough to maintain your body's needs.
- Eat only a small amount of fruit a day, preferably no more than half a cup. Eat the fruit only after you have finished a meal. This prevents hypoglycemia, a sudden drop in blood sugar, which can be quite severe in some people. (Until your cancer is under control, I would recommend avoiding fruits altogether.)
- If you cook your vegetables in water, use only distilled water or water purified by a reverse osmosis filter.

Keep the following points in mind about food in general:

- Avoid red meats such as beef and pork, which are high in two powerful cancer promoters. Choose chicken or turkey that has been minimally processed and has not been painted or injected with broth, hydrolyzed protein, or other monosodium glutamate (MSG)–containing products. Also, if using chicken, remove the skin and wash the meat thoroughly, since most chicken is sprayed with chlorine bleach at the processing plant.

- Avoid all commercially prepared foods. Try to make all your foods from fresh ingredients. Do not use commercial sauces, mixes, or seasonings unless they are made with pure herbs or spices.
- Avoid cow's milk, cheese, and other milk-based products, especially if low in fat. Low-fat milk products have a higher concentration of glutamate (an excitotoxin). In addition, milk allergies, which can be subtle, will impair your immune system. Allergies to milk are some of the most common food allergies.
- Avoid foods containing aspartame, MSG, hydrolyzed vegetable protein, soy protein, or the additive carrageenan. Carrageenan, commonly used in ice cream and baked goods, is an especially powerful promoter of cancer growth and spread. The name will be listed on the product label. Also, avoid all of the newer sweeteners, since they have not been adequately tested for safety. Sweet'N Low can be used, but only in limited amounts. Stevia can also be used.
- While in today's world this can be very difficult, try to avoid all foods and drinks in plastic containers, especially if the plastic has a pungent odor. Plastic releases estrogenic-like compounds, which can promote estrogen-sensitive cancers such as breast cancer, colon cancer, some brain tumors, renal cancers, and possibly prostate cancer. If possible, use only glass containers. Granted, these are harder and harder to come by.
- Avoid sugar, no matter what the source. Honey is sugar. Sure, there are a few flavonoids included, but it is still sugar and can be used by the cancer. Fructose, while it does not promote insulin release, is not a good choice. For one thing, it increases the free radical damage to cells, thereby increasing the risk of cancer.
- Avoid fruit juices. While fruit juices contain many anticancer flavonoids and vitamins, especially folate, they also are high in sugar and many have high levels of fluoride. This is especially true for most commercial grape juices.

Excitotoxins, such as MSG and hydrolyzed protein, can cause nausea, diarrhea, and stomach cramping, especially in people who are undergoing, or who have undergone, chemotherapy or radiation treatments.[18] In addition, they can cause irregularities of the heart beat (arrhythmia). This is important when taking chemotherapy drugs that are known to damage the heart, such as adriamycin, daunorubicin, Ara-C, Doxorubicin, Mitoxantrone, cyclophosphamide, and Taxol.

JUICING AND BLENDERIZING YOUR FRUITS AND VEGETABLES

As I discussed previously, one of the best ways to release the 10,000 phytonutrients in fruits and vegetables is to mechanically break open the cells.

Most people have heard of juicing. Juicing entails loading fruits and vegetables into a machine that grinds them up, separating the juice from the pulp, which is usually discarded. As many people who have tried juicing know, it takes a countertop of vegetables to make one 10-ounce glass of juice. I always feel that by throwing away all that vegetable bulk, we discard important nutrients and phytochemicals—which, in fact, we do.

In addition, there is the cleanup. With many juicing machines, this is a daunting task, to say the least. After each use, you have to take the machine apart, clean it thoroughly, lubricate its parts, and reassemble it. To do that even twice a day usually discourages most people, especially if they have busy lives. Shop around when looking for a juicing machine. Some are much easier to use and maintain than others.

Despite the cleanup necessitated by many juicing machines, however, it has been obvious to me that this process of mechanically breaking down fruits and vegetables is responsible for more miraculous cures of advanced cancers than any other thing people can do. But if you truly do not have the time to devote to cleaning up a juicing machine, there is a wonderful alternative: the vegetable blender.

Vegetable blenders have two real advantages over juicers. First, they do not waste anything. In addition to the thousands of nutrients inside them, plants contain numerous, often powerful phytochemicals on the outside of their leaves and stems. Among these phytochemicals are glycoproteins and polysaccharides, which regulate immunity. Furthermore, plant pulp contains a lot of fiber. Second, vegetable blenders are a snap to clean. Not any blender will do, however. Rather, the machine must be powerful enough to turn vegetables and fruits into liquids. The vegetable blender that I have in my kitchen is the Vita-Mix 5000.

When juicing or blenderizing fruits or vegetables, of even more importance than using the right machine is choosing the right ingredients. In addition, you need to thoroughly clean the fruits and vegetables with a vegetable wash before putting them in the machine.

One of the common mistakes people make when preparing juice is using only their favorite vegetables or fruits, usually based on taste. For example, many people use only carrots. They will drink carrot juice until they turn orange—not that turning orange is bad, even though it may attract rabbits.

Using only one vegetable, such as carrots, is wrong for two reasons. First, some vegetables are very high in sugar, which, as we have seen, can stimulate tumor growth. Second, you miss important phytochemicals found in other plants. Some special anticancer flavonoids are found only in certain vegetables and not others. Only by mixing various types of vegetables can you take full advantage of these potent anticancer chemicals.

For example, onions, teas, and apples contain a powerful cancer inhibitor called quercetin. Parsley and celery contain an anticancer flavonoid called apigenin, while green tea has a series of chemicals, including epigallocatechin gallate, catechin, and epicatechin, that not only suppress tumors, but also protect the heart and blood vessels. The more of these vegetables you mix together, the more likely your cancer will be either suppressed or eliminated, especially if you combine this dietary therapy with conventional treatments.

Something I often do personally is to make myself a salad with a large variety of vegetables, but instead of eating it, I throw it into my vegetable blender, blenderize it, and drink it. That way, I get a much higher intake of the salad's healthful phytochemicals than if I simply ate it. I find I can juice my salad and drink it quicker than I could just eat it in the normal way.

To blenderize or juice vegetables, first clean them thoroughly with a vegetable wash, then put them in the machine. Add a cup of distilled water and process on a low setting. Slowly increase the speed to full. Most machines have a special power switch that significantly boosts the speed; turn this switch on for a few seconds several times during the mixing procedure. You can keep adding water until the mixture is a consistency you can drink.

When preparing your own salad to drink, choose at least five vegetables from the list below. If possible, use all the vegetables on the list. In general, especially when first starting your conventional therapy, avoid fruits, or at least use just a minimum amount. For a list of good fruits to use, see page 31. If you wish, empty the contents of a multivitamin capsule into the blender as well and mix with the juice. Some vitamins are bitter and can affect the taste; experiment until you find a good balance.

For people who do not eat enough fiber, drinking vegetables may cause diarrhea or bloating. To avoid these effects, first start off with a dilute solution of vegetable juice—a good combination is half vegetable juice and half distilled water. Drink this for a week. Slowly increase the percentage of vegetable juice and decrease the percentage of water, until you are drinking almost 100 percent juice. (You may still need water just for consistency's sake.) Drink one 10-ounce glass of vegetable juice twice a day.

What to Include in Your Fresh Juice

Vegetables

Beets	Kale
Broccoli	Parsley
Brussels sprouts	Purple cabbage
Carrots	Spinach
Cauliflower	Tomatoes
Celery	Turnip greens

Fruits

Blackberries	Oranges
Blueberries	Raspberries
Cranberries	Red currants
Grapefruit	Strawberries
McIntosh apples	

Fresh Versus Frozen Juice

One of the major controversies regarding juicing or blenderizing fruits and vegetables is whether the juice needs to be consumed right away or can be stored in the refrigerator. Both sides have good arguments. Purists say that only freshly made juice is effective, since it preserves the enzymes. This means you would have to make juice twice daily.

The problem is that some people just don't have the time or desire to prepare fresh juice twice a day. Over time, they stop doing it altogether. In reality, many enzymes are preserved if the juice is kept cold in the refrigerator. Enzyme survival and activity are temperature dependent. Add heat, and they will quickly be destroyed.

For cancer patients who are unable to make juice daily, I suggest preparing a large batch over the weekend, when most people have more time. Freeze half of the juice and keep about a three-day supply available in the refrigerator for immediate use. Another option is to divide the prepared juice into daily amounts and keep all but a day's supply in the freezer. You just have to remember to thaw out your day's supply every morning. When juice is frozen, all of its phytonutrients and enzymes are preserved.

The Importance of Nutrition Before Surgery

Most cancer patients have as their primary treatment the surgical removal of the tumor. Sometimes this can be a relatively minor procedure, as with a skin cancer, but more often it is complicated, entailing the surgical removal of the cancer and any surrounding lymph nodes. The more complicated and prolonged surgeries can be extremely stressful, both physically and psychologically.

For more than forty years, we have known that malnutrition greatly increases surgical mortality, with malnourished patients being ten times more likely to die soon after surgery.

Most of us think of a malnourished person as looking like someone from Ethiopia. In fact, you can be malnourished and obese at the same time. The new term is undernutritous. It has been shown that people with even a single vitamin deficiency can have a poorly functioning immune system. Looks, indeed, can be deceiving.

A most enlightening study was done some years ago. The study included a careful survey of surgical patients admitted to the hospital and found that 44 percent of the patients had general malnutrition on admission. This means that the patients were malnutritous long before coming to the hospital. Even worse, 75 percent of the patients admitted to an intensive care unit were malnutritous. This put them at an even greater danger because they were under much greater stress. Stress is a tremendous drain on nutrition, and survival depends on nutritional status. Yet even more shocking was the finding that 69 percent of the patients underwent a deterioration in nutritional status while in the hospital, which is an indictment of hospital nutrition.

Another study involving a number of hospitals found that 38 percent of patients had obvious vitamin deficiencies and even a larger percentage were marginally deficient. Patients with marginal deficiencies are at a significantly higher risk of complications, especially of poor wound healing and infections.

For cancer patients, not only is wound healing and avoiding all the complications associated with surgery important, but so is making sure the immune system is functioning at peak activity. The status of a person's nutrition is critical to the immune system. Again, I emphasize that even a single nutrient deficiency can severely impair the immune system. For example, a vitamin B_6 deficiency alone can lower immunity, even when the levels of all the other vitamins are perfectly normal.

Most bleeding tendencies following surgery are minimal two days after the operation. This means you can safely resume taking your nutritional supplements. The only contraindication would be if you were receiving blood-thinning medications. In that case, I would avoid using vitamin E in doses over 200 international units, even though blood-thinning effects are rare below 1,000 international units. Several supplements can thin the blood (affect coagulation). They include ginkgo, garlic extract, quercetin, curcumin, and high-dose vitamin E (greater than 1,000 international units). In general, the blood-thinning effect of these supplements is no more than that of taking one aspirin a day.

Maintaining adequate magnesium levels is especially important in preventing surgical and postsurgical complications. Magnesium is one of those nutrients that seem to have an unlimited list of benefits. In addition to playing a role in more than 300 enzymes, it regulates blood flow, protects brain cells, protects the heart muscle, reduces the risk of cardiac arrhythmia, improves lung function, improves kidney function, and prevents one of the most frightening complications of major surgery: blood clots.

I have used magnesium in my neurosurgical patients for more than fifteen years and have never had a patient develop postoperative blood clots in the legs or lungs. In most cases, the blood clot forms in the veins of the legs or pelvis, where it can suddenly enter the bloodstream, producing a fatal clot in the lungs called a pulmonary embolism.

Sudden cardiac arrest can be another catastrophic event during surgery, leaving the patient with a stroke or myocardial infarction (heart attack). Magnesium significantly protects against these complications as well. Several studies have shown that magnesium infusions can reduce the severity of a stroke or heart attack by 50 percent. What is important is that your tissue magnesium level be normal before surgery. An ounce of prevention is truly worth more than a pound of cure.

People who take diuretics or birth control pills, or whose diet is low in fruits and vegetables, are at a very high risk of magnesium depletion. Teenagers often drink large amounts of carbonated soft drinks throughout the day. These drinks significantly lower the tissue magnesium levels. All of these individuals have a higher risk of surgical complications. Magnesium is also essential for normal immune function.

The bottom line is that the better your nutrition is before surgery, the less likely it is that you will have a major complication and the faster, and more completely, you will recover from surgery. Over the years, I have noticed that patients who take these supplements regularly have significantly less pain and fatigue after surgery as well. Postoperative fatigue has always been a problem for patients and one for which surgeons usually have little to offer.

We are becoming increasingly aware of the fact that even nutrient deficiencies too small to be recognized by clinical examination can impair the body's functioning. We call these deficiencies subclinical. A large number of people living in industrialized countries suffer from these subclinical deficiencies, and the number is continuing to grow.

VITAMIN BLOOD LEVELS VERSUS REAL DEFICIENCIES

When doctors want to know if you have adequate amounts of a certain vitamin in your body, they usually draw your blood and have it tested for the vitamin in question. When they want to assess the adequacy of your nutrition in general, they frequently have your blood tested for your folate and vitamin B_{12} levels. Newer studies, however, have shown this method to be very inaccurate. In one study, doctors compared the usual blood levels of the vitamins folate, B_6, and B_{12} to the actual levels in the tissues as measured biochemically. What they discovered was quite shocking.

When they measured the conventional vitamin levels in a group of healthy elderly, they found that approximately 19 percent of the study subjects had deficiencies. Yet, when they used the more accurate biochemical method, they found that 63 percent of these same individuals were significantly deficient in one or more of these critical vitamins. A similar comparison of sick elderly subjects found that 60 percent were deficient using conventional measurement and a whopping 83 percent were deficient when the biochemical method was used.

This study clearly demonstrates that measuring vitamin blood levels by the conventional method can result in a false assurance that all is well, when in fact severe deficiencies may exist. This is especially true for the chronically ill.

It is well known that surgery and especially anesthesia are powerful suppressors of immune function. This is especially so for surgeries lasting longer than two hours and in cases where more than a unit of blood is lost during the procedure. This immune suppression can last for several weeks and can be made even worse if the patient has to receive blood during or after the surgery. Immune suppression caused by blood transfusion, especially multiple transfusions, can equal that caused by acquired immune deficiency syndrome (AIDS).

This profound level of immune suppression can give cancer a chance to invade and spread. A combination of poor nutrition, the trauma of surgery, blood transfusion, and anesthesia can temporarily wipe out the immune system. It also puts you at a much higher risk of postoperative wound infection and pneumonia.

It has been shown that this immune suppression caused by surgery, anesthesia, and blood transfusion can be reversed or even prevented by proper nutrition. It will, of course, require special immune stimulants, but it can easily be done.

Of special concern are patients who undergo preoperative chemotherapy—that is, who receive a dose of chemotherapy before surgery. It is well recognized that most chemotherapy drugs cause significant immune suppression and interfere with wound healing, thereby significantly increasing the risk of infections after surgery.

Several studies have shown that nutritional immune enhancement can significantly reduce complications, especially infections, following major surgeries. In one study, almost 70 percent of immune-deficient cancer patients undergoing surgery developed postoperative complications as compared to 25 percent with functioning immune systems. This is a dramatic difference. It should be appreciated that the patients in the group with a functioning immune system did not have specific nutritional immune stimulation. My experience, as well as that of others, is that immunity not only can be restored in patients, but can also be maximized with special supplements.

CONCLUSION

We have seen in this chapter that nutrition plays a vital role not only in preventing cancer from occurring but also in allowing the body to control the growth of cancer that has already developed. In addition, we have learned that certain foods, especially fruits and vegetables, contain special chemicals that act powerfully to inhibit the growth and spread of cancers of various types. While nutritional supplements can offer highly concentrated anticancer biochemicals, they work much more efficiently and powerfully when combined with these food components.

The question of natural supplements versus artificial supplements, as we have seen, is not as clear-cut as some would have us believe. While some artificial forms of vitamins, such as vitamin E acetate, have poor anticancer effects, others, such as vitamin E succinate, have extremely potent anticancer effects. In fact, as we have seen, even foods themselves can vary considerably in their anticancer effectiveness, depending on how they are grown, harvested, and prepared.

Of particular importance in this modern world of pharmaceutical wonders is the effect of medications on nutrition. Most of the cholesterol-lowering drugs have been shown to dramatically deplete the body's supply of CoQ_{10}, a nutrient essential for cellular energy generation. In fact, low levels of CoQ_{10} have been associated with a poor prognosis.

One of the more frequently overlooked factors when considering the effectiveness of anticancer nutrients found in specific foods is how the food is prepared. We have learned that the vital anticancer nutrients in fruits and vegetables are contained within the plants' cells and that they cannot be released for absorption except by vigorous chewing, juicing, or blenderizing.

Finally, we have seen that cancer patients undergoing surgeries, especially radical, extensive surgeries, have an increased demand for nutrients, and that failure to supply these nutrients can greatly increase their risk of major complications, including poor wound healing, infections, and more rapid spread of the cancer.

2

The Cancer Process

As I mentioned in Chapter 1, you need to understand, at least to some degree, how a normal cell becomes a cancer cell in order to appreciate not only how nutrition protects you during your conventional treatments but, equally important, how it enhances the effectiveness of your treatments. This will require some understanding of how normal cells function and of the many ways cancer cells differ.

In general, when you understand why a particular treatment works, you feel better about putting your faith in it. In the past, nutrition seemed too much like voodoo. When we thought of herbs, we often had visions of an ancient, cronelike woman with a twisted spine, a face full of deep wrinkles, and one opacified blind eye, standing beside a black pot whose contents she was slowly stirring with a gnarled stick.

Today, herbal and medicinal plant science occupies some of the most high-tech laboratories in the world. In many instances, however, our science has taken decades, even centuries, to catch up to what is common knowledge among so-called folk medicine practitioners. For nutrition, it has taken even longer. But because of our deeper understanding now of how cells function and of the numerous chemical components in plants, we better understand why nutrition is so important to maintaining health and, especially, how this knowledge can be used in treating disease.

The main difference between cancer cells and normal cells is that cancer cells are immortal. Well, not in the literal sense; they can be killed. However, unlike normal cells, which divide only fifty or sixty times and then stop, cancer cells can divide forever. Some of the cancer cells used in laboratories, such as the HeLa cells, have been alive for more than three-quarters of a century after their owner died. These cells have reproduced so many times that, if put together, they would make a whole new person many times over.

Normal cells have a little cap on the end of their DNA strands called a telomere. A telomere is sort of like the plastic cap on a shoestring. In fact, it has a similar function: to keep the string from unraveling. Every time the cell divides, a little piece of the telomere is clipped off, until eventually none is left. At that point, the cell quits dividing and eventually dies.

A cancer cell, on the other hand, continues to make more of the telomere substance by using a special enzyme, called telomerase, that is rarely found in normal cells. This allows the cancer cell to divide forever, filling your body with uncontrollable cells. Even here nutrition can help. It has been shown that an extract of green tea called epigallocatechin gallate powerfully inhibits this enzyme, even in low concentrations—that is, in amounts equal to just several cups of green tea.[1] That brings us to the next difference between cancer cells and normal cells: a failure to communicate.

WHEN CELLS STOP TALKING

Normally, cells are always talking to one another by a system called gap-junction intercellular communication. By keeping the lines of communication open, cells keep each other from getting out of line—that is, they regulate each other's growth. If a cell starts to grow too fast, producing more and more cells (a tumor), its neighbors send a signal over telling it to quiet down. As with many things in nature, the conversation is by way of chemical messengers, called connexin 43.

We now know that one of the earliest changes during the transformation of a normal cell into a cancer cell is the loss of this communication system. Once cut off from its neighbors, the damaged cell begins to reproduce faster and faster, ignoring the panicked screams of its neighbors. In fact, some carcinogenic chemicals induce cancer by interfering with this communication system.[2]

Genes are what control the communication system. So, in the case of cancer, the problem is with the genes. Something has mixed up the signals coming from the genes so that the cell no longer manufacturers the necessary chemical messengers. As we shall see, if we catch this problem in time, we can use several nutrients to restore the communication system, averting the formation of a cancer. So now let us look at what happens to the genes.

Cancer and Genes

It now appears that all cancers begin with faulty genes. Cells that divide often are more likely to develop into cancers than cells that divide rarely, if ever. For example, the cells lining the colon divide frequently and more often develop into cancers than do the neurons (brain cells), which do not divide after the teenage years. In fact, tumors arising from the neurons themselves are quite rare. The most rapidly dividing cells are in the bone marrow and lymph nodes, accounting for the higher frequency of such cancers as leukemias and lymphomas.

The reason a rapidly dividing cell is more likely to become a cancer is that with each division, a cell runs the risk that its DNA will be damaged. The more times a cell divides, the more chances there are for an injury to develop. If the DNA is damaged, the injury is carried on to the newly formed cells. Over time, unless repaired, these injuries will accumulate. Eventually, the genes that control the cells' growth-regulating instructions—that is, the instructions that tell the cells not to overgrow or get out of hand—will be damaged.

Many cells have special growth genes, called protooncogenes, that remain asleep. This puts the brakes on the cells' dividing. If, for some reason, the protooncogene switch is accidentally turned on, the cell can go wild, producing millions, and eventually trillions, of offspring cells. This is a cancer.

So what turns on these sleeping growth genes?

WAKING UP CANCER GENES

We know that many things can cause cancer: viruses, chemicals, foreign bodies, chronic infection, radiation, and even nutritional depletion. How can all these different things cause the same event to occur—that is, cause the development of cancer? What they all have in common is the production of an increasing number of free radicals.

So what the heck is a free radical? Without going into a lot of chemical jargon, free radicals are very reactive chemical particles that can burn most things they touch through a process we call oxidation. Inside a cell, they can oxidize the fats (cell membranes are made of fats), proteins (especially the cell enzymes), and DNA. When a free radical collides with a cell's membranes, it sets off a destructive chain reaction in the fat molecules (polyunsaturated fats) called lipid peroxidation. It is these two processes—free radical generation and lipid peroxidation—that do all the damage.

Most free radicals are formed during the normal process of energy production, which we call metabolism. In fact, 95 percent of all free radicals come from our own metabolism. If we slow our metabolism, we produce fewer free radicals. This might explain why animals fed low-calorie diets live longer and have fewer cancers: they are producing fewer free radicals. The opposite is also true. If you increase your metabolism, you produce more free radicals—a lot more. This explains why animals on high-calorie diets have more cancers and overall shorter life spans. You might want to keep this in mind the next time you eye that dessert.

Yet, even things we do to improve our health can sometimes be harmful. Engaging in extreme exercise is an example. When we exercise intensely, our metabolism not only increases dramatically while we are working out, but remains increased for hours afterward. In essence, we are producing a storm of free radicals. Recent studies have shown this to be true in extreme athletes. Should their supply of antioxidant nutrients be short, the damage will be even greater. There is some evidence that such extremes of exercise are associated with an increased risk of disease, including cancer.

Many diseases are associated with significant free radical generation. For example, people with diabetes, arthritis, lupus, or another autoimmune disease all produce huge amounts of free radicals.[3] In fact, it is the free radicals that account for most of the complications associated with these diseases, including the increased risk of cancer seen in all of them.

A fairly recent study reported in the journal *Cancer* emphasizes the importance of this connection between diseases associated with increased free radicals and cancer risk.[4] In this study, researchers looked at the number of cancer patients who also had chronic diseases such as arthritis, cardiovascular disease, or diabetes. They found that almost 69 percent of the cancer patients also had one of these degenerative diseases. The highest incidence of these diseases in cancer patients was in African-American women, with some 76 percent associated with chronic disease. In African-American men, the incidence was 70.6 percent.

The really interesting finding was that the average time between the onset of one of these degenerative diseases and the appearance of the cancer varied from nine years to twelve years. This means that it took almost twelve years for the free radicals to be able to damage the DNA enough to produce a cancer. The interval was shorter for smokers, who we know produce enormous numbers of free radicals throughout their bodies. This, interestingly enough, was the first study to carefully demonstrate the strong connection between chronic disease and cancer.

We also know that cancer patients who have a chronic disease, such as diabetes, do much worse than cancer patients free of other diseases. This is most likely true for several reasons, including cancer patients having a high incidence of immune suppression and poorer nutrition, as well as free radical damage to their cells. Cancer patients with other diseases also do not tolerate chemotherapy or radiation treatments as well.

Earlier, I said that all cells have special genes containing instructions for the cell to divide and grow. Normally, these genes, called protooncogenes, are turned off, even in cells that divide frequently. They are turned "on" only for very brief periods of time during cell division and then are quickly turned off again.

As free radicals bombard the DNA, they cause the long strands of DNA to break. Sometimes just one strand is broken, but occasionally both strands break. The latter is more serious. Over a long period of time, even decades, the free radicals manage to damage the growth genes in a particular sequence that turns the growth process on full blast—that is, that causes all the signal switches on the gene to become stuck in the "on" position, screaming for the cell to keep making more cells. The cell ignores the signals from its neighbors to stop, since its communication system has been turned off. At this point, a gene is called an oncogene, or cancer gene.

The bottom line is that the more free radicals you produce, the greater the likelihood will be that you will eventually develop cancer. It is now evident that even after you have developed cancer, these same free radicals can cause the cancer to become more aggressive and more likely to metastasize.

WHY SOME PEOPLE ARE MORE LIKELY TO DEVELOP CANCER

Most of my cancer patients want to know why they developed cancer, rather than someone they know who eats a worse diet or smokes heavily. We all know someone who smoked four packs of cigarettes a day since age nine and lived to be ninety years old without ever getting cancer, or who never ate a vegetable in his or her whole life but escaped the feared disease. These are very unusual people. Most of us will pay dearly for our dietary and vice-related indiscretions.

On the other end of the spectrum are those people who seem to do everything right and still get cancer. Part of the answer to this mystery is how well we are able to protect our DNA. Built into our cells is an elaborate system of protection involving several antioxidant enzymes as well as nutrient-derived antioxidants, most of which come from our food.

Poor Antioxidant Defenses

Because DNA is so vital to life, our bodies include numerous protective systems to prevent severe damage to our genes. One of the most important systems involves the antioxidant enzymes and proteins. While all are important, glutathione, a special molecule found in all the cells, is vital. We know that people with low glutathione levels have a greater cancer risk than people with higher levels of glutathione. The same thing has been shown in animal experiments.

What makes this so important is that the glutathione level in cells is easily increased by special foods and nutritional supplements. For example, the amino acid L-cysteine, found in high levels in garlic, directly increases the level of glutathione in the cells. However, while L-cysteine is safe in foods, it can be a brain toxin (excitotoxin) when taken as a supplement. A safer alternative is N-acetyl-L-cysteine (NAC) because it enters the cell first before releasing the cysteine. Cysteine is toxic only outside the brain cells. The natural product alpha lipoic acid not only dramatically increases cellular glutathione, but is also a very powerful antioxidant itself. Most of the flavonoids from fruits and vegetables also increase the cell glutathione levels.

Magnesium plays a critical role in glutathione levels. Low magnesium levels in the tissues, something that is very common, has been shown to double the number of free radicals being formed and to dramatically lower the cell glutathione levels.[5]

The other antioxidant enzymes are also dependent on our diet and can be increased simply by eating the right foods or using the correct supplement, as we shall see. Some chemotherapy agents can cause a dramatic deficiency in several of these DNA-protecting antioxidants, making our normal cells very weak and putting them at high risk for damage.[6] This is especially so during prolonged chemotherapy cycles and extensive radiation treatments.

Unlike our antioxidant nutrients, the antioxidant enzymes depend on heredity to a large degree. If we are born with an impaired ability to make these special antioxidants, our risk of disease, including cancer, is greatly increased. For instance, if a person is born with an impaired ability to make glutathione and smokes the same amount as someone who has a very powerful ability to manufacture the antioxidant, the first person will more likely develop cancer, and will do so much sooner.

You have no idea if you have a very strong antioxidant enzyme system or a very weak one, since there are no available tests for these enzymes. In addition, the stress of surgery, chemotherapy, or radiation treatments can significantly weaken your antioxidant systems if you do not provide these vital nutrients in your diet.

Glutathione has an added advantage of reducing the toxicity of several chemotherapy agents, including the muscle toxicity of cyclophosphamide and the neurotoxicity of cisplatin.

From numerous studies, we have learned that antioxidants, especially those very efficient at protecting the DNA, significantly reduce the risk of developing cancer, and for people who already have cancer, they can slow the growth of the tumor and cause it to be less aggressive.[7] In addition, they protect the DNA of the normal cells against the damaging effects of other treatments, such as chemotherapy or radiation. This significantly reduces the risk of secondary cancers caused by the treatment itself.

Faulty Repair Processes

The repair of damaged DNA is critical to our survival. While free radicals continuously bombard our DNA, chipping away at the long strands of genetic material, more than a half-dozen repair enzymes scurry along its length repairing the damage. In fact, these repair enzymes correct about 98 percent of the damage. It is the 2 percent they don't repair that can eventually accumulate to a degree that will turn on the growth switches I mentioned earlier. When you consider the frequency of this damage during a lifetime, it's amazing that even more people do not develop cancer. However, most cells with severely damaged DNA merely die.

As we age, the repair process becomes less and less efficient. This helps explain why cancer is significantly more common after age sixty-five. For colon cancer, we are a thousand times more likely to develop cancer at age eighty than at age thirty. As we shall see later, the health of these repair enzymes is strongly dependent on our diet. Antioxidants also protect these special enzymes. Some specific nutrients can actually increase the number of these enzymes and assist in the repair process. For example, L-carnitine, zinc, vitamins B_6 and B_{12}, folate, and niacinamide all improve the repair process.

It is now becoming evident that impairment of this repair process plays a major role in why some people are much more susceptible to cancer than others. Sometimes, people inherit a defect in the repair enzymes. For example, in the condition xeroderma pigmentosa, the risk of developing skin or eye cancer is 2,000 times higher than normal. People with this condition also have a twelvefold increased risk of developing a cancer deep in their body.

A study reported by the M.D. Anderson Cancer Center emphasizes the importance of DNA repair ability.[8] Researchers measured the DNA repair capacity in a group of patients with basal cell skin cancer and compared the results to those of normal people, used as controls. The people having basal cell cancers were found to have a repair capacity of only 3 to 15 percent of what was seen in the normal controls. Those having a DNA repair capacity below 30 percent had a 200 percent increased risk of basal cell cancer. In addition, the patients having this defect had multiple cancers 39 percent of the time.

Women who have other damaged DNA repair proteins called breast cancer 1 (BRCA 1) and breast cancer 2 (BRCA 2) have an increased risk of breast cancer. In fact, these two mutations account for most premenopausal inherited breast cancers.[9] It may be that defects in DNA repair in cases of cancer are much more common than is presently realized. It is difficult to measure subtle impairment in these enzymes, so it could be missed.

We also know that the degree of malignancy of a cancer depends on the number of genetic mutations—that is, the extent of the damage to the DNA. Low-grade malignancies may have as few as six mutations, whereas highly malignant tumors can have as many as fifty mutations.

This indicates that the better we can protect our DNA, using antioxidants, the lower our risk will be of developing cancer.

Furthermore, if a cancer should develop, it is more likely to be less malignant. Newer studies have shown that many of the substances found in fruits and vegetables can cause cancers to become less malignant.[10]

The presence of defects in DNA repair means that a person is much more likely to develop cancer following diagnostic X-rays, such as chest X-rays, a barium study, or computed tomography imaging (CT scans). This raises the question: Should women with a strong family history of breast cancer have yearly mammograms? After all, it is these women who are much more likely to have defective DNA repair enzymes in the first place and therefore are more vulnerable to X-ray damage.

Some studies have shown a 3 percent per year increased risk of breast cancer caused by the mammogram itself. This figure is even higher in women with DNA repair enzyme defects. An alternative method of breast examination, such as a thermal scan or ultrasound examination, should be used in place of the mammogram.

People unlucky enough to be born with, or later develop, DNA repair defects should not only avoid risky behavior, such as smoking, drinking alcohol, eating seared meats, living with stress, and working around carcinogenic chemicals, but should also dramatically increase their intake of antioxidants. This will add protection in place of the weak DNA repair system.

Years of Toxic Exposures

Throughout our lives, we experience many events that seem beyond our control, such as colds, bacterial infections, pollutants, stress, and even chronic illnesses. All of these events cause a dramatic increase in our free radical production. Normally, our cells' DNA may be exposed to 10,000 free radical impacts per cell every day. With disease, or even fever, this can increase to 100,000 impacts. That's a lot of damage to repair.

Most people living in the industrialized countries are exposed to thousands of carcinogenic risks, including industrial and household chemicals, pesticides and herbicides, viruses, fluoride, toxic metals (such as lead, mercury, and cadmium), cigarette smoke, and food additives. In addition, they often do things that dramatically increase free radical production, such as performing extreme exercise, working at a stressful job, getting reduced sleep, and eating a diet high in free radical–generating foods.

As we shall learn, certain types of fats can dramatically increase free radical production by promoting inflammation. A diet high in sweets, especially in sweetened soft drinks, can also greatly increase free radical production. Foods high in absorbable iron or copper not only can lead to free radical production, but also have been shown to dramatically increase the risk of developing cancer and of increasing the growth of cancers that already exist.

Combine this with a typical Western diet devoid of fruits and vegetables, good fats, and other antioxidants, and you have all the makings of a high risk for cancer. Cancers usually do not develop in a month or even in two years. In most instances, it takes decades for a cancer to form. Estimates indicate that prostate cancer, for example, may take up to forty-five years to fully develop.

This gives us a tremendous window of opportunity to stop the process. I have noticed that when I give a lecture on cancer, the audience usually includes very few young people, yet it is young people who would benefit the most from the information I'm providing. Most of the people in the audience have reached the age where they either have already developed a cancer or they are worried they might. Most young people feel invulnerable. In truth, however, cancer prevention should begin at birth.

I am astounded when I see what mothers feed their children. Chicken nuggets, soft drinks, potato chips, and other assorted forms of junk food are the usual fare. Not only are these children's eating patterns being directed to a lifetime of similar trash foods, but the damage that will eventually lead to cancer is being established at a tender age. Yet it's just too convenient for mothers to stick a bag of chips in their children's hands to satisfy them. Few mothers are aware that the type of oils used in chips strongly promotes cancer, among other diseases.

Inflammation

We have known for a long time that people suffering from certain chronic inflammatory diseases, such as rheumatoid arthritis, lupus, or a parasitic infection, have a much higher risk of cancer than the general public.[11]

We also know that people infected with the hepatitis B or C virus have a higher incidence of liver cancer than uninfected people. Certain parasitic infections, such as schistosomiasis, are associated with a high incidence of bladder cancer. Further proof of the link to chronic inflammation comes from the testing of numerous inflammatory chemicals on animals. Not only will these inflammation-causing chemicals promote cancer, but once a cancer has developed, the inflammatory chemicals will cause it to become more malignant.[12]

We now know that several cancers, including breast, prostate, colon, brain, and lung cancer, are related to inflammation, and that using drugs that reduce inflammation can slow, and occasionally even shrink, these tumors. Incredibly, numerous nutrients are found in fruits and vegetables that also dramatically reduce inflammation and thereby accomplish the same goal without the side effects of drugs.[13]

Most likely, the connection between inflammation and cancer is that the biochemical pathways causing inflammation, such as eicosanoid formation, free radical generation, and lipid peroxidation, also dramatically increase the activation of cancer genes, angiogenesis, and the production of the enzymes needed by the cancer to grow and spread.

The first carefully controlled demonstration that inflammation increases the aggressiveness of cancers appeared in the February 2000 issue of *Cancer Letters*, a major cancer research journal.[14] In this study, researchers injected varying concentrations of the food additive carrageenan into the vicinity of a growing tumor. The carrageenan caused the tumor to become much more aggressive in its growth. The effect was dose dependent—that is, the higher the dose of carrageenan, the more malignant the tumor behaved. Even very dilute solutions, below the amount necessary to cause obvious inflammation, increased the tumor's growth.

Iron Deficiency

Numerous studies have shown that cancer is highly iron dependent. This is because rapidly dividing cells require iron for DNA replication. The cancer cells' need for iron is so great that they will steal iron from normal cells and from iron stores.

One way to deprive cancer of iron is to use a special iron-chelating agent, such as deferoxamine. Animal studies have shown that it is indeed possible to block iron utilization by a cancer using this method without excessive toxicity to the animal itself.[15] This same iron-chelating drug has been used successfully, both in tissue cultures and in animals, to inhibit neonatal acute leukemia.[16]

More evidence of the connection between cancer and iron comes from studies of iron inhalation. Mice made to inhale iron oxide dust had a significant increase in lung cancer.[17] Increased lung cancer has been seen in iron miners as well. In general, it takes from a few months to fourteen years for a lung cancer to develop using this method.

Higher dietary iron intake has also been associated with an increase in cancers stimulated by the powerful estrogen estradiol.[18] For example, one study found that renal tumors were two to four times more likely to develop in estradiol-exposed mice fed an iron-enriched diet than in mice fed either a low-iron diet or a diet with a normal iron content.

A recent study showed that the protective effect of calcium in preventing colon cancer may be secondary to the ability of calcium to precipitate iron within the colon, thereby blocking the iron from inducing cancer in the colon cells.[19] Previously, I mentioned that calcium reduces colon cancer incidence by binding with fats.

One of the best sources of absorbable iron is meat. The specific form it contains is called haem iron. In one carefully controlled, well-conducted study, the subjects who ate the most red meat had significantly higher rates of lung cancer than the subjects who avoided red meats. In fact, the lung cancer rate was 300 percent higher in the red meat eaters than in the abstainers. The smokers who ate red meat had a 490 percent greater chance of developing lung cancer than the smokers who ate little red meat.

It is interesting to note that the people who ate large amounts of yellow and green vegetables in addition to red meats experienced significant protection against lung cancer, with their lung cancer rates some 60 percent lower than normal. This demonstrates not only the tremendous ability of vegetables to inhibit cancer directly, but also their ability to remove the iron from cancer cells. Even though broccoli and spinach contain as much iron as a comparable amount of beef, only a small amount of the iron is absorbed from the vegetables, whereas 60 to 70 percent of the iron is absorbed from beef.

Because iron is so destructive to the cells and tissues when it is allowed to float around freely, most of the iron in the body is bound to special proteins. Free iron, you will recall, is a very powerful generator of free radicals and lipid peroxidation. Iron entering the bloodstream is quickly bound to a special transport protein called transferrin. This protein carries the iron to a cell, where it attaches to a special transferrin receptor on the cell's membrane. The iron is then escorted into the cell's interior. But even here it can cause mischief, and once again, it becomes linked to another protein, called ferritin, to prevent cell damage.

It is vital that cancer patients avoid iron supplements and high iron–containing foods with significant absorbability, such as red meats.

THE IMPORTANCE OF DETOXIFICATION

Most people I talk to think of detoxification as a way of flushing poisons out of the body, almost like flushing a car's radiator. In truth, the body has its own, very efficient detoxification system. While most detoxification takes place in the liver, the cells have their individual detoxification systems. This is because toxins can build up in the cells and cause severe damage long before the liver gets a chance to remove them.

While most of us worry about toxins introduced into our body through the air, water, or food, many are generated within the body itself. This is especially true during chemotherapy and radiation treatments. As the cancer cells die and break down, they release a load of very toxic debris into the blood and lymph. These toxins can cause severe damage to other tissues and organs. In fact, sometimes the damage is so extensive that it can be fatal.

If the body's detoxification system is weak, these toxins will quickly build up. Chemotherapy often damages the liver directly, but of even more importance is the effect of poor nutrition on the liver's detoxification ability. Evidence shows that people with poor detoxification ability have a higher incidence of cancer than people with normal detoxification ability.

The liver uses a two-phase system to break down toxins so that they can be safely eliminated.

Phase One Detoxification

Upon its presentation to the liver, a toxin is first acted on by what are known as the p-450 enzymes, a system of some seventy-five different enzymes. A number of these detoxification enzymes are specific to a particular toxin. Many drugs, pesticides, and herbicides are neutralized by this system. On occasion, instead of making a chemical pollutant less harmful, the system will make it more harmful. When this happens, a cancer-causing substance can be formed. In essence, the chemical, called a procarcinogen, is inadvertently converted by the detoxification enzymes into an active carcinogen.

By inhibiting the p-450 detoxification enzyme system, some nutrients prevent this from happening. The flavonoids, especially hesperidin from oranges and naringenin from grapefruit, do this very efficiently.[20] This is one way that fruits can prevent cancer.

Another way inhibiting these detoxification enzymes is beneficial is when certain drugs are prevented from converting to chemicals that are much more toxic when detoxified. Take, for example, the pain medication acetaminophen, which normally is not very toxic. However, when the phase one system tries to detoxify the drug, inadvertently it produces a very toxic by-product that damages the liver and kidneys. Eating a lot of grapefruit or oranges significantly reduces the toxicity of acetaminophen.

For other toxins, such as caffeine and some drugs, this inhibition of detoxification enzymes is harmful, since grapefruit and oranges can reduce their detoxification, causing their effects to last a lot longer. Mixing grapefruit juice and a cup of coffee will make the caffeine "high" last a lot longer.

Phase Two Detoxification

To prevent phase one from harming you with the toxins it may have created, a second detoxification system works to bind (conjugate) the toxins to various other substances. This conjugation process is very dependent on your nutrition. Deficiencies in the sulfur compounds (such as the amino acid taurine), glutathione, and substances created by fermentation in your colon can cause this vital detoxification system to work poorly.

We also know that many other nutrients can boost phase two's efficiency, greatly enhancing your protection against numerous toxic agents, including chemotherapy drugs, pain medications, antinausea medications, and antibiotics. I will discuss ways to enhance the phase two detoxification process using nutrition in Chapter 6.

CANCER CELLS ON THE MOVE: INVASION AND METASTASIS

One of the big differences between cancers and benign tumors is that the latter do not invade their neighbors. Instead, benign tumors will just push the normal cells to the side. Cancer cells, on the other hand, will slither between their neighboring cells like long probing fingers. This explains the origin of the name *cancer,* which is Latin for "crab." The crab's body is the main tumor, and its legs are the invading tentacles of the tumor.

The Importance of Cell Glue

Normally, cells are held in place by a gluelike substance lying between them. This glue, called integrin or E-cadherin, also helps to keep invading organisms, such as bacteria, viruses, and fungi, from making their way deep into tissues. It also forms a barrier to invading cancer cells. The stronger this barrier, the less likely the cancer will invade. Removing the barrier will allow even normal cells to invade surrounding tissues, just like cancer. Adding it back will stop the invasion.

One of the main ways cancer cells are able to penetrate the glue around normal cells, walls of blood vessels, and other barriers is by secreting a powerful set of protein-dissolving enzymes called matrix metalloproteinases (MMP), which erode the surrounding connective tissue like an advancing wall of lava. Recent studies have shown that cancers with high levels of these enzymes are more likely to invade and metastasize.[21] The exciting news is that several nutrients have been shown to inhibit these protein-dissolving enzymes.

How Cancer Cells Prepare for Invasion

Over the past twenty years, we have learned an enormous amount about how cancer cells prepare themselves to invade surrounding tissues. Of special importance are a number of enzymes, normally present in cells, that suddenly increase dramatically. For example, the enzyme ornithine decarboxylase increases about thirtyfold in benign tumors and more than a hundredfold in cancers. This enzyme, along with several others, such as tyrosine kinase and protein kinase C, plays a major role in the invasion and spread of cancers. The good news is that several flavonoids from vegetables powerfully suppress these vital cancer enzymes, slowing the growth and invasion of the cancer considerably.

One of the key factors in cancer invasion is a set of special protein-dissolving enzymes called proteases, mentioned above. Within this group of tissue-dissolving enzymes are two special types called matrix metalloproteinase-2 (MMP-2) and matrix metalloproteinase-9 (MMP-9). These enzymes are especially effective at dissolving the collagen surrounding blood vessels (collagen IV), called the basement membrane.

Studies of highly invasive cancers, such as melanomas, fibrosarcomas, carcinomas, and lymphomas, have all shown that these tumors contain high levels of these proteinases. One of the most dramatic demonstrations of the importance of these enzymes in tumor invasion was made when a breast cancer progression was analyzed from its early benign changes until it became an obviously invasive cancer. As the tumor became more invasive, the level of MMP-2 increased significantly.[22]

Recent studies of women with breast cancer have also shown that the presence of high levels of MMP-2 in the primary tumor indicates an increased relapse rate and a shorter survival, despite the use of antiestrogens (tamoxifen) postoperatively.[23] This is especially so in postmenopausal women having small tumors but positive lymph nodes.[24] Dr. Garth Nicolson and his coworkers at the Institute for Molecular Medicine in Irvine, California, have isolated several different proteinase enzymes that promote tumor invasion and metastasis.[25] They have also isolated a gene, called mouse transplantation antigen homolog 1 (MTA1), that when activated promotes metastasis in breast cancer and possibly in other cancers.[26]

One of the body's defenses against tumor invasion is to build up the connective tissue barriers around the tumor. This includes blood vessels. The more difficult it is for a tumor to get through the collagen barriers around the normal cells and blood vessels, the less likely the cancer will spread. Several nutrients improve the strength of these barriers. They include vitamin C, zinc, magnesium, the flavonoids, and procyanidins (grape seed extract and Pycnogenol).

There are several nutritional steps you can take to reduce tumor invasions. They include:

- Decrease your intake of the omega-6 oils, found in corn, safflower, soybean, sunflower, peanut, and canola oil.
- Increase your intake of the omega-3 fatty acids, especially docosahexaenoic acid (DHA).
- Take supplemental magnesium ascorbate, citrate, or citramate every day to bring your total daily intake up to 1,000 milligrams.
- Take 25 milligrams of zinc every other day.
- Take 100 milligrams of grape seed extract three times a day.

Grape seed extract prevents the destruction of blood vessel barriers and is a powerful antioxidant.

- Instead of grape seed extract, take 50 milligrams of Pycnogenol three times a day. Pycnogenol also increases the strength of the blood vessel barrier walls and is a powerful antioxidant.
- Take 100 milligrams of bilberry extract three times a day. Bilberry extract strengthens the walls of the blood vessels.
- Take horsechestnut extract every day. While aescin, a component of this extract, is known to strengthen the blood vessel walls, it is difficult to calculate the appropriate daily dose of the extract itself. Most horsechestnut extracts come in 300-milligram capsules, with the recommended dose being two to three capsules a day. Because of its blood-thinning effect, horsechestnut extract should not be used with anticoagulant drugs, such as aspirin or coumadin, or herbs with anticoagulant effects, such as ginger, garlic, or curcumin.
- Take 500 milligrams of curcumin three times a day. Dissolve the contents of one capsule in one tablespoon of extra virgin olive oil. Curcumin has a slight anticoagulant effect, so it should not be combined with aspirin or anticoagulant drugs.
- Take 500 milligrams of luteolin (artichoke extract) twice a day.
- Take 500 to 1,000 milligrams of quercetin every day.
- Eat at least ten servings of fruits and vegetables (mostly vegetables) or drink about three to four servings of blenderized fruits and vegetables every day.

A particularly interesting finding is that the chemotherapy agent cisplatin inhibits one of the proteinases most associated with a poor prognosis in malignant brain tumors, whereas the drug bischloroethyl nitrosourea (BCNU) does not.[27] This may explain why cisplatin is more effective than BCNU against this particular tumor.

Angiogenesis: Making New Blood Vessels

Until recently, scientists thought that because cancers grow so rapidly, they soon outgrow their blood supply and, as a result, quickly die. Rather, in response to this need, a cancer stimulates the growth of a whole bundle of new blood vessels to supply it with the badly needed nutrients. This process is called angiogenesis. Animal and culture studies have shown that interfering with this process will cause a tumor to starve and die.

Before a recent study appearing in the *Journal of the National Cancer Institute*, it was thought that the tumor started the process of angiogenesis once it reached a size of a few millimeters (about one million cells). Using a special observation method, scientists at Duke University Medical Center found that the process starts much earlier, when the cancer consists of only three or four cells. By the time the cancer reaches the size of 100 to 300 cells, the new blood vessels are already fully developed.

The blood vessels formed by a tumor are not like normal blood vessels. The main difference is that there are gaping holes in the basement membrane of tumor vessels. Normally, the barrier tries to keep cancer cells out of the lumen of the blood vessels. In this case, the cancer cells can easily slip their way into the vessels, to whisk down the lumen of the vessels in search of a new home.

On some occasions, cancer cells invade normal blood vessels. They do this by inducing the same invasion enzymes they use to erode their way through the walls of the normal cells surrounding them. The stronger the basement membrane wall around the blood vessel, the more difficult it is for cancer cells to enter the vessel and the less likely metastasis will succeed.

A plant flavonoid called catechin, found in grape seed extract and Pycnogenol, significantly increases a basement membrane's resistance to the eroding proteinase enzymes.[28]

Pharmaceutical companies are working on several promising new drugs that inhibit angiogenesis. One older drug, thalidomide, has been found to significantly inhibit angiogenesis in some tumors, such as Kaposi's sarcoma (associated with AIDS), prostate cancer, glioblastoma multiforme, and multiple myeloma. Thalidomide was banned several decades ago because of severe limb malformations in babies born to women who had taken the drug during pregnancy.

In Chapter 6, I will discuss new findings on nutritional ways to inhibit angiogenesis without the side effects of drugs. Once an antiangiogenesis drug is released for general use, combining it with nutritional antiangiogenesis supplements should make the drug much more effective.

Metastasis: Finding a New Home

Once cancer cells are able to erode their way into blood vessels, they can separate and float through the bloodstream. Depending on the particular direction of flow of the blood, the cancer cells will be carried to various other sites in the body. Because certain organs, such as the lungs and liver, act as blood filters, they are some of the more frequent sites of metastasis. Colon cancers tend to metastasize to the liver. Many cancers will metastasize to the bones as well. There is some evidence that certain cancer cells are attracted to particular tissues by chemical attractants, like bees to a flower.

While in the bloodstream, some cancers will induce clotting of the blood. This has two effects. First, it increases the survival of the floating cancer cells, and second, it releases growth factors from the platelets (platelet-derived growth factor) that increase tumor cell growth. This phenomenon explains the observation that anticoagulants, such as coumadin and aspirin, often reduce metastasis.

Some tissues are particularly resistant to invasion by cancers. For instance, the brain and cartilage are both highly resistant to tumor invasion. At first, this seems strange, when you consider that one of the first places in which lung cancers appear to produce symptoms is the brain. Yet, while the cancers end up in the brain arterioles and capillaries, they do not invade the brain itself. As they enlarge and grow, they push the brain tissue aside, but they do not invade it—that is, in the brain, they act like benign tumors in terms of their invasiveness.

Within the bloodstream, cancer cells are very vulnerable to immune attack and death. In fact, fewer than 1 in 10,000 cancer cells in the bloodstream will survive. To ward off immune attacks, cancer cells use two clever ploys. First, they secrete a product called prostaglandin E2 (PGE2), which powerfully suppresses the immune system. Second, they produce proteins that cover up the antigen recognition sites that allow the immune system to recognize them as an enemy.

Cancer cells floating around in the bloodstream really do no harm. They become harmful only when they attach to the wall of a microscopic blood vessel and bore their way into the surrounding new tissue. When cancer cells finally attach to the walls of a blood vessel, they once again must mobilize the proteinase enzymes in order to erode their way through the blood vessel wall and invade the new tissue.

Immediately we see several opportunities to stop the cancer from metastasizing. First, we can inhibit the eroding proteinase enzymes that allow the cancer to get into and then back out of the blood vessels. Second, we can thin the blood so the cancer cells cannot attach to the walls of the vessels. And finally, we can beef up the immune system to kill the cancer cells during their trip. Nutritional supplements and components of fruits and vegetables can do all of these things.

DELAYED CANCER DEVELOPMENT

Most carcinogens produce cancerous changes in cells after a very prolonged lag period, usually five to more than forty years. Why there is such a long gap between exposure to the carcinogen and development of the cancer is not completely known. This makes identification of specific carcinogens very difficult. For example, did a person develop lung cancer because thirty years ago he worked in a furniture factory dense with chemical fumes?

This lag period between exposure to the carcinogen and appearance of the cancer is determined by many factors, the most important of which are the DNA repair enzymes and inborn DNA fragility. Scientists have now identified numerous diseases associated with fragile DNA or impaired DNA repair, including Bloom syndrome, Fanconi anemia, and ataxia telangiectectasia syndrome. In all of these syndromes, we see an increased incidence of spontaneous breakage of the chromosomes and chromatids, and a high incidence of cancers of various types.

When individuals with fragile DNA or an impaired DNA repair system are exposed to even mild carcinogens, they are much more likely to develop cancer than the normal population. And they will do so much quicker. Instead of taking twenty years to develop a cancer, they may develop a cancer in two years or even in months.

Nutritional status plays a major role in a person's sensitivity to and likelihood of developing a cancer following chemical carcinogen exposure. The health of our DNA is very nutrient dependent, as is our ability to repair DNA damage from any cause.[29]

No matter what the cause of the cancer is, people with low folate levels, fragile DNA syndrome, or a poor DNA repair system have an increased sensitivity to carcinogenic agents, whether viral, chemical, or radiological. Likewise, the lag time between exposure to the carcinogen and appearance of the cancer is much shorter for them. This is often overlooked when evaluating the potential of suspected carcinogenic agents.

What is also often overlooked is lesser degrees of impairment of the DNA repair enzymes. We know that with many disorders, for every obvious full-blown case, there may be millions of subclinical cases, which are not so easily recognized. Individuals with subclinical cases of disorders such as Bloom syndrome, Fanconi anemia, and ataxia telangiectectasia syndrome are at greatly increased risk without knowing it.

Virtually all of the frequently used chemotherapy agents also cause cancer themselves—that is, they are mutagenic. The question is: How long of a lag time exists between exposure to the chemotherapy drugs and the development of the cancer? Another unanswered question is: Could it be possible that recurrences of cancers are caused by the chemotherapy agents themselves? We really don't know for sure because no one has looked into these questions. It may be that the immune suppression and overall cellular damage caused by the chemotherapy set the stage for the later recurrence.

There is good reason to believe that many cancers that are thought to be cured are instead lying dormant, waiting to be awakened by immune suppression or procarcinogenic dietary stimuli, or triggered by free radical generation. This could easily occur two or even five years after the cancer was considered to be cured. I have seen this many times. Patients go for five years after conventional treatment of their cancer completely free of obvious disease and then suddenly are found to have extensive metastatic cancer growth.

I firmly believe if cancer patients begin to follow a strict diet and basic supplement regimen at the time of their original diagnosis and continue to follow them for life, most recurrences of cancer will be avoided. In reviewing the dietary habits of patients following treatment of their original tumor, I have found virtually all had diets known to promote cancer growth and spread. The problem is that their oncologists did not tell them about the importance of diet and nutritional supplementation during, and especially following, cancer treatment.

THE CAUSES OF CANCER

Because cancer has a central mechanism, the free radical injury to genes, many things can cause it. In most people, more than one factor leads to the development of a cancer. For example, we know that asbestos is linked to a rare cancer called a mesothelioma, yet smokers exposed to asbestos are at a much higher risk than nonsmokers. We see the same relationship between heavy alcohol use and tobacco use in the case of esophageal cancer risk.

This synergism holds true for inherited cancer risk as well. You may inherit a high risk for colon cancer, for example, yet escape the disease unless you eat seared meats every day, avoid fruits and vegetables, eat lots of bad fats, and eat little fiber.

Women with a high familial risk for breast cancer who also have a low intake of the omega-3 oils and a higher intake of the omega-6 oils have a much greater breast cancer risk than women with the same hereditary risk who follow a good nutritional diet. If you add low folate, selenium, and vitamin E intake to this, the risk goes even higher, especially with a daily intake of alcohol and seared meats.

Now let us look at some of the known causes of cancer.

Chemicals in the Environment

More than two centuries ago, it was recognized that repeated exposure to certain chemicals could result in cancer. We call these cancer causing chemicals carcinogens. As we have seen, chemicals that cause a mutation of the DNA (called mutagens) also frequently cause cancer. Basically, chemicals cause cancer in two ways. First, they damage the DNA, and second, they selectively stimulate cell growth and proliferation by their effects on the growth-control processes in cells.

One of the better known chemical carcinogens is tobacco smoke. It is believed that 30 percent of cancer deaths are related to the use of tobacco. Not surprisingly, tobacco smoke contains numerous cancer-initiating chemicals. Like most carcinogens, tobacco smoke affects only selected tissues in terms of cancer causation. These selected tissues include the lungs, upper respiratory tract, esophagus, pancreas, bladder, and probably the kidneys, liver, and stomach.

Some carcinogens act only if they are combined with another chemical, called an initiator or cocarcinogen. For example, as I just pointed out, while asbestos can cause chronic lung inflammation (asbestosis), it seems to cause cancer (mesothelioma) only in smokers. In fact, the heavier the smoking habit, the greater the risk. The recent effort to remove every vestige of asbestos from workplaces and schools was undertaken only to protect smokers, not people who follow good health habits. (It also enriched a large number of politicians, consultants, lawyers, and asbestos-removing companies.)

In many cases, even small exposures to combined carcinogens can cause significant increases in cancer incidence, whereas exposures to the individual carcinogens usually pose little or no risk. The problem of synergy of toxins is something that has been overlooked by health officials and agencies, not only in cancer epidemiology, but also in the relation to the many degenerative diseases.

Most Food and Drug Administration (FDA) examinations of chemicals for safety and cancer risk do not include tests for these combined toxicities. As a result, they give false assurances to the unwary public. In addition, there are so many additives combined with foods, as well as industrial chemical combinations, that the Food and Drug Administration and Environmental Protection Agency (EPA) are unable to adequately test most of them for safety. The only tests being conducted are on millions of unaware citizens the world over.

Chemicals Hiding in the Body

Some carcinogens accumulate in the body. In most studies, the ability of a chemical to induce cancer is directly proportional to its concentration. Yet, an often overlooked fact is the ability of some chemicals to linger in the body for decades, or even for a lifetime. For example, fat-soluble chemicals such as those found in many pesticides and industrial chemicals are stored in the body's fat cells and therefore tend to accumulate over time, eventually reaching very high concentrations in these tissues. We see this with dichlorodiphenyltrichloroethane (DDT), in which breast tissue levels have been measured to be as much as 700 times higher than blood levels.[30]

In 1976, the EPA began measuring the levels of pesticides, herbicides, and industrial chemicals in fat tissues obtained by autopsy and by biopsy during surgery. More than twenty different potential carcinogens were found in 75 percent of the samples. Other studies of biopsied fat from women's breast tissue found pesticide and herbicide residues in virtually all the samples.

A similar process of toxin accumulation can occur within the cells themselves. For example, formaldehyde, one of the breakdown products of the sweetener aspartame, has been shown to attach to DNA nucleotides resulting in serious DNA strand breaks.[31] Even more frightening is the fact that this carcinogen accumulates in the nucleus of the cell and is difficult to remove. This means that drinking even a single cola sweetened with aspartame can eventually result in significant damage to the DNA and finally cancer cell development. This would explain the very high incidence of tumors, especially brain tumors, seen in the original experiments using aspartame.[32]

The accumulation of carcinogens in our fat tissues can greatly increase our risk of developing cancer later in life. Unfortunately, this process can be completely silent, leaving us unaware that it is happening. With these carcinogens, or even cocarcinogens, working silently to transform cells into cancer, another event, such as a viral infection, stress, or exposure to diagnostic X-rays, can, in essence, be the straw that breaks the camel's back.

Viruses

That infectious diseases may be the cause of cancer has been suggested many times in the past—as far back as the time of chemist Louis Pasteur (1822–1895), developer of the germ theory, and cancer researcher William F. Koch, M.D., Ph.D. (1885–1967). Renewed excitement over the possibility that infectious agents can cause cancer periodically recurs with the appearance of "cancer clusters." Cancer clusters are sudden appearances of numerous cases of cancer of a particular type within a confined area, almost like an epidemic. Careful studies of these cases have concluded that they are mere coincidences. After reviewing these studies myself, I feel that these assurances are premature.

Some of the oncogenic viruses, like cancer cells in general, have devised clever ways to prevent the immune system from finding and destroying them. One method they use is to alter the membrane recognition system that the immune cells use to identify cancer cells. The membrane recognition system is sort of like a bar code. Once they alter the system, the cancer cells resemble stealth aircraft in enemy radar: they are virtually invisible.

It is often the ability of an oncogenic virus to suppress the immune system and to subvert other protective mechanisms that determines its power to cause cancer transformation. For example, some sixty-four species of human papilloma viruses (HPV) have been isolated from benign or malignant lesions of the oral cavity, larynx, and anogenital region. Of these, only a few are associated with cancer.

HPV types 5 and 8 have been associated with a rare disease called epidermodysplasia verriciformis. In this condition, the skin is very sensitive to the mutagenic effects of sunlight, resulting in numerous skin cancers. This is an example of a cocarcinogen (sunlight) activating a carcinogenic virus.

This same virus is associated with cancers of the anogenital region, with more than eighteen types of viruses having been isolated. Of these, some (HPV types 16, 18, 31, and 33) are much more likely to result in cancer development than others. These types of the HPV virus are also seen in 85 to 90 percent of all cervical cancers.

We also know that many factors can affect the tumor-inducing ability of oncogenic viruses. For example, animals infected with the Bittner's virus are more likely to develop breast cancer if they are given estrogen hormones.[33] More convincing is that males infected with the virus will not normally develop breast tumors, but those given estrogen hormones will. It is also known that certain chemicals, radiation, and irritation in the face of infection by certain viruses can significantly increase the likelihood of cancer transformation.

One of the most obvious relationships to cancer induction by oncogenic viruses is the status of the immune system. For example, we know that animals infected with mouse leukemia virus are much more likely to develop the disease if they have had their thymus gland removed or if they are given immunosuppressing drugs. Likewise, persons suffering from AIDS-induced immune suppression also have a much higher incidence of cancerous tumors, as do people purposefully immunosuppressed for organ transplantation.

So we see that there is a complex interplay between oncogenic viruses and a number of environmental and homeostatic factors. This accounts for the tremendous variation in the susceptibility to cancer and why it is so difficult to define why one person is more likely to develop cancer than another person, even though both people are exposed to virtually the same harmful carcinogens. One may be infected with a cancer virus and not the other.

Oncogenic virus research is ongoing. Of special interest are the so-called stealth organisms, which may include not only viruses, but also rickettsia (a type of bacteria), mycoplasma (a type of parasite), fungi, and bacteria. These are normal microorganisms that have the unique ability to lose their cell walls, enter a host cell, and hide from immune detection. They are also invisible in terms of the usual laboratory detection techniques, such as media cultures, microscopic examination, and immunological detection. These organisms have become a special problem with the widespread use of vaccinations, since there is increasing evidence that several vaccines may be contaminated with them.

Because of their stealth characteristics, these organisms are very difficult to detect in human cancers and require special detection methods. This is one of the reasons it is so difficult to connect infectious organisms to various cancers.

Radiation

Most people are aware that prolonged or repeated exposure to radiation can result in cancer in both experimental animals and humans. We know that high-energy radiation passing through a cell interacts with the water in the cytoplasm of the cell to produce a very reactive and damaging free radical called a hydroxyl radical. Hydroxyl radicals damage the DNA of cells, often producing double strand breaks, which are difficult to repair. Oxygen in the cell aggravates the damage considerably.

As with the chemical or viral induction of cancer, specific genes controlling cell growth and cell death (apoptosis) must be altered by the radiation before a cancer cell can be formed. This is why there have been so few cases of cancer among the people of Hiroshima and Nagasaki, Japan, relative to the number of people exposed to the radioactive fallout following the atomic bombing of World War II.

These same factors determine the latency period between exposure to the carcinogen and the development of cancer. While it may take thirty to forty years for some cancers to develop following exposure, others develop in less than three years. This is especially so when other carcinogenic factors, such as weakness of the DNA repair mechanism, are in play. One factor often overlooked is that the radiation may activate a sleeping (latent) carcinogenic virus hiding in the cells. Once activated, the virus will have its own latent period for cancer cell development.

All of this becomes important when considering routine radiological examination or extensive radiological testing. Take as an example a woman with a strong family history of breast cancer. The woman is advised by her physician that because of her increased risk, she should have yearly mammograms, and that after age forty, she should have these exams every six months. There are several problems with such a program. For one, we know that mammograms themselves increase breast cancer risk by 3 percent per year because of the radiation exposure.

We also know that women with strong family histories of breast cancer have a high likelihood of defective DNA repair enzymes.[34] This makes them even more susceptible to radiation-induced breast cancer. Such studies would indicate that instead of resorting to frequent mammograms, these women should use other methods of breast lump detection, such as careful breast exam, thermograms, or ultrasonography.

Further evidence comes from the now discontinued use of medical radiation to treat a variety of benign problems, including ankylosing spondylitis, tonsilitis, ringworm of the scalp, and "thymus tumors." Long-term follow-up of children treated for these disorders disclosed that they had a high incidence of cancerous tumors develop years later in the area of the radiation exposure. Young girls treated with radiation for ankylosing spondylitis, an arthritic condition of the spine, had a high incidence of breast cancers as adults. This is because the radiation passed through their breast tissue on its way to the spine.

At the turn of the nineteenth century, it was standard practice to radiate children suffering with ringworm of the scalp, a fungal infection otherwise difficult to treat. This often included numerous treatments. These unfortunate children had very high incidences of thyroid and brain cancers.

One of the problems in dealing with radiation-induced cancers is appreciating the fact that humans are biological individuals and that their responses to radiation are also individual. Some people will be excessively sensitive and others will be quite resistant. While we know some of the reasons for this difference in sensitivity, there is still much we do not know. Yet it is obvious that individuals differ considerably in the latent period between exposure and development of a cancer.

(For a discussion of the safety of X-rays, see page 69.)

Are X-Rays Really Safe?

As we have seen, in some individuals, there may be a forty- or even fifty-year latency period before a cancer develops. However, most of the studies that are conducted on the safety of even diagnostic radiation are based on follow-ups that are shorter than this. A study that extends only ten years will miss most of the more delayed cancers, giving physicians a false sense of safety, which they then pass on to their patients. We know that unborn babies exposed to radiation during pelvimetry (X-rays to determine the mother's pelvic size) have a considerably higher incidence of leukemia compared to babies not irradiated while in the uterus. Few mothers are told this.

The issue of radiation-induced cancers takes on a special importance in the cancer patient being treated with high-energy radiation. One of the early problems in the radiation treatment of cancers was the damage it inflicted on the surrounding normal tissues. I can remember well as a medical student seeing a large number of patients with extensive burns of the skin caused by their treatments. If these patients survived the primary cancer, there was a dramatic risk of secondary cancer arising, essentially caused by the radiation treatment itself.

Because of this problem, radiotherapists worked hard to devise new technologies and methods to avoid as much as possible radiating normal tissues. Today, radiotherapy is much less likely to produce severe radiation damage to surrounding normal tissues, but the problem is still not totally solved. Fractionation of radiation, so that smaller doses are given over a longer period of time, as well as dividing the fields of exposure, has helped. Newer techniques using highly focused gamma radiation beams have even been given such names as the Gamma Knife, implying surgical precision.

Despite this, we still see damaging scatter radiation reflected throughout the body from the beam having bounced off bones and metal appliances implanted during surgery. This means that even parts of the body far away from the area of treatment can be irradiated. For example, during treatment of a tumor in the chest, the pelvic organs are irradiated. Using lead-containing aprons will not help because the scattering beams are inside the body.

In addition, even though the beams are reduced in strength by dividing them into converging fields, they are potent enough to injure normal cells, especially when combined with chemotherapy. It is the cells in your body that are the most sensitive to the damaging effects of radiation that are also injured the most by chemotherapy treatments and the ones most likely to transform into cancer cells.

Chronic Undernutrition

Besides their effect as antioxidants, many nutrients play a major role in cell health. For example, several nutrients, such as vitamins B_6 and B_{12}, folate, choline, and methionine, are vital to DNA synthesis. Several studies have shown that chronic deficiencies in these nutrients greatly increase the risk of developing cancer. In addition, other nutrients, especially the oils, are essential in maintaining the cell membranes.

Among these nutrients, most of the research regarding cancer has been done in relation to folate deficiency. Several studies have shown that when folate is deficient in the diet, not only is it easier to induce cancers in animals, but the deficiency causes the tumors to grow faster and act more aggressively.[35] When we look at the genes of folate-deficient animals, we see numerous injuries to the DNA that closely resemble what we see in many cancers.[36]

When combined deficiencies exist, as we commonly see in patients receiving chemotherapy and/or radiation treatments, the risk of aggravating tumor spread also increases significantly, as does the risk of developing secondary cancers.

It has also been shown that women who take drugs that deplete folate, such as the antiseizure medication phenobarbitol or phenyltoin, have a very high risk of their children developing a nervous system tumor (neuroblastoma) sometime after birth.

Deficiencies in vitamin B_{12} and methionine are also associated with increased cancer risk. You might be wondering at this point that if you already have cancer, how will this information help? There are several things that should concern you. First is that folate deficiency can increase the malignancy of some cancers and promote their spread. Second, as we have seen, it also greatly increases the risk of developing a second cancer sometime after recovery from the original cancer.

So, why are drugs such as methotrexate, which blocks folate activity, used to treat cancer? While it is true that severe deficiencies of folate can inhibit the growth of some cancers, several studies have shown that giving folate with the methotrexate not only does not interfere with the drug's effectiveness, it actually enhances its anticancer activity. It may be that cancer recurrence, even years later, may be related to chronic folate deficiency caused by a combination of the treatment and a poor diet.

So, we see that diet can make a dramatic difference in the ability to overcome cancer, just as a poor diet can dramatically increase the risk of being overcome by the disease.

Conclusion

We have seen that there are many ways to initiate the conversion of a normal cell into a cancer cell. In addition, nutritional depletion, even when subclinical, can significantly increase the risk of developing a cancer. This is logical when you realize that all of a cell's defenses depend on a constant supply of energy, special molecules, vitamins, and minerals. Later in this book, I will explain how special complex molecules in fruits and vegetables can prevent cells from undergoing malignant change and how they can even slow or stop abnormal cell growth should a cancer develop.

3

Chemotherapy: Poisoning Cancer (and You)

The use of chemotherapy has become so common in the treatment of cancer that it is now considered a standard part of the regimen. Dr. Ralph Moss, who has written extensively on the subject of cancer treatment, has noted that while chemotherapy has definite benefits for several selected cancers, in many cases it is used inappropriately. I have found the same thing in my observations over the past thirty years in medicine.

Before deciding on chemotherapy, there are several important things you should know and discuss with your oncologist. Of critical importance is the fact that most chemotherapy agents can also cause cancer themselves and may do so many years after your therapy has been completed. You should be informed of this risk before you make any decisions.

You should also be aware of the difference between "cure" of cancer and "control" of cancer. In the past, a cancer was considered "cured" if the patient had no evidence of disease five years after the treatments were finished. Some feel the cancer-free period should be extended to ten years, and I agree. Despite this optimism, there is evidence that some cancers may never be cured in the literal sense. Rather, the cancer cells are placed in a dormant state—that is, put to sleep.

Often oncologists imply that their treatment will cure your cancer, when in fact they know that it may merely control your cancer. When a cancer is under control, it means that an obvious residual tumor remains but is not growing. Usually, your doctor will order repeat studies to make sure the tumor does not begin to grow again. Another point of confusion for patients is the term "tumor response." Your oncologist may tell you that your tumor should respond to a particular chemotherapy program. Response is not synonymous with cure. A tumor is responsive if it either stops growing or shrinks, even if just temporarily.

If your cancer is more advanced, you need to know if the treatment is merely palliative rather than intended to cure or control your cancer. A palliative treatment is usually done to relieve some symptom, such as pain, or an obstruction caused by the tumor. In many instances, especially with pain, nutritional treatments are a much better alternative, since they cause no unpleasant side effects and, in most cases, help the patient's energy levels to improve, sometimes dramatically.

If your tumor is well localized, you have negative lymph nodes, and you have no evidence of local invasion or metastasis, your oncologist may recommend a cycle of chemotherapy and/or radiation treatments to eradicate any cancer cells that may have escaped. Several studies have shown that such adjunctive chemotherapy may reduce the incidence of tumor recurrence. The problem with these studies is that the results were never compared to those of a carefully constructed nutritional program. My experience is that a good nutritional program is just as effective as, and possibly even more effective than, chemotherapy or radiation. When combined with these conventional treatments, a nutritional program greatly enhances their effectiveness and reduces complications.

You should thoroughly discuss all the possible side effects and complications of your treatment program with your oncologist. Do not let the doctor brush them off as nothing to worry about. As we shall see, properly selected nutritional supplements and a good diet can greatly reduce and even eliminate many of the side effects and complications.

Before beginning your chemotherapy or radiation treatments, you should begin your nutrition program. In most instances, the nutrients will work best if started before the conventional treatments, yet they will also be effective if started afterward as well.

While you can tell your oncologist about your nutrition program, do not expect him or her to understand the scientific basis of its effect on your cancer and how it aids in your treatment. Remember that your doctor may have had no training in nutritional biochemistry and may be unaware of the research in this area. An oncologist's expertise is with the conventional cancer treatments: surgery, chemotherapy, radiation therapy, and biological response modifiers.

A Little Sleight of Hand

Because of the huge investment in the chemotherapy business—by supporters such as the pharmaceutical industry, many universities, the editors of major journals, the major media outlets, and even your oncologist—all the individuals involved in this area of cancer treatment have been working overtime to make the public think chemotherapy works better than it really does.

At the heart of the problem is the clinical trial, a study involving groups of patients using different treatment protocols. The only way to adequately test the efficacy of chemotherapy is with a randomized clinical trial (RTC). Here, patients are chosen at random to prevent selecting patients who will artificially support one idea or hypothesis.

To see if the treated group of patients really does fare better and that the results are not a "placebo" effect, or just the natural course of the disease, the researchers compare the treated group to another group of patients serving as a control group. The control group is either given a "placebo," which in theory is an inactive substance, or it is just followed along with the treated group. Unfortunately, placebo substances are often assumed to be inactive when in truth they may have some indirect effect. For example, sugar can affect the immune system.

To prevent intentional or unintentional bias from affecting the outcome, some researchers do double-blind studies. This simply means that neither the people receiving the pills (the subjects) nor the people giving the pills (the researchers) know who is getting the real medicine and who is getting the placebo until the end of the experiment. While all this seems pretty foolproof, there are still ways to bias the experiment.

One of the recently exposed deceptions of oncologists is the fact that cancer is now being diagnosed at an earlier stage of the disease than in most earlier reported studies, thereby giving the impression that people are living longer due to their treatment. For example, if a cancer is diagnosed five months earlier than was possible ten years ago, it will appear the patient lived five months longer due to the treatment. Earlier diagnosis also allows oncologists to move patients into a higher staging of the disease, so that it appears the treatment works even for more serious stages of the disease. It's all smoke and mirrors.

Another deception is to compare high-dose versus lower-dose treatments and conclude that the high-dose treatments work better because more patients survive longer. In truth, patients are selected for high-dose groups because they are in better physical condition. If they are not in better physical condition, they will not be able to survive the higher dose of the drug regimen.

Likewise, some patients in high-dose groups drop out from the study because of severe side effects. The result is that only the healthiest patients, and the ones who would live longer even with no treatment, are left in the high-dose treatment group. This artificially makes the treatment look more effective than that of the low-dose group. It is an illusion.

The bottom line is that all of this data manipulation may be masking the true conclusion that some forms of therapy may actually be causing patients to die earlier. We may never know because none of the studies compare chemotherapy treatment to treatment by other means, such as phytochemical treatment, surgical treatment alone, or no treatment at all, in a like manner.

They also do not take into consideration the improvements in general care of the person with cancer, such as better nursing care, more effective antibiotics, better cardiac support, and better control of associated conditions such as diabetes and hypertension. When these factors are considered, patients may well do better without chemotherapy, especially when taking into consideration the cancers that either respond poorly or not at all to such treatments.

IGNORING COMPLICATIONS

One thing we must always remember is that chemotherapeutic drugs are extremely toxic to numerous tissues and cell types, including brain cells. Oncologists assume that the brain cells are not affected because they do not reproduce, but the brain contains many types of cells that do reproduce, including astroglia, oligodendrocytes, and microglia. In addition, we now know that the nervous system contains numerous stem cells that play a vital role in brain regeneration and plasticity. All of these cells can be seriously damaged by many of the chemotherapeutic drugs. Many chemotherapeutic drugs also damage cells that do not divide, such as the neurons in the nervous system.

In addition, chemotherapeutic drugs are toxic to the liver cells, which play a critical role in protecting the body from the toxins released by the dying tumor cells and from other cellular waste products. Patients who are severely nutrient deficient at the time of their treatment run a much higher risk of toxic reactions, which can further impair the immune system. The greater the immune suppression and general debilitation of the body, the more likely the treatment will fail. In addition, a person made toxic by these drugs is more likely to suffer recurrences of the cancer later on. Unfortunately, most of these considerations are ignored by oncologists during the ongoing care of cancer patients.

Combining Toxicity

Some chemotherapy agents are much more toxic than others. In general, the alkylating agents, such as carmustine, melphalan, and busulfan, are among the most toxic. Adriamycin, 5 fluorouracil (5-FU), doxorubicin, and taxol also carry significant toxic risk. More than twenty different chemotherapy drugs have been shown to cause cancer in humans.[1]

As with most toxins, when chemotherapy drugs are combined as a "cocktail," the total toxicity of the combined drugs can exceed the toxicities of the individual drugs simply added together due to synergy, which I spoke about earlier. Again, through synergy, two plus two could equal twelve.

In his book *Questioning Chemotherapy*, Dr. Ralph Moss quotes a study of patients who survived ovarian cancer for one year that showed that the patients who took the drug melphalan were a hundred times more likely to develop nonlymphocytic leukemia or preleukemia than the patients who received no chemotherapy.[2]

In another study quoted by Dr. Moss and originally published in the 1995 issue of the *Journal of Clinical Oncology*, a drug combination called ICE (ifosfamide, carboplatin, and etoposide) was examined, with the incidence of complications found to be astronomical, even for the lowest doses used.[3] Damage to the mucous membranes of the mouth (mucositis) and the lining of the gastrointestinal tract (enteritis) in the patients receiving the low-dose cocktail was 67 percent and 39 percent, respectively. Even more shocking was the finding that 50 percent of the patients receiving the moderate dose had nervous system toxicity and lung damage. The high-dose patients suffered even more, with 61 percent having liver toxicity, 81 percent hearing damage, 70 percent kidney injury, and 92 percent pulmonary difficulties. Especially frightening was the finding that 94 percent of the patients demonstrated heart muscle damage. Some 13 percent of the patients receiving this toxic cocktail actually died as a result of the drug combination itself.

As pointed out by Dr. Moss, what made the article so incredible were the author's conclusions—that is, that the drug combination was well tolerated with acceptable side effects and organ toxicity. I hardly think these figures represent acceptable risk, especially the 13 percent mortality.

Besides the synergistic toxicities, some evidence also exists that these chemotherapy combinations can cause cancers to grow and spread much faster than would ordinarily occur.

In one study of women having relapsing breast cancer, it was shown that the women who received chemotherapy had progression of their cancer much earlier than the women given endocrine treatment alone.[4] In addition, the effectiveness of the treatments differed considerably, with 47 percent of the women treated without chemotherapy showing a favorable response versus only 23 percent of the chemotherapy group responding favorably.

The probability that chemotherapy makes tumors more aggressive, inhibits the immune system, and damages vital organs was reviewed in the medical literature as far back as 1987.[5] It has been my impression as well, from following cancer patients for thirty years, that in many instances, chemotherapy makes the cancer more aggressive and more likely to metastasize.

How Chemotherapy Works

When oncologists attempt to scare their patients away from using nutritional supplements, they always resort to the idea that their treatments work by creating large amounts of free radicals, which kill the cancer cells, and that antioxidant supplements would neutralize these free radicals. While it is true that some chemotherapy agents kill cancer cells by generating free radicals within them, most also have several other mechanisms of action. Several of the mechanisms are also used by phytochemicals to combat cancer, but the difference is that phytochemicals do not affect normal cells.

Alkylating Agents

Alkylating agents act much like radiation and are often referred to as radiomemics. They cause cancer cells to die by attaching to their DNA molecules at several sites resulting in DNA breaks. If enough DNA breaks occur and are serious enough, the cancer cell will die. Normal cells are less affected if they have adequate DNA repair enzymes. But as we have seen, there is growing evidence that people who develop cancer often have defective DNA repair mechanisms to begin with. This means that alkylating agents would also cause considerable damage to these patients' normal cells, possibly leading to secondary cancers after a variable latent period. Secondary cancers are cancers caused by the treatment. And in fact, alkylating agents are more often associated with secondary cancers than are other treatments.

It is well known that alkylating agents easily produce cancer in normal animals. Furthermore, the longer the exposure and the higher the dose, the greater is the likelihood more cancers will be produced. Alkylating agents may increase the likelihood of degenerative diseases as well, since the injured normal cells will have impaired functioning.

Little research has been done into the effect of chemotherapy agents on mitochondrial DNA, which is much more susceptible to damage. This is because mitochondrial DNA normally contains very few repair enzymes. Damaged mitochondrial DNA would severely impair the ability of even normal cells to function. We see this type of damage in the brain cells of people with Alzheimer's or Parkinson's disease.

Examples of alkylating agents are cyclophosphamide, thiotepa, busulfan, mitomycin C, and chlorambucil.

Antiestrogens

Antiestrogens are compounds that bind with the estrogen receptors on estrogen-sensitive cancer cells, thereby blocking the action of the hormone. This is vital in, for example, estrogen-sensitive breast cancers. Tamoxifen, derived from the Pacific yew tree, is one of the newer drugs of this class. It has been shown to bind with the estrogen receptor and thereby effectively block the binding of the more powerful estrogen called estradiol.

As we shall see, several natural plant compounds have been found to have the ability to bind with estrogen receptors and thereby inhibit the growth of estrogen-sensitive tumors. While breast cancers are the most obvious of these, some brain tumors also contain estrogen receptors that, when stimulated, enhance their growth. Antitestosterone agents, as well as other hormone-blocking drugs, are also available.

Antimetabolites

Antimetabolites are a class of drugs that imitate a major cellular metabolite, thereby interfering with the cancer cell function (as well as with normal cell function). For example, methotrexate closely resembles folate, but cells cannot use the drug to function.

Examples of antimetabolites are 5-FU, 6-mercaptopurine, Ara-C, and fludarabine.

Antitumor Antibiotics

Antitumor antibiotics are drugs that started out intended for use as antibiotics but were found to be too toxic. They damage cells by inducing free radicals and interfering with cell reproduction.

Examples of antitumor antibiotics are bleomycin, daunorubicin, epirubicin, and mithramycin.

Plant Alkaloids

Plant alkaloids are chemicals that are actually derived from plants. They inhibit cell division by binding to a protein called tubulin. This protein forms the microscopic strands that pull the chromosomes toward the new cell during cell division. When the plant alkaloids bind to the tubulin proteins, they prevent the proteins from lining up, which prevents cell division.

Examples of plant alkaloids are vinblastine, vinorelbine, paclitaxel, and docetaxel.

Toposiomerase Inhibitors

Toposiomerase inhibitors are a class of drugs that also interfere with cell division. Normally, when a cell begins to divide, its DNA strands are pulled apart, but the process requires that the DNA strands be temporally broken as other strands pass through. A special enzyme called topoisomerase repairs the temporary breaks.

Toposiomerase inhibitors interfere with the reparative enzyme, leading to cell death. As with the other chemotherapeutic agents, it also does this in normal dividing cells. Fortunately, most cells in the body are not dividing at the time the drug is given. But rapidly dividing normal cells, as we have seen, will be affected.

Examples of toposiomerase inhibitors are doxorubicin, daunorubicin, and camptothecin-11 (CPT-11).

Cytotoxic Agents of Unknown Mechanism

Some chemotherapeutic agents have a mechanism that has not yet been defined. For example, dacarbazine (DTIC-Dome), used to treat metastatic malignant melanoma and Hodgkin's lymphoma, kills these cells by one of three possible mechanisms, none of which has been proven. Gemcitabine is known to block cell division in its early phase, but the exact mechanism by which it does this is unknown. The same is true for the hydrazine derivative procarbazine.

COMPLICATIONS AND SIDE EFFECTS OF CHEMOTHERAPY

Complications and *side effects* are two terms that are often confused when patients and doctors discuss the effects of chemotherapy. A side effect is an expected reaction to taking a drug or even a nutritional supplement. Sometimes, side effects are wanted. For example, taking an aspirin will relieve your headache, plus it will help prevent colon cancer and possibly lower your risk of Alzheimer's disease as well.

Most of us think of side effects as bad. The majority of pharmaceutical drugs have harmful side effects, whereas nutritional supplements more often have helpful side effects. To appreciate this difference, just listen to the drug advertisements on television with the idyllic country setting and a beautiful woman telling you how wonderful she feels now that she has NasalBlow, a new drug for allergies. At the end of the ad, a rapidly speaking voice tells you that the drug may cause explosive diarrhea, blindness in one or both eyes, heart failure, collapsed lungs, intense vertigo, and a possible loss of memory.

On the other hand, a complication is an unexpected reaction to taking a drug. For example, a complication of using aspirin is severe bleeding from the stomach. What is important to you is the percentage of the risk and the severity of the complication. If a "cocktail" of chemotherapy drugs has a complication rate of 65 percent and the main complication is development of a second cancer more lethal than the one you have, the risk is not justified.

Now let us look at some of the common side effects and complications of the chemotherapeutic drugs, and what you can do about them.

Fatigue

Fatigue is the most common complaint from patients receiving chemotherapy treatments. Because it is so common, I will address it in a special section in Chapter 8.

Nausea and Vomiting

Of all the side effects of chemotherapy, nausea and vomiting are the most dreaded by patients. Oncologists tend to play this down, claiming they have new, powerful antinausea drugs that can treat these symptoms, which is true to an extent.

Nausea and vomiting are caused by two properties of chemotherapy drugs. The first is stimulation of the chemoreceptor trigger zone (CTZ) in the brain stem (the nausea center), and the second is irritation of the lining of the stomach. Both of these events can be significantly reduced by following carefully designed dietary guidelines and by using special supplements.

Many nutrients have powerful anti-inflammatory properties, which may explain why patients on a nutritional program have dramatically less nausea. These same properties protect the stomach lining.

There are several supplements that soothe the stomach lining, including ginger extract, deglycyrrhizinated licorice root, slippery elm, gamma-oryzanol, and marshmallow root. They do this by increasing the mucous produced by the stomach, something that is lost during chemotherapy treatment. Several companies make combination supplements to help nausea and vomiting. Check the labels for the ingredients that work the best for you.

Patients having gastritis or an ulcer will benefit greatly from these supplements, much more than they would from prescription drugs. Not only will these supplements calm the stomach, but they will also improve digestion. This will decrease bloating.

While nausea and vomiting are less of a problem today, a substantial number of cancer patients still suffer from uncontrollable nausea and/or vomiting. Fortunately, we now have some very powerful drugs to combat this, such as the 5H3 receptor antagonists including ondanestron (Zofran) and granisetron (Kytril). Nausea and vomiting fall into two categories in cancer patients: acute (immediate) and delayed. Acute nausea or vomiting develops during chemotherapy treatment and usually subsides when it ends, whereas delayed symptoms can occur months after the treatments have been completed. The 5H3 receptor antagonists work very well for the acute type of sickness, but not for the delayed.

There are several risk factors for developing nausea and vomiting with chemotherapy, including being female, being between the ages of six and fifty, and having drunk little or no alcohol in the past. (This is not an excuse to go pour yourself a stiff one!) As we shall see, nutritional supplementation is a better way to avoid chemotherapy-related nausea and vomiting. In fact, there are several things you can do to reduce your risk of developing nausea and vomiting, including the following:

- Avoid spicy or acidic foods. Acidic foods include oranges, lemons, and tomatoes.
- Avoid greasy foods.
- Drink a mixture of vegetables, as described in Chapter 1. It will buffer the excess acid in your stomach and other irritating foods as well.
- Eat smaller meals several times a day. Avoid eating too much at any one time.
- Start your nutritional program and supplements at least one week before beginning your chemotherapy treatment. If you have already started your treatment, they will still work, but less well.
- On the day before your treatment begins, eat very lightly and drink clear liquids (distilled water) only.
- Avoid foods with strong odors.
- Stay out of the kitchen while foods are being cooked. The smell of foods cooking can bring on nausea and vomiting.
- Eat relaxed meals in comfortable settings.
- Avoid all food additives, especially MSG (all forms), aspartame, and carrageenan. All of these are known to irritate the gastrointestinal tract and induce nausea. MSG frequently causes diarrhea.
- Avoid eating around strong perfumes, cosmetics, and other odors.

By eating a diet composed mostly of vegetables and low-fat protein sources, you will avoid many of the food components that stimulate nausea. In addition, many of the phytochemicals in plants, especially the flavonoids, reduce inflammation, buffer the blood, and directly inhibit the factors known to stimulate nausea and vomiting.

Some chemotherapy drugs are more associated with nausea and vomiting than others. The worst include dacarbazine (DTIC-

Dome), streptozocin, cisplatin, mechlorethamine (Mustargen), and high-dose Ara-C. Less serious nausea and vomiting are seen with CCNU, BCNU, cytoxan, semustine, procarbarzine, mithracin, and cosmegen. In about 50 percent of patients, 5-FU, daunorubicin, L-asparginase, mutamycin, and adriamycin cause significant nausea and vomiting.

Remember that everyone is different. Some drugs will cause severe problems for some patients and little or nothing at all for other patients.

Food Aversion

One of the really bad effects of chemotherapy is the development of food aversions. This is a reaction to foods eaten either just before or during the beginning of chemotherapy treatment. Some doctors will tell you to avoid eating the foods you like before starting your chemotherapy treatments because afterwards you will not be able to enjoy them. In some patients, even the thought of the food can precipitate feelings of nausea and vomiting.

Food aversion can be a problem because it can include aversions to some of the more nutritious foods. Taking nutritional supplements for several weeks before the start of your treatments may prevent this reaction. The same precautions described for nausea and vomiting also help minimize food aversions.

Sore Mouth and Throat

Sore, inflamed tissues of the mouth and/or throat can lead to numerous problems besides the immediate pain and suffering. Infection, malnutrition due to an inability to swallow, dehydration, and bleeding can all result from this condition.

Many chemotherapy agents, and especially combinations, as well as radiation treatment to the head, neck, or upper chest area, can cause this agonizing condition. The cells lining the mouth and esophagus are included in the list of cells that divide rapidly and that are thus very vulnerable to these treatments.

Several things can be done to minimize the symptoms caused by this condition:

- Avoid hot foods. Eat only foods that are slightly warm or cold.
- Avoid spicy foods and drinks.
- If you have dentures or other dental appliances, make sure they fit well and do not rub against your gums or the inside of your mouth.
- Do not smoke, chew tobacco, or drink alcohol.
- Avoid mouthwashes that contain alcohol, peroxide, fluoride, or another powerful astringent.
- Use a soft toothbrush and brush gently. If you use an electric or battery-powered toothbrushing appliance, use it on the gentle setting.
- To prevent infections, use a mouthwash compounded from grapefruit seed extract. Because grapefruit seed extract is extremely bitter, have a compounding pharmacist mix it with the natural sweetener stevia. Add one teaspoon of the concentrated liquid to four ounces of distilled water and use it as a mouthwash. It can be swallowed. Grapefruit seed extract is a very powerful antibacterial, antifungal, and antiparasitic that soothes inflamed tissues.
- Take 100 milligrams of CoQ_{10} three times a day. Make sure the oil in the capsule is rice oil. CoQ_{10} protects the gingiva from infection and irritation. In addition, it plays a major role in protecting the heart. Another way to relieve the inflammation is to mix 100 milligrams of CoQ_{10} powder with one tablespoon of extra virgin olive oil and swish it in your mouth until the membranes are well coated.
- Dissolve the contents of one capsule of vitamin E succinate in two ounces of distilled water and swish it in your mouth for thirty seconds, then swallow. Do this three times a day. Vitamin E has been shown in clinical studies to relieve the irritation of oral mucous membrane inflammation.
- Take 4 grams of the amino acid glutamine twice a day. Glutamine has been shown in clinical studies to significantly reduce stomatitis associated with chemotherapy. Mix the glutamine with four ounces of distilled water, swish it in your mouth for thirty seconds, and swallow.[6] Note, however, that people with a glioma type tumor of the brain (astrocy-

toma or glioblastoma) should avoid glutamine, since it is converted in the brain to glutamate, which has been shown to dramatically increase the growth of these tumors. For a complete discussion of this, see page 152.

In most cases, the mouth and throat soreness associated with chemotherapy will subside in two to three weeks following completion of the treatments. These measures will allow you to deal with the discomfort much more effectively.

Hair Loss

The neurosurgery department to which I belonged, the same as all neurosurgery departments, believed that the answer to a loss of hair associated with radiation treatment or chemotherapy was a wig. There are better answers. The reason these treatments cause the hair to fall out is because hair cells reproduce very rapidly, just like cancer cells.

I noticed early on that using a high dose of antioxidant vitamins prevented hair loss in a significant number of my patients undergoing chemotherapy or radiation treatment. The patients using antioxidant supplements who lost their hair found that it grew back faster and healthier than the hair of other patients. This is because antioxidants protect the hair follicle cells from being damaged by the treatments. In addition, they promote hair growth and health.

One of the key nutritional factors in stimulating hair growth and preventing hair loss is biotin. Combining biotin with the antioxidants brings maximum protection. Many of the flavonoids protect against several types of powerful free radicals normally resistant to the vitamin antioxidants.

There are several things you can do to reduce hair loss, including the following:

- Avoid harsh shampoos, especially those containing sodium lauryl sulfate.
- Dry your hair either naturally or with a blow dryer set on low heat.
- Wash your hair every other day rather than daily.

The following supplement program will help to reduce hair loss and speed its healthy regrowth:

- Take 3 milligrams of biotin twice a day throughout your treatment and for two weeks afterward. Then cut back to 3 milligrams once a day thereafter.
- Take a multivitamin-and-mineral capsule every day.
- Take 400 international units of vitamin E succinate three times a day.
- Take 500 milligrams of quercetin three times a day with meals.
- Take 500 milligrams of hesperidin three times a day with meals.
- Take 500 milligrams of curcumin three times a day. Dissolve the contents of one capsule in one tablespoon of extra virgin olive oil.
- Take 100 milligrams of decaffeinated green tea extract with each meal.

Depressed Production of Blood-Forming Cells

The depressed production of blood-forming cells is most often described as "bone marrow depression," but in truth it involves much more. As I stated earlier, chemotherapy suppresses the reproduction of all rapidly dividing cells, normal or cancerous, and increases their death. The body's demand for red blood cells, immune cells, white blood cells, and platelets is so enormous that these cells normally reproduce as fast as many cancerous tumors. Billions of these cells can be produced every minute.

The immune cells are produced in the bone marrow, intestinal wall (Peyer's patches), lymph nodes, spleen, and a few other tissues, collectively called the hemopoietic system. When all of these cell types are depressed, as is common with the use of chemotherapeutic drugs, the results can include an increased risk of infections, increased spread of the cancer, abnormal bleeding, and severe states of anemia.

The vast majority of the chemotherapeutic drugs cause varying degrees of depression of the blood-forming organs, with some affecting particular types of cells more than others. For example, the drug vinorelbine, a vinka alkaloid, specifically produces granulocytopenia, a loss of granulocytes such as the neutrophils, eosinophils, and basophils.

Despite advertising claims and news media reports of its smart bomb–like effects, the new drug Gleevec has as one of its consistent findings a suppression of normal blood cells, especially the neutrophils and thrombocytes (platelets). On occasion, the suppression will require that the treatment be discontinued, either temporarily or permanently.

Hemopoietic system suppression is one of the most common reasons cancer patients need to discontinue their chemotherapy treatment. This is very important, since it has been shown that discontinuing chemotherapy treatment, even temporarily, or lowering the dose of the chemotherapy agent, is a common cause for failure of the treatment. Again, treatment success relates to tumor-free survival, not to permanent cure.

In one survey of 1,500 chemotherapy patients, 45 percent had treatment delays of more than five days due to side effects, while 28 percent required a reduction in the dose of their drugs.[7] In another survey of 500 patients undergoing chemotherapy, 25 percent had to stop or delay treatment following the first dose of the drugs because of complications.[8]

In addition, a significant number of patients receiving chemotherapy require blood transfusions or medications to increase a depressed blood count caused by the treatment itself. Several medications have been developed to stimulate the production of blood cells of various types. For example, when the neutrophils are depressed by chemotherapy drugs, a granulocyte-colony-stimulating hormone can be prescribed. Another product, epoetin alfa (Epogen, Procrit), acts like the natural substance erythopoetin, which stimulates red blood cell production.

Like all drugs, these blood-stimulating medications have some significant side effects associated with their use. For example, as many as 57 percent of patients experience nausea and 11 percent develop significant fatigue when taking colony-stimulating factor. Epoetin alfa produces fatigue in as many as 25 percent of patients and fever in 38 percent of patients. One particular problem associated with this latter drug is hypertension, seen in up to 24 percent of patients.

A return of the blood cells to normal levels may take several weeks; occasionally, it can take several months. When their blood counts are very low, patients are at a high risk of infection, anemia, relapse of their disease, and hemorrhaging. When a drug known to cause severe bone marrow depression, such as carboplatin, is used in conjunction with other such drugs or following radiation treatments, abnormalities of the blood cells are often more severe.

Several nutrients have shown an ability to protect the bone marrow and to stimulate a return of normal cells. Because of the enormous number of cells produced by the haematopoietic system, many nutrients are needed. Following are my recommendations:

- Take 500 milligrams of curcumin three times a day. Dissolve the contents of one capsule in one tablespoon of extra virgin olive oil. This flavonoid, extracted from the spice turmeric, has been shown not only to protect the bone marrow cells, but also to stimulate their regeneration. I have found it to work very well, even with drug combinations known to severely suppress the bone marrow.
- Take 800 micrograms of folate every day. Folate plays a major role in haematopoietic cell reproduction. Large amounts of this vitamin are needed to produce these cells.
- Take 1,000 micrograms of sublingual methylcobalamin three times a day during your treatment. Dissolve the tablet under your tongue. Methylcobalamin also plays a major role in blood cell reproduction. Cut back to one tablet twice a day when your treatments are finished.
- Take 50 milligrams of pyridoxal-5-phosphate every day. Pyridoxal-5-phosphate is the form of vitamin B_6 used by the blood cells.
- Take a multivitamin-and-mineral capsule every day. It is best to take this supplement between meals, but if it causes stomach upset or nausea, take it with meals.

- Take 500 milligrams of vitamin C (buffered as magnesium ascorbate) three times a day between meals.
- Take 400 international units of vitamin E succinate three times a day. This vitamin helps protect the bone marrow cells when used in conjunction with the other supplements.
- Take 500 milligrams of niacinamide twice a day. This vitamin plays a major role in DNA synthesis, a process used by the blood cells to reproduce. Niacinamide is the form of niacin used by the body. It is safer than niacin and does not cause flushing.

Cardiac Toxicity

Cardiac toxicity is a major cause of death for cancer patients, either during or following chemotherapy treatments with certain agents. It is a problem especially with doxorubicin (adriamycin), an antibiotic that is frequently used to treat breast cancer. Doxorubicin's mechanism of action involves not only inhibition of DNA and RNA replication, but also blocking of the topoisomerase II enzyme, cell membrane binding, and production of the extremely toxic hydroxyl free radical. It is the last action that is the suspected cause of the heart damage done by the drug.

According to the *Physicians' Desk Reference* (*PDR*), a guide to medications published by Medical Economics Company and updated annually, doxorubicin is associated with irreversible myocardial toxicity, which in its worst form can lead to fatal congestive heart failure. The truly frightening thing about this drug is that the heart failure may occur during treatment (acute toxicity) or even years later (delayed toxicity). In fact, delayed heart failure is more common in children treated with the drug. This is because the drug poisons the heart muscle during the child's development, preventing it from reaching its required size in later life.

According to *PDR*, as many as 40 percent of pediatric patients suffer from subclinical cardiac dysfunction—that is, they have weakened hearts—and 5 to 10 percent develop congestive heart failure. When used in combination with other chemotherapeutic drugs, doxorubicin can result in even higher incidences of heart damage. The amount of damage inflicted is dose dependent—that is, the higher the dose of the drug, the greater the damage.

The delayed type of heart damage is particularly frightful because it does not respond to the heart medications usually used to treat congestive heart failure, such as digitalis. Biopsies of the heart muscle in such cases demonstrate swelling of the mitochondria, the main energy source in the heart muscle cells.

Another, newer drug associated with severe degrees of heart muscle injury is Herceptin. This drug acts by suppressing the overactive human epidermal growth factor 2 (HER2) receptor, which is a growth factor protein found in 25 to 30 percent of breast cancers. The congestive heart failure associated with Herceptin can be very severe and can lead to strokes and fatal heart failure. Patients taking this drug must be followed closely with cardiac function tests.

Several drugs, such as Taxol and Taxotere, can complicate preexisting cardiac disease and must be used cautiously. People with cardiac disease may not be able to tolerate the more cardiotoxic drugs, such as doxorubicin and Herceptin.

While not a major complication, heart toxicity is also a problem with 5-FU. The drug has been known to cause sudden death mimicking a heart attack.[9] More often, the side effects are angina, pulmonary edema, or arrhythmias, but even these are fairly uncommon. Cardiac toxicity is also a major complication of cyclophosphamide, cytarabine, daunomycin, actinomycin D, and mitoxantrone.

Oncologists have searched for a way to prevent the damage caused by drugs such as doxorubicin and cyclophosphamide. The most extensively studied method has been the supplemental use of vitamin E. Most of the studies have shown that vitamin E, when started just before the onset of therapy, can significantly reduce acute heart muscle damage, but not delayed damage.[10] Of real importance is the fact that the vitamin E did not interfere with the effectiveness of the doxorubicin against the cancer.[11] Vitamin C can also protect the heart against the acute toxicity of doxorubicin without compromising the effectiveness of the chemotherapy. In fact, vitamin C significantly increased the tumor-killing effectiveness of the doxorubicin and of several other chemotherapy drugs as well.[12] Two other supplements, selenium and NAC, have also been shown to significantly protect against the acute cardiac injury caused by doxorubicin. The dose of selenium used was very high: 4,000 micrograms a day in four divided doses for eight consecutive days, starting four days before the chemotherapy was begun.[13] Selenium in this dose can be toxic and should not be taken for more than eight days.

NAC is a supplement compound containing the amino acid cysteine, which is used by the cells to produce glutathione. In clinical studies, NAC has been shown to protect against the acute cardiac toxicity of doxorubicin, but not against the delayed toxicity.[14] The problem with most of these studies is that the supplement was given, usually in huge doses, starting just days before the treatment or on the first day of treatment. Lower doses can be used if the supplement is started several weeks before the treatment is begun. This gives the cells more time to produce glutathione.

So what about delayed cardiac injury? So far, all the nutrients I have mentioned prevent only acute heart damage. One supplement has been found to significantly protect against delayed damage: CoQ_{10}.[15] This may be because doxorubicin causes the CoQ_{10} levels in the heart muscle to fall, eventually leading to damage of the muscle cells. In addition, CoQ_{10} binds with the free iron in the heart muscle. Free iron is a powerful generator of free radicals.

There are many nutritional steps that you can take to protect your heart against damage by the chemotherapeutic drugs. Central to this protection is supplying the heart muscle with adequate levels of the antioxidant nutrients:

- Take 400 international units of vitamin E succinate three times a day.
- Take 500 milligrams of magnesium ascorbate three times a day.
- Take 500 milligrams of curcumin three times a day. Dissolve the contents of one capsule in one tablespoon of extra virgin olive oil.
- Take a bioflavonoid complex with quercetin every day. Make sure the product contains rutin, quercetin, and hesperidin,

all of which are powerful antioxidants that protect against free radical cardiac damage by the chemotherapeutic drugs.
- Take 100 milligrams of decaffeinated green tea extract every day. This extract has been shown to protect the blood vessels, including those of the heart. In addition, it protects the heart muscle against free radical damage.
- Take 400 milligrams of propolis extract twice a day during treatment and for three weeks afterward. Propolis extract is a cement material produced by bees that contains very high concentrations of the flavonoids. In one study, it was shown to strongly protect mice against doxorubicin-induced cardiac muscle injury.[16]
- Take 500 milligrams of NAC three times a day starting at least one week before beginning your therapy and continuing for three weeks after completing it. Then take 500 milligrams twice a day.
- Take 200 micrograms of selenium twice a day starting at least one week before beginning your therapy and continuing for one week into the treatment. Then take 200 micrograms once a day.

In addition, there are a number of nutrients that improve cardiac muscle strength, thereby improving heart function. I recommend the following:

- Take 500 milligrams of acetyl-L-carnitine three times a day on an empty stomach. Acetyl-L-carnitine significantly improves cardiac muscle energy, which is depleted during chemotherapy. An alternative is L-Carnitine Fumarate. This supplement's advantage is the fumarate, which is a major metabolite used in the Kreb's energy cycle. The combination of L-carnitine and fumarate improves cardiac function even more.
- Take 200 milligrams of CoQ_{10} four times a day starting at least one week before beginning your therapy and continuing for three weeks after completing it. Then take 100 milligrams three times a day. The heart muscle utilizes large amounts of CoQ_{10}, a mitochondrial energy molecule. Several studies have shown the nutrient combats congestive heart

failure, especially when caused by doxorubicin. It is also a powerful antioxidant and improves cellular glutathione levels.

- Take 150 milligrams of magnesium citrate plus malate every day. Magnesium is essential for heart protection and the prevention of arrhythmias (irregular heartbeats), which are often caused by the chemotherapeutic agents. Citrate and malate are Kreb's cycle energy metabolites.
- Increase your intake of the omega-3 fatty acids. The omega-3 fatty acids protect against arrhythmias. In addition, they improve coronary blood flow and cardiac muscle function. Most brands contain no more than 30 percent of these protective oils. Do not take more than the highest recommended dose of your chosen brand, however, since higher doses increase the risk of bleeding tendencies.
- Take 500 milligrams of hawthorne extract one to three times a day. Hawthorne extract has been shown to improve the blood flow through the coronary arteries and to increase cardiac muscle strength. It may also lower blood pressure in hypertensive people. Use hawthorne extract only under the supervision of a physician and never combine it with cardiac or blood pressure prescription medications.

In addition to taking the above supplements, avoid all products containing MSG in any form, since MSG can overstimulate the heart's electrical conduction system, resulting in sudden cardiac failure or arrhythmia. Overstimulating of the heart's electrical conduction system is a special risk for patients using cardiotoxic chemotherapy agents. Most hospital foods contain MSG in some form.

Pulmonary Complications

The alkylating agent busulfan is associated with a form of lung damage called pulmonary fibrosis. Though fairly rare, when pulmonary fibrosis develops, it does not respond to medical treatment and is uniformly fatal within six months. Like the delayed cardiac toxicity seen with doxorubicin, "busulfan lung" can develop within eight months to ten years after treatment, with the average onset being four years.

Again, combining radiation treatments to the chest area with chemotherapy using several agents simultaneously increases the risk of pulmonary damage. Protection should be aimed at the prevention of free radical damage to the lungs. The scarring of pulmonary fibrosis develops as a result of the damage caused by free radicals.

There are several nutrients and nutrient combinations known to protect the lungs from busulfan toxicity. The flavonoids rutin, quercetin and hesperidin, taken together, strongly protect the lungs from free radical damage, as well as from injury from iron excess.[17,18,19]

One supplement of special usefulness is Bioflavonoid Complex with Quercetin. This product combines the anticancer flavonoid quercetin with the other antioxidant flavonoids in a capsule form. Take two capsules three times a day with meals throughout your treatment period and for three additional weeks. Then take one capsule three times a day thereafter. At the first sign of pulmonary symptoms (shortness of breath), return to the higher dose and maintain it until all the symptoms subside.

Another powerful anticancer flavonoid-containing supplement, green tea extract, has numerous properties beneficial to the cancer patient. Green tea is high in the flavonoids catechin and epigallocatechin gallate, which not only inhibit cancer by several mechanisms, but are also very powerful antioxidants, chelate iron, and strengthen the walls of the blood vessels as well as of the air passageways in the lungs. I recommend taking only the decaffeinated form of the extract to avoid jitteriness and insomnia. Take 300 milligrams three times a day with meals.

Commanding a lot of attention in the field of cancer research is curcumin, a flavonoid found in the spice turmeric. As we have seen, curcumin contains many properties beneficial to the cancer patient. Because of its powerful anti-inflammatory and antioxidant properties, it offers considerable protection against pulmonary injury secondary to the conventional treatment.

Vitamin E has been known for some time to prevent scarring following injury of any sort. It also reduces scarring of the lungs associated with chemotherapy and radiation injuries. To maximize effectiveness, combine two types of vitamin E: the natural (mixed tocopherols) and vitamin E succinate. Natural vitamin E contains several forms of the tocopherol molecule, all of which play a role in cell protection. Vitamin E succinate, as we have seen, is the most potent antioxidant form of vitamin E and appears to have the greatest anticancer effect.

Finally, boswellia, an herb demonstrating powerful anti-inflammatory properties, also strengthens the connective tissues, which play a vital role in the lungs. It usually comes in 300-milligram capsules, one of which should be taken twice a day between meals. Because of its low complication rate, boswellia can be taken long term.

Gastrointestinal Complications

The cells lining the gastrointestinal tract, especially those concerned with the absorption of foods, have a high turnover rate, which means they are very vulnerable to the vast majority of chemotherapeutic agents, especially when these agents are combined. The alkylating agents seem to cause the greatest problems. In addition, one of the antibiotic chemotherapy drugs, Actinomycin D, is known to cause severe gastrointestinal toxicity at the higher doses.

Damage to the epithelial cells lining the gastrointestinal tract is especially harmful to cancer patients, since this not only can cause severe malabsorption problems but can also open “holes” in the intestinal lining that allow whole food proteins and large carbohydrate molecules to enter the bloodstream (leaky gut syndrome). This can trigger an immune reaction leading to food allergies, driving the already weakened immune system away from its primary job of fighting cancer cells.

In addition, the chemotherapy drugs are all immune suppressants and can therefore lead to an overgrowth of yeast organisms, such as *Candida albicans*, not only in the gastrointestinal tract, but also throughout the body (systemically). Many cancer patients receive one or more courses of antibiotics during their treatment, which further increases the risk of yeast overgrowth as well as the loss of “beneficial” colon bacteria.

The same as food allergies, yeast overgrowth in the blood

and tissues diverts the immune system away from attacking the cancer cells, since it must also attack the yeast cells. In addition, yeast organisms secrete toxins that cause fatigue, mental fog, and muscle and joint pains. Intestinal and systemic yeast overgrowth are universally ignored by physicians treating cancer patients.

Normally, the colon contains trillions of bacteria and viruses, and a small amount of fungi. The exact mix of these organisms has been shown to play a major role in health. We refer to the mix as our gut ecology. When our ecology is disrupted, the condition that results is called dysbiosis. Of particular importance is a group of bacteria referred to as the "beneficial" bacteria. These beneficial bacteria serve many useful purposes, including immune regulation, suppression of pathogenic (disease-causing) organisms, manufacture of nutrients, and metabolism of various hormones.

The beneficial bacteria consist of three types of organisms: several species of *Lactobacillus,* several species of *Bifidobacterium,* and *Escherchia coli.* Each of these species has a special function in the gastrointestinal tract. Not only should all be present, but they must exist in amounts sufficient to maintain a healthy colon environment. Bacteria are measured in quantities from NG (no growth) to plus 4, with the latter being the highest growth concentration. All beneficial bacteria are vulnerable to the chemotherapy drugs, radiation, and antibiotics.

Replacement of these crucial bacteria is vital, not only during chemotherapy treatment, but long term. The supplements used to replace these bacteria are called probiotics. There are many brands available. While most of the products can be kept at room temperature, I recommend storing them in the refrigerator. Most studies have shown that the organisms live much longer when refrigerated.

Because the beneficial bacteria are live organisms, they must have food available to survive. This is especially critical in the brands that are kept at room temperature. One of the most common bacteria foods is fructooligosaccharide (FOS). In most instances, FOS will feed only the "beneficial" bacteria, but in some instances, it will also feed the pathogenic species. Several foods for bacteria are commercially available.

Because FOS can stimulate the budding of Candida yeast organisms, I prefer other forms of prebiotics, which is another name for these beneficial bacteria products. Stool and possibly blood cultures for Candida infections are vital to detect such infections early. Early treatment increases the likelihood of successful control of the cancer.

Another frequent problem seen in cancer patients exposed to multiple chemotherapy courses or combined chemotherapy and radiation treatments is a loss of the digestive enzymes. This includes the enzymes secreted from the stomach, pancreas, and intestinal wall. Unless you digest your food well, you will not be able to absorb its nutrients properly. In addition, you will experience bloating, cramping, and impaired bowel function.

Stomach acidity is also vital to gastrointestinal function. When stomach acidity is low, many enzymes cannot function properly. For example, the protein-dissolving enzyme chymotrypsin must be converted to trypsin to work. However, it cannot be converted if the stomach does not have adequate amounts of hydrochloric acid. As we age, our stomach acidity falls (hypochlorhydria). Chemotherapy can also damage the cells that produce stomach acid.

Vigorous nutritional treatment of an intestinal injury will also greatly improve your comfort level, as well as your ability to overcome your cancer. Because the gastrointestinal tract includes over 50 percent of the immune system, protecting it becomes essential to successful cancer treatment. In addition, for the nutrients you ingest to work, they must be able to get to your cells and tissues. The gastrointestinal system is the key to successful treatment.

Liver Injury

Liver damage is common with many chemotherapy agents, since it is the liver that must detoxify these agents. In advanced cancer patients, metastasis to the liver is also frequently seen, especially with colon cancers. The more chemotherapeutic drugs that are combined, the greater is the risk of liver toxicity. In some cancer treatment programs, six or more drugs are used.

Another important consideration is the detoxification load

put on the liver during intense chemotherapeutic treatment. When large numbers of cancer cells are killed, the debris released as the cancer cells die can produce a severe toxic reaction, which in some instances can be fatal. It is the liver that must detoxify these cellular toxins.

In most instances, liver injury is indicated by elevations in specific enzymes, such as serum glutamic oxalacetic transaminase (SGOT), serum glutamic pyruvic transaminase (SGPT), alkaline phosphatase, serum bilirubin, lactic dehydrogenase, and ornithine carbamyl transferase. Taxol can be particularly damaging to the liver, especially in cases of preexisting liver damage.

Busulfan has been reported to cause esophageal varices in patients who are receiving long-term (continuous) doses of the drug combined with thioguanine for treatment of chronic myeologenous leukemia. This condition is caused by an obstruction of the venous system in the liver, resulting in gross dilation of the veins of the esophagus. This not only interferes with swallowing, but can lead to fatal hemorrhages.

Note that elevations in the liver enzymes are not a sensitive measure of liver injury. Cellular damage can occur, especially in the detoxification ability of the liver, without causing an elevation in liver enzymes. The ability of the liver to detoxify these poisons can be measured by a special test. In addition, there are many ways to enhance the liver's detoxification ability using nutraceuticals.

Several of the supplements used to improve the liver's detoxification process are used to prevent and treat cancer as well. For example, curcumin, indole-3-carbinol, the carotenoid vitamins, and D-glucarate all perform both functions. In addition, curcumin improves the removal process by which dead cells are eliminated from the body (reticuloendothelial system). Methyl sulfonyl methane (MSM) is an excellent source of sulfur molecules, which are used by the liver in detoxification. Another good souce of sulfur for the liver is the amino acid taurine.

Kidney Injury

The administration of combined chemotherapeutic agents is often limited by the existence of kidney damage, since most of these compounds are excreted by the kidneys. Because of the high concentration of these compounds in the urine, damage to the kidneys is common. Severe kidney damage can prevent the use of many of these agents.

In most instances, kidney function is tracked by testing the level of serum creatinine or blood urea nitrogen (BUN) to avoid severe kidney damage. One way to protect the kidneys is to utilize nutrients known to protect the kidneys. For example, quercetin has been shown to protect renal cells in culture from the toxicity of cisplatin.[20] Curcumin has also been shown to powerfully protect the kidneys from injury.[21]

Extracts from the herb Panax ginseng have demonstrated a very powerful ability to protect the kidneys from cisplatin toxicity in experimental studies using mice.[22] The only real drawback to Panax ginseng is that it can increase your energy to such a high level that you will be nervous and jittery. It can also cause insomnia.

Several studies have shown that intravenous glutathione can significantly reduce the kidney toxicity of cisplatin.[23] The glutathione works by interacting with the cisplatin, blocking its ability to kill cells. The reason the glutathione doesn't interfere with the cisplatin's ability to kill the cancer cells is that normal cells take up a lot of the glutathione, whereas the cancer cells take up very little. In fact, studies have shown that patients treated with glutathione plus cisplatin have a better cancer remission rate than those treated with cisplatin alone.[24]

Another supplement, NAC, has been shown to prevent or significantly reduce the incidence of hemorrhagic cystitis (bleeding in the bladder) caused by the chemotherapy drug cyclophosphamide and its chemical cousin ifosfamide.[25] The bleeding is caused by a metabolic product produced by these drugs called acrolein, which depletes the antioxidants, especially glutathione, from the bladder cells. Large doses (9 grams a day) of NAC were used in these studies. At these high levels, most cancer patients will experience nausea and vomiting. Again, by taking lower doses (1 to 2 grams) over a longer period of time (several weeks), the same effect can be attained without the side effects. NAC does not interfere with the anticancer effectiveness of the drugs.[26]

Other supplements that protect the kidneys during cancer treatment and stimulate their healing are magnesium citramate, vitamin E succinate, magnesium ascorbate, calcium-AEP, and asparagus extract. In addition, be sure to take a good multivitamin-and-mineral supplement every day.

Neurological Complications

I believe that all chemotherapy agents cause some degree of brain injury. As I have already stated, most oncologists believe that the brain is rarely affected by these drugs because the brain cells (neurons) do not divide after birth. In fact, the brain cells do divide after birth and may do so for several years after birth. The brain reaches only 80 percent of its growth by the age of four. During this critical period, the brain grows rapidly, not only in terms of brain cell production, but also in terms of the trillions of connections between the neurons, dendrites, and synapses.

Drugs that affect DNA function, which include most of the chemotherapy drugs, can alter the formation of these pathways. DNA toxins can affect both neuron reproduction and the growth of dendrites and synapses. Ultimately, this can result in miswiring of the developing brain and a loss of critical cells in the temporal lobes, both of which can result in impaired higher cognitive functions such as reading, comprehension, logic, and emotional development.

These effects may vary from obvious to quite subtle. In addition, they can be delayed by years or even decades. Unfortunately, very few studies have been done on the long-term consequences of chemotherapy treatments in children—that is, by evaluating children when they have reached adulthood.

In addition to the brain continuing to grow for several years after birth, it constantly changes and remodels itself throughout life by a process called plasticity. Basically, plasticity is the growth of new connections between the neurons and the repairing of old connections. Furthermore, the brain contains millions of stem cells, which change to mature neurons when needed. All of these cells and connections in the adult brain can be injured by chemotherapy agents and radiation treatments.

The studies that have been done show a definite increase in

the long-term complications as well as in second malignancies. For example, both chemotherapy and radiation treatments can result in infertility, pulmonary injury, hypertension, and endocrine disorders many years following the treatment.[27] The development of secondary cancers caused by chemotherapy drugs and radiation treatments is triple that seen in normal youths. In the case of Hodgkin's lymphoma treatments, the incidence of secondary cancers is as high as 17 percent.[28]

Another recent long-term follow-up study of young men who had nonseminomatous testicular cancer treated successfully with cisplatin found that 28 percent suffered polyneuropathy symptoms, with the symptoms severe in 6 percent of the subjects.[29] In addition, 23 percent had reduced hearing, 37 percent had pulmonary toxicity, and 35 percent had vascular disorders. An earlier study found that 30 percent of the subjects experienced abnormal heart function.[30]

It is important to remember that secondary cancers are not recurrences of a previous cancer but entirely new cancers caused by the treatment. Most often, the secondary cancer is much more resistant to treatment than was the original cancer.[31]

As far as I am aware, no one has looked into the effects of these treatments on the brain's system of stem cells. Stem cells are primitive cells in the brain, especially in the temporal lobes, that function as replacement cells when mature cells are damaged. If we lose these reserve cells early in life, or at any time, we lose a major protection system.

Even though we know that most chemotherapeutic agents act by damaging the DNA, no one has looked at the effect of chemotherapy on cellular mitochondrial function, especially in the nervous system. The mitochondria are the energy factories within the cells that supply virtually all of the cell's energy needs. It is known that mitochondrial DNA is ten times more sensitive to free radical injury than is nuclear DNA.[32] The reason is that the mitochondria have very few DNA repair enzymes.

Damaged mitochondrial DNA is suspected to be a major cause of neurodegenerative diseases such as Alzheimer's disease, Parkinson's disease, and Lou Gehrig's disease.[33] For example, it has been shown that one of the earliest changes in Parkinson's disease is a 42 percent loss of mitochondrial energy production in the part of the brain responsible for the disease. No one has yet looked to see if there is an increased incidence of one or more of these degenerative brain disorders in the survivors of chemotherapy regimens.

One chemotherapy agent that causes significant nervous system toxicity is procarbazine, a component of the MOPP combination of drugs (which also includes mechlorethamine, vincristine, and prednisone) used to treat Hodgkin's disease. It can cause somnolence (sleepiness), confusion, and cerebellar ataxia (loss of balance). One of the most notorious drugs for causing neurological side effects is cisplatin. Ototoxicity—that is, damage to the inner ear—is commonly seen with this drug and can present as ringing in the ears (tinnitus), a loss of high-frequency hearing, or even complete deafness. And as we have seen, it can cause other neurological injuries as well.

Some experts argue that chemotherapy is not dangerous to the brain because many of the drugs used cannot pass the special protective system called the blood-brain barrier. The problem is that many conditions make this barrier permeable. An example is fever. Brain tumors, hypertension, certain medications, the presence of neurodegenerative diseases (such as Parkinson's disease), radiation treatments to the head, and aging itself can break down this barrier, allowing the drugs to enter.

We also know that many substances normally excluded by the blood-brain barrier will enter the brain if they are given over a long period of time. Many chemotherapy cycles last for months or even for as long as a year.

So, what can be done to protect the nervous system from these treatments? The main things from which you want to protect the brain are free radical damage and DNA damage. Within the brain, many types of free radicals can be produced, requiring a multitude of antioxidants for protection. A good nutritional program to follow is:

- Take 200 milligrams of alpha-lipoic acid twice a day with meals throughout your treatment and for three weeks afterward. Then take 100 milligrams twice a day thereafter.
- Take 500 milligrams of curcumin three times a day. Dissolve

the contents of one capsule in one tablespoon of extra virgin olive oil. Curcumin has a slight anticoagulant effect, so it should not be combined with aspirin or anticoagulant drugs.

- Take 500 to 1,000 milligrams of quercetin three times a day with meals.
- Take 175 milligrams of milk thistle every day.
- Take 160 to 320 milligrams of ginkgo biloba every day on an empty stomach. Ginkgo has been shown to increase brain blood flow. Do not take ginkgo with blood thinners.
- Take 400 international units of vitamin E succinate three times a day.
- Take 750 milligrams of magnesium ascorbate three times a day.
- Take 300 milligrams of magnesium citramate three times a day. Magnesium plays a major role in protecting the brain and heart.
- Take 120 to 240 milligrams of CoQ_{10} twice a day starting at least one week before beginning your therapy and continuing for three weeks after completing it.

In addition to taking the recommended supplements, discuss with your doctor the possibility of receiving reduced glutathione, which has been shown to significantly protect the nerves from cisplatin toxicity. Reduced glutathione must be taken intravenously, however, since the oral product is poorly absorbed and does not reach a high enough concentration in the body to be effective. Intravenous glutathione can be prepared by a compounding pharmacist and given by your doctor or other healthcare practitioner.

CONCLUSION

It is obvious that chemotherapy drugs, especially when used in combination, can cause injury to numerous organs and tissues. Of particular importance is damage to the liver, gastrointestinal tract, and immune system. Combining radiation therapy with chemotherapy magnifies these damaging effects. As we have seen, nutraceuticals and dietary changes can significantly reduce the damage to the normal tissues and organs, thereby greatly increasing the chances of a favorable outcome.

As you read through the lists of recommended supplements, you may have been overwhelmed by the large number noted. Notice, however, that many of the supplements are listed repeatedly for different conditions, demonstrating their versatile protective usefulness. In addition, many of the supplements that are later recommended to enhance the effectiveness of your conventional treatments are also among those recommended here. It is not necessary to take all of the supplements recommended. They are listed to give you a choice among the many available.

4

Radiation Therapy: Burning Cancer

Most cancer patients, upon first learning they will face radiation treatments, have an image of lying down under a death ray. Most know that radiation is dangerous and can cause burns, nausea and vomiting, loss of hair, and even additional cancer. Their fears are not unfounded.

Authorities in the field of radiation biology do not even agree on the safety of diagnostic X-rays, which involve infinitely lower doses of radiation than radiation therapy.

Today, many doctors recommend that their cancer patients undergo radiation treatments following surgery just as a precaution. In my estimation, this is not good science. Despite the fact that we have many sophisticated ways to determine who should have postoperative radiation and who shouldn't, we are not using many of these tools with the majority of cancer patients.

Yet even more shocking is the fact that many of the complications associated with radiation treatments can be avoided simply by using what we know about certain radioprotectant nutrients. As we shall see, we can avoid most of the complications associated with radiation treatments, including the production of new cancers, by changing the diet and using certain nutritional supplements. First, let us take a brief look at how radiation first came to be used in the treatment of cancer.

A Brief History of Radiation Therapy

By the early 1920s, X-rays were used primarily for diagnostic purposes, since they had very little penetrating ability. However, they were also used to treat external conditions, such as skin cancers, keratoses, plantar warts, and even ringworm. In fact, thousands of children had their scalps irradiated for ringworm, a common fungus infection. Unfortunately, a significant number of these children later developed cancers of the head, neck, or thyroid.

One of the early observations was that X-ray particles could not only kill cancer cells, but also cause cancer. In fact, Marie Curie and her daughter, Irene Joliot-Curie, both died of leukemia caused by their prolonged exposure to radium.

As the power of X-ray-generating machines was increased, more and more attempts were made to treat cancer. In the 1930s, Maurice Lenz used high-intensity X-rays to treat thirty-eight patients with inoperable breast cancer. He used doses of 6,000 to 8,000 rads, which are very high, over a two-to-three-month period. Examinations of the breasts of these women revealed surviving cancer cells. These early attempts at using radiation treatments before surgical removal of breast cancers were short lived because of disappointing results and complications.

One of the important early observations was that tumor cells exposed to abundant oxygen are much more vulnerable to radiation damage than are cells deficient in oxygen (hypoxic). In the mid-1950s, Dr. R. H. Thomlinson and his associate Dr. L. H. Gray proposed the idea that tumors contain populations of hypoxic cells.[1] John Reed, a clinical physicist, had already confirmed their suspicions in 1952, when he demonstrated that stem cells from broad beans, when made hypoxic, needed two and a half times more radiation to be killed than cells exposed to oxygen. Later studies indicated that large tumors may contain up to 30 percent hypoxic cells and smaller tumors may contain from 1 to 2 percent hypoxic cells. This means that deep within, cancers hide cells that are highly resistant to radiation, and these cells can survive to later grow and spread.

Based on these observations, several attempts were made to improve the effectiveness of radiation treatments by putting patients in hyperbaric 100 percent oxygen chambers. Unfortunately, doing this also increased the damage to the surrounding normal tissues, resulting in numerous complications. As a result, the method was abandoned. (For a discussion of mild hyperbaric oxygen chamber treatment, see below.)

Mild Hyperbaric Oxygen Chamber Treatment

While high-oxygen hyperbaric treatments are fraught with complications, a better and safer approach may be what is referred to as mild hyperbarics. In mild hyperbarics, normal room air, or lower levels of oxygen, are used under higher barometric pressures using a small, even portable, chamber. It has been shown that the oxygen content of the tissues is definitely elevated using this method, but not to the toxic levels seen when using 100 percent oxygen hyperbaric chambers. This new method allows us to raise the oxygen levels in tumors beyond what is possible by other methods. The raised oxygen level makes the tumor more susceptible to radiation therapy, as well as to chemotherapy. When using mild hyperbarics, it is vital to protect the normal tissues by using antioxidant vit amins, minerals, and flavonoid supplements during treatments.

Certain drugs, called radiosensitizers, have also been found to make cancers more sensitive to radiation. One of the early drugs was metronidazole, normally used to treat a protozoan infection (trichomonas). Several newer drugs have since been developed.

During the 1950s and 1960s, postoperative irradiation was used in breast cancer patients, but since it seemed to offer little, it was used only sporadically. Later studies indicated that irradiating the lymph node chains that most likely contain tumor cells does reduce recurrence.

Over time, the precision of the X-ray beam has been greatly improved, as has the sophistication of the X-ray tubes. Scandinavian researchers Dr. G. Forssell and Dr. R. Sievert refined and advanced the dosage schedules (dosemetry) used in the clinical treatment of tumors, making radiation treatments safer and more effective.

Our knowledge of the biological effects of radiation has also improved dramatically. We have learned that the young are more sensitive to the damaging effects of X-rays than are the old. Of critical importance is the fact that radiation damage to the cells is cumulative—that is, it is not necessary to give a full dose of radiation all at once. Instead, it can be divided into small exposures and spread out over several weeks, significantly reducing complications.

One of the great advances made in radiotherapy for cancer is the removal of the alpha and beta particles from the beams. Removing these particles prevents one of radiotherapy's greatest complications: damage to the skin. Severe and often disfiguring burns were commonplace in the early days of cancer treatment.

Over the last thirty years, dramatic improvements have been made in the dosemetry and methods of administering radiation, resulting in reduced complications. We have also witnessed the introduction of radioactive implants and radioisotopes, used to treat special cancers with particles that penetrate only a few centimeters to millimeters of tissue. Recent advances have also been made experimentally in directing the radiation selectively to the cancer cells by using antibodies linked to the radioisotopes. The antibodies carry the radiation to the specific cancer cells.

Unintended Radiation Injury

As I mentioned above, one of the major problems in the early years of radiotherapy for cancer was the damage to the normal tissues surrounding the cancer. Because no way existed to really concentrate the X-ray beam on the cancer, the result was often a wide zone of damage, including to the overlying skin. The effects of this damage were not always immediate.

Today, as discussed, the ability to target a tumor to limit scatter radiation has been greatly improved, yet radiotherapy still carries danger. Even when the treatments are fractionated, the damage can accumulate and produce injury to the tissues in the path of the beam. In addition, the beam continues to reflect off hard surfaces, such as bone and surgical implants, with the result being delayed damage.

Delayed damage was recognized as a major problem soon after radiotherapy was first used for cancer. Because the effects of radiation on the cells are accumulative, it may take decades for the complications to occur. As you will recall from Chapter 1, a cancer resulting from radiation treatment may not appear for as long as twenty to forty years following the exposure. Some cells are more likely to undergo malignant change than others. For example, bone marrow cells are more likely to undergo malignant transformation and to do so sooner than, say, lung cells.

In addition, people with inborn defects in their DNA repair mechanism or with fragile chromosomes are significantly more likely to develop cancer following radiation exposure than are those with normal repair mechanisms. In addition, their cancers appear much earlier. This is especially so when the radiation treatments are combined with chemotherapy.

Not all of the complications caused by radiotherapy are related to the development of cancer. Often, patients who undergo radiation treatments experience degeneration of tissues months or even years after their treatments end. For example, delayed radionecrosis can occur following penetration of the brain or spinal cord by X-rays. This penetration may have occurred intentionally, as during the treatment of a brain or spinal cord tumor, or unintentionally, as when the nervous system is in the line of fire. Radionecrosis of the nervous system has the appearance of a tumor and the consistency of rubber.

Delayed radionecrosis of the brain is a problem I saw far too frequently in my neurosurgical practice. Usually, the patient had been treated elsewhere for his cancer and was referred to me because of the rather sudden onset of neurological symptoms. A quick review of the patient's history revealed that he or she had been treated with radiation within the last two years and that the radiation beam had been allowed to pass through the spinal cord or brain.

Patients undergoing radiation treatments of the brain for brain tumors risk this complication as well. Because the necrotic part of the brain within the radiation beam is localized, the damaged brain swells much like a brain tumor. Before the development of magnetic resonance imaging (MRI) and positron emission tomography (PET), the condition could be differentiated only by biopsy.

Subsequent studies have shown that the risk of radionecrosis of the brain can be greatly reduced simply by giving the person specific antioxidants during the radiation treatments and for several months afterwards. The condition results because of free radical and lipid peroxidation damage precipitated by the radiation.

Some damage, however, is not as obvious as radiation necrosis. For example, we know that people with Alzheimer's disease, when exposed to cranial radiation, are much more likely to suffer damage to their brain DNA than people of the same age without Alzheimer's. We also know that long before a person's Alzheimer's disease becomes obvious, his or her brain cell DNA is being damaged by free radicals. We have good reason to believe that cranial radiation in these people could precipitate the rapid onset of Alzheimer's disease or even Parkinson's disease.

PROTECTING AGAINST RADIONECROSIS

While the radiation damage to normal tissues can be greatly reduced by using specific combinations of antioxidants, oncologists fear that this will also reduce the effectiveness of the radiation against the cancer. As this book demonstrates, there is little evidence to suggest this and a lot that says otherwise. In fact, numerous studies have shown that selected antioxidant combinations can actually enhance the effectiveness of radiation treatments against cancer, while at the same time significantly protecting the surrounding normal tissue from radiation's harmful effects. The following supplements have been shown to do just that, but they must be taken in combination and not alone. Here are the guidelines:

- Take 25,000 international units of mixed carotenoids (extracted from the algae *D. salina*) twice a day.
- Take 1,000 milligrams of magnesium ascorbate three times a day on an empty stomach (between meals).
- Take 400 international units of vitamin E succinate three times a day.
- Take a multivitamin-and-mineral capsule without iron or copper every day.
- Take 500 to 1,000 milligrams of quercetin three times a day with meals.
- Take 500 milligrams of curcumin three times a day. Dissolve the contents of one capsule in one tablespoon of extra virgin olive oil.
- Take 200 milligrams of alpha lipoic acid twice a day with meals throughout your treatment and for three weeks afterward. Then take 200 milligrams once a day thereafter.
- Take 5 milliliters of ashwaganda (*Withnia somnifera*) 1:2 extract in water once or twice a day. Ashwagandha, also known as Indian ginseng, has been used to protect the DNA and cell integrity. It has been shown to safeguard the bone marrow from damage by radiation. In addition, it increases the number of cells within the bone marrow following radiation treatments. *Caution:* Do not use ashwagandha with amphetamines or central nervous system (CNS)–depressant drugs.

Accumulation of Radiation Damage

Another problem I have never seen discussed is the damage caused by using diagnostic X-rays in conjunction with radiation therapy. Remember, radiation's harmful effects are accumulative—that is, they add up, even when given over time.

Let's say you have a lung tumor. Before your surgery, you may have several CT scans, at least one series of chest X-rays, a radioactive bone scan, and several other diagnostic X-rays, all within a few days to a few weeks. Altogether, these studies add up to a significant dose of radiation. Of course, scout X-rays will need to be done for your radiation therapy. To this, add the radiation treatments themselves and then all the posttreatment follow-up X-rays. Further, add all the X-rays you had earlier in your life, even as a child.

Estimates indicate that a single chest CT scan is equivalent to 400 chest X-rays. It is not uncommon for chest CT scans to be repeated every three to four months in cases of lung tumors. Therefore, the cumulative dose of radiation for the average cancer patient, counting all the diagnostic X-rays and radiation treatments, is enormously high.

Of special concern is the woman who has had yearly mammograms for five to ten years before her cancer was recognized. The accumulative damage to the cells in both of her breasts can be quite substantial. We know that the risk of cancer developing in the remaining breast is already higher—even without the radiation exposure—once the disease has developed in one breast. This is because of the impaired DNA repair enzymes. Yet, the accumulative damage to the DNA in the cells in the remaining breast will greatly increase the likelihood of cancer developing in that breast as well. Women are rarely told this.

Most women cringe at the thought of getting their yearly mammogram because of memories of having their breasts crushed during the study. The radiological technologist, in an attempt to get clearer pictures, will compress the breasts as flat as possible, often bringing tears to the poor woman's eyes. Unfortunately, the pain and humiliation are not the least of her worries. During my training, I was taught that even feeling tumors (palpation) too frequently or too vigorously can send millions of cancer cells coursing through the lymph channels and blood vessels—that is, the examination could cause the cancer to spread. As a result, I was cautioned to limit the number of examinations I performed.

Recently, an alarmed cry has been expressed at what is being done to the breasts when they are crushed during mammography. The pressure on the breast is so high that if a cancer is present, spreading it beyond the confines of the original tumor is almost assured.

Little appreciated, even by doctors, is the fact that some patients are at greater risk than others. For example, patients who have a chronic disease, such as diabetes or an autoimmune disease, have normal cells lying outside the cancer that are much more vulnerable to the effects of radiation than are the cells of a person without a chronic disease. Aged patients are also at greater risk, as are those who have been given chemotherapy before or during their radiotherapy.

In general, poor nutrition greatly increases a person's susceptibility to radiation injury. Nutritional deficiencies, even of a single nutrient, further endanger those with one of the other risk factors, especially defective DNA repair enzymes. Quercetin and vitamin C, especially when taken together, play major roles in protecting the DNA. Other flavonoids—such as hesperidin, fisetin, curcumin, and luteolin, all commonly found in fruits and vegetables—can also play major roles in cell protection.

As we saw earlier, people who have inherited fragile genes or poorly functioning DNA repair enzymes are much more likely to develop cancer. In addition, the exposure to radiation is much more likely to damage their normal cells than it would the cells of a person without these defects. Unfortunately, as stated, these are the very people who are at the highest risk of developing cancer in the first place. This means that they are at higher risk not only during radiation therapy, but also during routine X-ray examinations.

Radiation and Nutrition

The nervous system is not the only tissue that can be damaged by scatter radiation. Most vulnerable are the cells lining the gastrointestinal tract, as well as the cells of the bone marrow, lymph system, spleen, and hair follicles. This is because these are all rapidly dividing cells, easily damaged by radiation.

Many factors can increase the risk of and sensitivity to radiation injury, including:

- Age, especially being very young or very elderly
- Smoking

- Illegal drug use, especially marijuana use
- Chronic illness, especially diabetes, autoimmune disease, chronic infection, or neurodegenerative disease
- Low intake of fruits and vegetables
- High intake of red meat or other sources of iron
- High intake of copper
- Chronic stress
- Chemotherapy
- Poor general health
- Impaired or fragile DNA repair system, inherited or acquired
- Extreme athletic exertion

The damage to the cells lining the intestine, colon, and rectum can range from defective absorption (malabsorption) to severe inflammation of the bowel wall with resulting bloody, mucus-filled stools. The cells lining the intestine are very complex and delicate. Damage to these cells can significantly alter the body's ability to absorb foods, vitamins, and minerals, leading to significant malnutrition, despite a healthy diet. The simple fact is that if food cannot be properly digested and absorbed, a healthy diet does little good. This is especially a problem when chemotherapy is combined with radiation.

Damage to the intestinal lining can also result in leaky gut syndrome, in which undigested food substances are able to pass into the circulation. Leaky gut syndrome can lead to food allergies with resulting immune diversion, in which the immune system is tied up reacting with food antigens instead of the cancer cells.

Abdominal radiation treatments, especially when combined with chemotherapy, also can kill off the helpful bacteria in the colon, such as the acidophilus and bifidus organisms. This, in turn, can result in an overgrowth of harmful microorganisms such as *Candida albicans* and pathogenic (disease-causing) bacteria. When such bacterial disruptions are severe, which in my experience is not uncommon, yeast and bacteria can enter the bloodstream, with significant negative consequences to the immune system.

In severe cases of radiation injury to the gastrointestinal

tract, the inner lining of the intestine can slough off, resulting in intense abdominal pain, cramping, and bloody diarrhea. Fortunately, these complications can be avoided by following the same supplement guidelines listed on page 113. It is vital to begin taking these nutrients at least several weeks before beginning your chemotherapy or radiation treatments. The nutrients are not ineffective after the treatments are under way; the only negative result of starting late is that you will not get their full protection. In addition, it is much more difficult to repair a damaged gut than to prevent the damage in the first place. "A stitch in time saves nine."

Radiation injury to the cells of the immune system, primarily to the cells of the bone marrow, is less likely, unless the skeletal radiation is extensive, as it frequently is in the case of leukemia, lymphoma, or medullablastoma. Most of our active bone marrow is located in the spine, the sternum, and long bones such as the femurs and the bones of the upper arm. Over half of all our immune cells are found in the gastrointestinal tract. In both cases, radiation protection by nutrients is vital.

It is important to remember that the nutrients listed on page 113 act one way with normal cells and in the opposite way with cancer cells, making the cancer cells more sensitive to the radiation and the surrounding normal cells more resistant to the radiation. This differential effect was dramatically demonstrated by Dr. Stanley Levenson and his coworkers at the Albert Einstein College of Medicine using mice implanted with tumor cells.[2]

First, Dr. Levenson established that supplementation with beta-carotene could dramatically increase the survival rate of normal mice exposed to whole-body radiation as compared to mice not given supplements. In fact, at the higher doses of radiation, the mice consuming a high-beta-carotene diet lived more than four times longer than the mice consuming a regular diet. The researchers then treated the mice with implanted tumors with 3,000 rads of radiation, a very high dose, to the area of the tumor. The mice that had been given high-dose beta-carotene or vitamin A demonstrated considerably more tumor killing than the controls. In fact, the tumors in the mice given the vitamins plus radiation all regressed completely, with less than 10 percent reappearing later. The tumors in the mice fed regular chow without beta-carotene also regressed, but all returned, eventually killing the mice.

The protective effect of the radiation plus beta-carotene or vitamin A prevented the return of the tumors throughout the experiment, which was terminated one year later. The beta-carotene was found to be more effective than the vitamin A. Of great surprise to the researchers was that in the mice given the vitamin supplements, the radiation caused all of the tumor cells to die or become dormant, but it barely affected the surrounding normal cells. This was not the case in the radiated animals not given the vitamin supplements. In these mice, the normal cells surrounding the tumors were damaged by the radiation.

At this point, you may be thinking that you have heard that beta-carotene may cause lung cancer. We will discuss this later. For now, you should just appreciate that for everyone but people who smoke and/or drink heavily, beta-carotene is a powerful inhibitor of cancer growth. Numerous experiments, even ones using human cancer, have shown this to be true.

INCREASING THE EFFECTIVENESS OF RADIATION TREATMENTS

As we have seen, beta-carotene and vitamin A can significantly enhance the effectiveness of radiation treatments. One of the big questions in considering the effectiveness of these two vitamins is: Do they cause the cancer to be completely eradicated or do they merely suppress its growth? From the study conducted by Dr. Levenson and his coworkers, it appears that they mainly suppress the cancer's growth—that is, they cause the cancer to become dormant. Dormant cancers cannot harm you.

In the mice in Dr. Levenson's study having combined vitamins and radiation, in which all the tumors regressed, 10 percent of the tumors later returned. This is still very impressive when compared to the animals that were not given vitamins and experienced recurrence of all their tumors. Yet, in the former group of animals, when the vitamins were later stopped, more tumors did recur. For example, in the animals given the vitamin A plus radiation, when the diet was changed to a regular chow without vitamin A, 67 percent of the mice experienced a recurrence of their tumors. The animals on the beta-carotene-enhanced diet fared a lot better, with only 20 percent of the tumors recurring. After two years, 40 percent of the animals still on vitamin A and 82 percent of the animals on beta-carotene were alive and without evidence of a tumor.

It, therefore, appears that the vitamins suppressed the cancer tumors rather than actually killing them. In fact, they suppressed the tumors quite effectively as long as the vitamins were continued. Again, I emphasize that the beta-carotene enhanced the ability of the radiation to kill or suppress the cancer, but protected the surrounding normal tissues and cells from the harmful effects of the therapy.

While the study done by Dr. Levenson and his coworkers used beta-carotene, there is evidence that the other carotenoids may be even more effective. So far, more than forty carotenoids have been identified in the human diet. The most powerful forms against cancer have been found to be the canthaxanthins, beta-carotene, alpha-carotene, lutein, and lycopene. This is why I recommend using only the carotenoids from the *D. salina* algae, now widely available. I also recommend combining the carotenoids with niacinamide. Good guidelines to follow are:

- Take 50,000 international units of mixed carotenoids twice a day with meals.
- Take 500 milligrams of niacinamide three times a day with meals throughout your treatment and for three weeks afterward.
- Take 10 milligrams of resveratrol three times a day. Resveratrol is a flavonoid extracted from the skins of grapes.

While the results seen with mixed carotenoids and niacinamide are best when the supplements are begun before starting the radiation treatments, it has been shown that they work even if started several days after radiation treatments have been initiated. The resveratrol should be started before the radiation treatments are begun.

Niacinamide, the form of niacin used by the body, has been shown to increase the blood flow through tumors, thereby increasing the oxygenation within the cancer cells. As you will recall, a high oxygen level in cancer cells makes the cells very sensitive to destruction by radiation. The niacinamide should be started several days before the radiation treatments are begun and should be continued throughout the treatment period.

Resveratrol has the opposite effect on cancer cells than it does on normal cells. Normal cells exposed to the extract are protected from radiation while cancer cells are made more vulnerable to it. This again demonstrates the difference between normal cells and cancer cells. Substances that inhibit the cyclooxygenase 1 (COX-1) enzyme, whether they are arthritis drugs or plant extracts, are known to protect the cells from the damaging effects of radiation. But blocking the same enzyme in cancer cells makes the cells more sensitive to radiation damage.

SPECIAL RISK TO BLOOD VESSELS

One hazard rarely considered, even by radiation oncologists, is the danger of blood vessel injury caused by the radiation passing through blood vessels, from small arterioles to larger arteries. We know that the cells lining the blood vessels, called the endothelia, are quite sensitive to the harmful effects of X-ray beams. The endothelial cells are vital to normal blood vessel function, and we now know that damage to these cells plays a major role in atherosclerosis, also called hardening of the arteries. (For a discussion of this, see below.)

Atherosclerosis Caused by Radiation

In a recent study in which doctors examined a total of seventy-one patients treated for nasopharyngeal cancers with radiation treatments, it was found that arterial stenosis was significantly more common than among nonradiated patients. The two groups of cancer patients—those treated with radiation and those not exposed to radiation—were carefully matched for other vascular risk factors. Of the radiated patients, fifty-six out of the seventy-one developed stenosis (narrowing) of the carotid artery, the main artery supplying blood to the brain, whereas only eleven of the fifty-one nonirradiated patients developed stenosis. Of the patients demonstrating severe stenosis (greater than 50 percent occlusion), all were in the radiated group. The artery most often damaged by the radiation was the carotid artery. The third most often injured was the vertebral artery, which supplies blood to the brain stem.

While this study sounds an alarm regarding the use of intense radiation beams to treat nasopharyngeal cancers, it issues an equal warning about the use of radiation to treat any cancer lying close to a vessel supplying blood to a critical area. For example, when the brain, one of the most vascular organs in the body, is irradiated, significant damage is done to an extensive collection of critical blood vessels. This damage can cause small blood vessels to suddenly occlude, leading to dementia or severe neurological impairment.

Often, major arteries course very close to a cancerous tumor, and sometimes they are encased by the tumor. This means that the blood vessels receive a large degree of the radiation dose. This is true in the case of cancer of the stomach, intestines, kidneys, and lungs (mediastinum), which lie near the aorta and its major branches. The arteries supplying blood to the brain are endangered by radiating tumors of the head and neck, as well as by the hundreds of miles of blood vessels within the brain itself.

While it is well known that the body's tissues differ considerably in their sensitivity to radiation, what is less well known is that the same tissue can vary in sensitivity depending on the state of the body. For example, researchers recently discovered that during pregnancy, a woman's chromosomes become exceedingly vulnerable to the effects of radiation.[3] This state of high vulnerability disappears as soon as the baby is born. The hypersensitive state appears to be related to the female hormones, especially progesterone. Apparently, the change in the hormone levels during the last half of pregnancy is what causes the increased sensitivity to radiation-induced DNA damage.

Unfortunately, women also have hormone fluctuations at times other than pregnancy. One example is during hormone replacement therapy. Progesterone creams are very popular these days, and their use could significantly increase the likelihood of DNA damage if diagnostic X-rays, including mammograms, are done. In addition, a woman undergoing treatment for a cancer that is not hormone-sensitive is not generally told to stop using her progesterone cream. Rarely do radiation oncologists even ask women about their hormone use, unless an obvious hormone-sensitive cancer, such as breast cancer or ovarian cancer, is involved.

It is obvious that there are many as-yet-unexplored physiological changes in both men and women that can affect sensitivity to radiation hazards. These include daily, monthly, and even seasonal variations.

PROTECTING AGAINST RADIATION INJURY

While there are numerous nutritional supplements that can protect the cells from the damaging effects of radiation, including garlic, melatonin, selenium, curcumin, alpha lipoic acid, and numerous flavonoids, there are some that serve a double function. Take, for example, beta-1,3-glucan, a polysaccharide extract from mushrooms and the outer wall of baker's yeast. Beta-1,3-glucan has been shown to offer significant protection against the damaging effects of radiation, especially the severe injury seen when the immune cells are irradiated. The immune cells include the cells of the spleen, bone marrow, and lymph nodes.

In addition, beta-1,3-glucan is a powerful immune stimulant, especially for the immune cells that primarily fight cancer cells. One of the more important cells in this battle is the macrophage, which is sort of the brains of the operation. The macrophage can be considered the general of the battle forces opposing the invading cancer cells. The T-lymphocytes can be viewed as the noncoms and privates. The T-lymphocytes, or noncoms and privates, go to the general, or the macrophage, for their orders. The macrophage can also call up more troops from the bone marrow. It is this latter function that makes the macrophage such an important player in the protection against the damaging effects of radiation on the bone marrow.

Mice exposed to high doses of whole-body radiation have been shown to be significantly more likely to survive if they are first treated with beta-1,3-glucan.[4] Not only does beta-1, 3-glucan protect the bone marrow cells from destruction, but it also prevents the infections that frequently follow extensive radiation exposure. It does this while increasing the killing of the cancer cells. Therefore, it provides a double benefit.

Another way to protect the normal cells from radiation while giving the therapy an additional boost in its cancer-killing effectiveness is to use supplements that block the cyclooxygenase 2 (COX-2) enzyme. COX-2 is a special enzyme that causes inflammation. Arthritis drugs, call nonsteroidal anti-inflammatory drugs (NSAIDs), block this enzyme. Later, we shall see that blocking this enzyme also inhibits the growth of several cancers.

Another effect of blocking the COX-2 enzyme is protection of the normal cells against radiation damage. This has been shown using such arthritis drugs as indomethacin.[5] Many of the plant flavonoids, such as curcumin, quercetin, hesperidin, and kaempferol, also powerfully block this enzyme. Of special interest is curcumin, the extract of the spice turmeric. Not only does curcumin block the COX-2 enzyme, offering radiation protection, it also strongly inhibits the growth, invasion, and metastasis of many cancers. This is truly targeted therapy, which oncologists claim to be seeking, with a major bonus protection of normal cells at the same time.

A study coming out of India has found that ashwagandha (Indian ginseng) not only protected mice exposed to high-dose radiation, but also increased their white blood cell counts.[6] In addition, the ashwagandha increased the number of blood-forming cells in the mice's bone marrow. With bone marrow depression being a major problem in cancer patients treated with radiation or chemotherapy agents, ashwagandha may be a most useful herb.

Another study has found that calcium channel blocking drugs, frequently used to control high blood pressure, can also dramatically protect normal cells from radiation damage.[7] In this study, to make sure the treatment did not interfere with the ability of the radiation to kill the cancer cells, the researchers implanted three types of cancers in mice, added the calcium blocking drugs, and radiated the tumors. The drugs did not reduce the efficiency of the radiation in killing the cancers. Again, the researchers noted a differential effect—that is, the calcium blocking drugs increased the killing of the cancer cells, but protected the normal cells exposed to the same radiation.

One of the most powerful natural calcium channel blockers is magnesium. This action is how magnesium protects the brain and heart during strokes and heart attacks. As we have seen, magnesium plays a major role in protecting many tissues and organs. Radioprotection is an added bonus.

As I have stated previously, beta-carotene has been shown to protect normal cells from radiation. For most tissues this is true, yet one study found that while it protected spleen immune cells, reticulocytes (scavenger cells), and spermatids, it did not protect bone marrow cells from damage by X-rays.[8] This again demonstrated the necessity of using several types of nutritional supplements together, since each nutrient plays a separate role in protecting the whole body.

One of the more interesting radiation protectants is the herb ginkgo biloba. Ginkgo contains not only the special components that we associate with memory enhancement, but also several very powerful antioxidant flavonoids, called apigenin, quercetin, and kaempeferol. All three of these flavonoids powerfully protect cells against radiation-induced damage, especially DNA damage.

A very interesting study on the effectiveness of ginkgo in protecting against radiation injury was conducted using recovery workers from the nuclear reactor disaster at the Chernobyl (Soviet Union) Power Plant in 1986. It was known that when people are exposed to high doses of ionizing radiation, they develop a special set of proteins in their blood called clastogenic factors, which are a reliable measure of the damage being done. These factors can persist in the blood for more than thirty years after exposure.

Examination of the Chernobyl recovery workers demonstrated elevated clastogenic factors in thirty-three of the forty-seven workers studied. The affected workers were then given ginkgo biloba extract three times a day for thirty days. On the first day, their clastogenic factors fell to normal levels and remained there throughout the period of observation. When examined one year later, only one-third of the workers showed a return of the clastogenic protein. The benefit from the ginkgo lasted at least seven months after the herb was stopped. This is incredible! The protection supplied by this herb not only began immediately, but also lasted long after the supplement was stopped.

Another advantage of the ginkgo herb is that it is especially efficient at protecting the blood vessels, and by slightly thinning the blood, it may reduce metastasis of tumors. The blood-thinning effect of ginkgo biloba taken at a daily dose of 240 milligrams is approximately equal to that of one aspirin taken daily. Stories of hemorrhaging after taking the herb are serious exaggerations.

In addition, there are a number of nutrients that help to strengthen the walls of the blood vessels. This action has the added advantage of preventing the spread of cancer, since it is difficult for a tumor to erode through a strong wall. Following is a good nutritional program:

- Take 300 milligrams of decaffeinated green tea extract twice a day with food. This supplement also helps prevent iron absorption.
- Take 500 milligrams of curcumin three times a day. Dissolve the contents of one capsule in one tablespoon of extra virgin olive oil. Curcumin has a slight anticoagulant effect, so it should not be combined with aspirin or anticoagulant drugs.
- Take 200 micrograms of selenomethionine every day.
- Take 25 milligrams of zinc every other day.
- Take 120 milligrams of ginkgo biloba every day. Ginkgo con-

tains several flavonoids that are very protective of the blood vessels. Do not take ginkgo with blood thinners.

- Take 300 milligrams of magnesium citramate three times a day. Magnesium plays a vital role in endothelial cell function. It also offers major protection of the brain and heart.

CONCLUSION

Most cancer patients fear their treatments because of the stories they have heard about terrible fatigue, nausea and vomiting, hair loss, and numerous other complications. Fortunately, most of these complications can be avoided without sacrificing the effectiveness of the conventional treatments. In fact, as we have seen, nutritional treatments and dietary changes can actually enhance the effectiveness of the treatments, making a true cure more likely.

The vast majority of the patients I have treated, including those who came to me long after their conventional treatments had been started, reported that they felt dramatically better after beginning their nutritional program. They had significantly more energy, little or no nausea, greater endurance, improved mood, and dramatic improvement in their symptoms, including pain.

Pain can be a special problem for patients with bone metastasis. I have noticed that many of my patients with metastatic pain improve, sometimes dramatically, once they are fully on the dietary and supplement program. In addition, they lose fat weight and gain muscle weight.

As we will see in the next several chapters, the fear expressed by oncologists that nutritional supplementation can interfere with the conventional treatments, or even make cancers grow faster, is totally unfounded and denies patients a major weapon in fighting, and ultimately defeating, their cancer.

5

Nutrition and Cancer: Facts and Fallacies

When you tell your oncologist that you want to start a nutritional program and that the program will involve taking antioxidant supplements, you may see your doctor's eyes grow as big as saucers, as if he has seen a ghost. With panic gripping his voice, he may tell you, with an ever reddening face, that you must not take any antioxidant supplements because they will do two things: one, they will make your cancer grow faster, and two, they will interfere with the effectiveness of your treatments. As you will see, neither of these beliefs is true when the nutritional program is carefully designed.

Most patients arrive at their oncologist's office in a state of panic. In their minds, they have been given the worst diagnosis a person could ever hear: You have cancer. Everything in their lives suddenly changes. It has been said that impending death sharpens the mind. It can also cloud the mind. Fear often makes it difficult to think rationally. When most people reach that point, their natural reaction is to turn to the person who is most likely to save them from this horrifying disease. The oncologist, dressed in his starched white coat, stern-faced, eyes either penetrating or evasive, represents a commanding presence. In essence, at that point, it is the oncologist who stands between you and a possible reality that you have been fighting so intensely to keep out of your mind: a slow, painful death from your disease.

Oncologists represent the best that medical science has to offer in the fight against cancer. They have trained for many years in some of the best medical institutions in the country and have access to the latest breakthroughs in cancer treatments.

Their world is a secret, often frightening universe dominated by strange words, powerful drugs, and *Star Wars*–looking machines that hum and destroy tumors. Their self-assurance and boldness fill you with a renewed hope of a favorable outcome. Success, you tell yourself, depends on doing all that the oncologist tells you to do. After all, your oncologist knows all that is known about cancer.

The look of shock that may cross your oncologist's face, and his uncompromising stance on avoiding all antioxidants, will break your confidence. In your mind, you will tell yourself that your oncologist must know something that the person who recommended the nutritional program does not know. This is a difficult conclusion to overcome. Some cancer patients will, at that point, abandon all thoughts of defying their oncologist. Success, some will conclude, will depend on absolute loyalty to the oncologist.

Other patients will abandon their nutritional treatments, despite their belief in their usefulness, because they will fear alienating their oncologist, possibly leading to the doctor's refusal to treat them any further. This is a terrifying thought with which many people cannot deal.

WHAT MOST DOCTORS DO NOT KNOW

Over the years, I have found that most patients believe that all doctors know the same things concerning medicine—that is, that all doctors are knowledgeable about all the illnesses they treat. Unfortunately, this is not true. One of the great intellectual vacuums in medical training is nutrition. The vast majority of doctors do not know a great deal concerning nutrition, especially in regards to particular illnesses. This is because most medical schools do not teach nutrition to their budding doctors, and the vast majority of residency training programs never mention anything other than the basics.

For example, neurosurgeons and neurologists, in general, know very little concerning the effects of nutrition on brain function or its use in treating neurological diseases. The same is true for most medical specialists, especially oncologists.

I have found that the vast majority of oncologists rarely give their patients good advice concerning nutrition. Despite the fact that it has been known for many years now that certain foods and food components can dramatically increase the growth and spread of cancers, oncologists frequently allow their patients to eat these very foods.

In fact, one otherwise excellent book on dealing with cancer recommends, as healthful snacks to keep on hand, cakes and cookies, cheesecake, ice cream, and dried fruits. All of these "healthful snacks," in fact, contain known cancer-promoting nutrients and additives. Even to the untrained, these snacks represent poor nutritional choices for anyone.

We also know, for example, that many types of fats and oils dramatically promote cancer growth and spread. All of these fats are the ones most commonly used in processed foods, again being promoted by oncology and hospital dietitians. The doctors themselves do not seem to be aware of these important relationships between cancer and nutrition.

In my own medical community, for instance, an annual report about the oncology services at one of the more prestigious cancer centers advertises the following nutritional services: "Nutrition services stocks the oncology floor with milk, ice cream, soft drinks, crackers and other snacks and nutritional supplements to encourage patients to increase caloric intake." Among the "nutritional supplements" are soft-serve ice cream, yogurt, and milkshakes. As we will see, many of these snack items contain components that promote cancer growth.

From the time doctors enter medical school all the way through their residency training, they learn to use three things: surgery, pharmaceutical medications, and radiotherapy. The remainder of their time is spent on the proper methods of making a diagnosis.

For the oncologist, the greatest emphasis is placed on the use of pharmaceuticals and radiotherapy. There is little question that oncologists know an awful lot about the pharmaceutical treatment of cancer. Unfortunately, as we have seen, successes with this treatment have been few and far between. The death rate for the major cancers has changed little over the past thirty years. In fact, little at all has changed, outside of the ability to make an earlier diagnosis.

Despite the tremendous advances made in the nutritional treatment of cancer, especially as a complementary enhancement of the conventional treatments, oncologists remain largely ignorant of this knowledge. As a result, they not only harm their patients by giving them cancer-promoting nutritional advice, but deny them nutritional treatments that would make their conventional treatments safer and more effective.

In the past, we did not know why cancer rates were lower in people who ate a diet of mostly fruits and vegetables. This left many oncologists skeptical. Determined to practice "scientific" medicine, the oncologists turned to the pharmaceutical and radiological treatments, things that had more "science" behind them. These therapies often failed as cancer treatments, but at least they were scientific.

All of this has changed over the past thirty years, especially over the past decade. We now have good scientific explanations about why and how nutrition inhibits cancer development, growth, and spread. In addition, we have many confirmed studies showing that a large number of nutrients enhance the effectiveness of the traditional treatments, while at the same time reducing their toxicity to normal cells. When we can make chemotherapy agents and radiotherapy less harmful to the normal cells, we can safely increase the dose of these treatments, possibly making the treatments more successful.

Because most oncologists know nothing of the vast scientific nutritional literature, much of which appears in their own journals, they continue to scare their patients away from these treatments with stories of harm, which appear in no valid scientific studies. While most doctors would never accept as truth information based purely on theory and hypothesis, they readily do so when it comes to the so-called dangerous complementary nutritional treatments. Their fears are based purely on hypothesis and not on scientifically verifiable facts. As we will see, the science is on the side of using nutrition to enhance the effectiveness of the traditional treatments.

What the Science Shows

To bypass the problems of food aversion, nausea, and malabsorption, doctors began to use highly concentrated intravenous infusions, called total parenteral hyperalimentation (TPH), to force the body to retain proteins and fats. Initially, glucose infusions were used alone, but it was found that they could actually cause tumors to grow faster and to spread more widely.

Early experimental results indicated that giving rats with tumors infusions of highly concentrated nutrition could increase their tumor growth, as well as cause them to gain weight.[1] More careful studies indicated that, in fact, the tumors were not abnormally stimulated by the nutritional supplementation, but rather increased in weight in proportion to the rat's gain in overall body weight—that is, the tumors gained only in proportion to what the rat itself gained.[2] Still, these early infusions contained very high concentrations of glucose (sugar), which we now know significantly increases tumor growth. This is because cancer cells, unlike normal cells, are restricted to using glucose as their main energy fuel.

More balanced infusions containing less glucose and additional proteins (or amino acids) and fats caused weight gain but did not appear to stimulate tumor growth and spread. The best results were seen with patients with advanced cancers and suffering from severe malnutrition. The controversy continued, however, concerning patients having lesser stages of cancer growth, as well as patients with poorer nutrition. In fact, earlier, many cancer specialists had advocated reduced-calorie diets as a way to "starve" the cancer. Unfortunately, they also starved the patient, and as we have seen, starvation at one time was the leading cause of death in cancer patients.

Armed with this knowledge, researchers tested low-calorie diets on animals having malignant tumors and found no effect on tumor growth. They then combined low-calorie diets with low-fat diets and found a significant reduction in tumor growth and spread.[3]

In one study in which tumor growth was carefully monitored using a high-tech method, no evidence of stimulation of tumor growth was discovered when using high concentrations of nutritional supplementation.[4] In fact, the nutritionally depleted patients were found to have the highest rates of tumor growth.

Nutrition, like so many other things in nature, can be a double-edged sword. Several studies have shown that, like the polyunsaturated fats and glucose, certain amino acids can also enhance tumor growth and spread. For example, the amino acid methionine has been shown in animal models to increase the development of colon cancers, and the amino acid arginine has been shown to stimulate certain experimental breast cancers (those producing nitric oxide).[5]

The conclusion of these studies was that supplying cancer patients with high concentrations of nutrients did not cause their tumors to grow faster or to metastasize more often. This is why oncologists and oncology dietitians today tell their patients that the most important consideration is gaining weight, no matter how you do it. They have failed to understand the studies that were done, especially later studies that clearly demonstrated that it matters very much how you gain the weight.

ANTIOXIDANTS AND CANCER PREVENTION

It is generally accepted that anywhere from 33 percent to 70 percent of all cancers are diet related.[6] Likewise, the amount of evidence demonstrating a protective anticancer effect with a high intake of nutritious foods, such as fruits and vegetables, is now overwhelming. For example, as I quoted in Chapter 1, one recent review of 206 human epidemiological studies and 22 of the best animal studies found that, overall, there was a 50 percent lower incidence of cancer of all types in the subjects eating the greatest amounts of fruits and vegetables.[7] For certain cancers, the figure was a 75 percent lower incidence.

Throughout history, the approach used by science has been to seek the one component that will possibly explain a beneficial effect. For example, most early studies assumed that the beneficial effect of citrus fruits against cancer development was due to the vitamin C content. While studies using vitamin C supplements met with some success, most of the human studies demonstrated little effect, save for certain cancers. The same can be said for vitamin E and the carotenoids when used alone.

Only recently have scientists begun to appreciate the concept of synergy in nutrition. In synergy, the dramatic effect of a particular food in preventing disease is due to the combined effects of its nutrients and not a single nutrient. Numerous studies have demonstrated this synergistic effect, not only regarding beneficial effects, but also with toxic effects. For example, many pesticides and herbicides have now been found to have profound synergistic toxicity when used in combination. Likewise, chemotherapy agents can also demonstrate synergistic toxic side effects.

Beneficial synergism is especially evident in the case of vitamins combined with flavonoids.[8] The flavonoids are a group of complex chemicals, some 5,000 in number, previously referred to as the bioflavonoids. Despite the identification of more than 10,000 chemicals in edible plants, there are thousands more that have not been identified, many of which may hold even more promise of health benefits.

While many of these compounds are antioxidants, they also have other properties that play a role in cancer prevention, as well as in the inhibition of cancer growth and spread. These properties are what cancer oncologists have ignored when warning their patients against taking antioxidants. These cancer-inhibiting effects are, in some cases, quite profound, as we shall see.

There is little dispute regarding the ability of a diet high in fruits and vegetables to prevent many cancers from developing in the first place. In terms of prevention, the antioxidant abilities of these nutrients appear to play a dominant role. This is because chronic free radical damage to the DNA of particular cells appears to be the central event in cancer causation, as we have seen previously.

Good Fats and Bad Fats

Like most things in nature, not all fats are created equal in terms of disease-causing potential. Some fats promote disease when consumed in excess, others inhibit disease, and some are neutral—that is, they do not prevent disease and they do not promote disease. This classification of fats is especially true when considering cancer risk. Because of this, I have chosen to call fats "good fats" and "bad fats," as have others.

Fats are very powerful biomolecules and not just something that hangs off your waist and hips. In fact, fats have the potency of most prescription medications and should be treated as powerful drugs.

Unfortunately, modern industrial societies have utilized far too many of the bad fats in food processing. These fats are referred to biochemically as the omega-6, or N-6, fats. While the omega-6 fats are all polyunsaturated vegetable oils, other polyunsaturated oils are quite healthy, such as the fish oils, flaxseed oil, and certain oils extracted from algae. The universal problem with polyunsaturated oils, even the good ones, is that they oxidize very easily. When an oil oxidizes, it becomes rancid. Rancid oils can produce harmful substances (lipid peroxides) and free radicals.

For instance, the omega-3, or N-3, oils enhance immunity, reduce inflammation, protect the nervous system, prevent cardiac arrhythmia, improve cell function, improve blood flow by reducing platelet adhesiveness, and inhibit cancer development, growth, and spread. The omega-6 oils have just the opposite effects: they inhibit immunity, promote inflammation, increase brain injury, impair cell function, promote platelet adhesiveness, and stimulate cancer induction, growth, and spread.

Because of the profound effects of these types of oils on health, careful control of the diet by the cancer patient is crucial. The average person consumes an enormous amount of these cancer-stimulating fats. How much of which fats is consumed becomes especially important for the cancer patient during traditional treatments and afterward. Just how important was emphasized by a study using mice that under normal circumstances would never have had metastasis of their cancers. When the mice were fed a diet high in corn oil, their tumors metastasized widely. This same powerful promotional effect of the omega-6 oils on cancer spread has been confirmed in numerous studies.

The truly upsetting thing is that few oncologists tell their patients to avoid the omega-6 oils in their diets. In fact, most oncologists promote these oils, as we saw in the example of the oncology center's dietary service. Cakes, crackers, cheesecake, chips, and other processed foods contain very high amounts of the omega-6 oils. Trusting patients have no idea that the diet being promoted by their oncologist is actually making their cancer grow faster and metastasize, as well as significantly increasing the likelihood that it will recur.

Another problem with a diet high in the omega-6 oils is that it significantly lowers the level of vitamin E in the body. This increases the damage by free radicals and also promotes the growth of the tumor and its spread.

So what are the omega-6 oils? They include safflower oil, sunflower oil, corn oil, peanut oil, soybean oil, and to a lesser extent, canola oil. As you are probably aware, these are the most commonly used oils in food processing and cooking recipes. All of these oils are extracted from plant seeds, which is important, since it means they have no protective flavonoids. Beginning in the late sixties, the American Heart Association heavily promoted these oils as being healthy for the heart and as a way to prevent atherosclerosis. One of the most heavily promoted oils was corn oil. Ironically, it is corn oil that has most often demonstrated the promotion of cancer growth and spread in experimental studies.[9]

The Bad Fats

Now let us look a little deeper into the subject of the bad fats and why they are bad. I think this is necessary because many people have to be convinced that favored foods truly are bad before they are willing to give them up, especially when virtually every processed food we buy contains these fats.

Several studies have shown that a diet high in the omega-6 fats increases the development and eventual spread of breast cancer in animals.[10] One study in which the data from ninety-seven different animal studies were analyzed found that a diet high in the omega-6 fats significantly increased tumor growth.[11] Studies have also shown that obese women with breast cancer, especially those on diets high in the omega-6 fats, had lower survival rates and more advanced disease than thinner women.[12]

A recent study of 217 men with prostate cancer found a strong association between a high intake of the omega-6 fats and the occurrence of this cancer.[13] This has also been confirmed in other studies. Many oncologists have noted that cancer of the prostate and cancer of the breast share many risk factors.

Interestingly, a diet high in the omega-6 fats has also been shown to increase the number of cancers caused by human papilloma virus (HPV) 16.[14] HPV is found in 90 percent of cervical cancer cases. The exact mechanism for this occurrence is unknown, but is in part related to the immune suppression caused by the high intake of omega-6 fats.

A diet high in the omega-6 fats has also been shown to suppress immunity by producing the powerful immune-suppressing substance prostaglandin E2 (PGE2).[15] Immune suppression may be responsible for the activation of latent (sleeping) cancers. Patients receiving intravenous fat solutions high in the omega-6 fats during hospitalization have been shown to experience significant suppresson of their cancer-fighting lymphocytes (total lymphocytes, T-helper cells, and natural killer cells).[16]

The omega-6 fats have been shown to significantly increase inflammation, which is closely correlated with the growth and spread of tumors.[17] As I discussed earlier, anything that increases inflammation also increases the risk of developing a cancer.

Fat cells themselves can produce estrogen (estradiol) independent of the ovaries.[18] Diets high in the omega-6 fats increase estradiol levels and thereby increase the risk of breast cancer and can increase the growth of prostate cancer at certain stages of the disease as well.

A diet high in the omega-6 fats has been shown to increase the level of insulin, which is a powerful stimulator of cancer growth and spread.[19] In addition, high insulin levels stimulate inflammation.

One study found that a diet high in the omega-6 fats dramatically increased colon cancer in experimental animals, but if the bad fats were combined with vegetables, fewer tumors resulted.[20] In addition, increased calcium intake was shown to reduce the cancer-causing effects of these fats.

Several studies found that diets high in the omega-6 fats were associated with much more aggressive cancers in men with prostate cancer.[21,22] There is evidence that the high levels of bad fats increased testosterone levels, thereby increasing the aggressiveness of the cancers.[23] Despite this observation, it has been shown that the omega-6 fats can stimulate prostate cancer even without testosterone.

To summarize, diets high in the omega-3 fatty acids, which are good fats:

- Stimulate immunity
- Decrease inflammation
- Suppress tumor growth and spread
- Decrease the 16-alpha hydroxyestrone levels
- Increase the 2-hydroxyestrone levels
- Decrease coagulation
- Improve brain function
- Decrease depression
- Increase the effectiveness of chemotherapy drugs

Diets high in the omega-6 fats, which are bad fats:

- Depress immunity
- Increase inflammation
- Increase coagulation
- Increase the 16-alpha hydroxyestrone levels
- Increase depression
- Increase tumor growth and spread

To improve your diet, there are a number of things you can do. Most important is to avoid all commercially prepared foods containing one of the omega-6 fats: safflower oil, sunflower oil, corn oil, peanut oil, soybean oil, and canola oil. Virtually all commercial foods made with oil contain one or more of these oils, even when the label says the product is based on olive oil.

Do not eat cookies, cakes, chips, commercial breads, crackers, or pies, all of which contain high levels of the omega-6 fats. In addition, some of these products, such as pies, cakes, and pastries, are also high in sugar, another promoter of cancer growth. You should also avoid all commercial salad dressings.

As a replacement, either make your own salad dressing using olive oil as the base or use spices. I prefer to eat salads either without a dressing or blenderized into a drink (see Chapter 1).

Use only extra virgin olive oil in cooking. As a monounsaturated oil, extra virgin olive oil is very stable and suitable for cooking. I would suggest adding turmeric to the oil. The curcumin in turmeric is a powerful anticancer, antioxidant, and antibacterial flavonoid. Several studies have shown that curcumin powerfully inhibits colon cancer.

One of the oil by-products associated with cancer development and growth is arachidonic acid. Diets high in the omega-6 fats are broken down into arachidonic acid in the cells, and this fatty substance is then metabolically converted into the inflammatory eicosanoids. A significant number of studies have linked diets high in arachidonic acid to increased tumor growth and spread. Some foods naturally contain high levels of arachidonic acid. Foods high in arachidonic acid include:

- Almonds
- Chicken
- Coconut
- Egg yolk
- Hazelnuts
- Macadamia nuts
- Peanuts
- Pecans
- Pistachios
- Walnuts

The Good Fats

In 1936, researchers reported for the first time that feeding experimental animals diets high in the omega-3 fatty acids inhibited the growth of tumors.[24] Since this early report, numerous studies have confirmed the finding. The mechanism by which the omega-3 oils suppress tumor growth is still incompletely understood, but we do have some answers. The omega-3 oils are truly remarkable.

Unfortunately, the consumption of the omega-3 type fats is

at an all-time low. During the process of preparing foods for market, most manufacturers remove these oils and replace them with the procarcinogenic omega-6-type fats. In the past, we could obtain some omega-3 oils from animal products. This is because animals that graze obtain some omega-3 fats from the grasses they consume. With today's corporate farming methods, however, food animals are fed grains, which contain little or no omega-3 oils.

Vegetables contain some omega-3 oils, but it is impossible to eat enough to meet your needs. Most of these beneficial oils come from seafood, flaxseed oil, and nutritional supplements. What is important is both the amount of the omega-3 oils you consume and the ratio of the omega-3 oils to the omega-6 oils.

Even though I refer to the omega-6 oils as bad, they are essential oils—that is, they are essential for life and must be supplied by the diet. Problems arise when we consume too many of these oils.

A common mistake people make when they learn of the beneficial effects of the omega-3 oils is to start taking a lot of fish oil supplements without cutting back on their omega-6 fat intake. While the ratio of good fats to bad fats is important, it is also vital to cut down on the total amount of bad oils you consume. This is because ingesting large amounts of the omega-6 type oils can suppress the entry of the omega-3 oils into the cancer cells' membranes. As you will recall, cancer cells that have a lot of omega-6 fats in their membranes are resistant to immune attack and are more likely to metastasize. It may take as long as two years to remove the omega-6 fats from cell membranes, whereas the omega-3 fats can enter the membranes within months. The sooner you start making dietary changes, the sooner you will reap the beneficial effects.

The omega-3 fats have numerous benefits. A number of studies have shown that the omega-3 oils, when added to the diet, improve immune function, especially the portion of the immune system that fights cancer, called cellular immunity.[25] In addition, animal studies have consistently shown that diets high in the omega-3 oils significantly suppress the growth of implanted human tumors, especially prostate and breast cancers.[26]

The omega-3 oils also suppress cancer growth and spread by

suppressing inflammation.[27] The mechanism by which they do this involves the suppression of the inflammatory eicosanoids. Recently, it was shown that the omega-3 oils suppress a powerful cancer growth–promoting protein (ras) often found in the cell membranes of cancer cells.[28]

Studies of large populations of men have shown that those who eat the most omega-3 oils have the lowest incidence of prostate cancer. In addition, the omega-3 oils have been shown to suppress the stimulation of prostate cancer growth by androgens (male sex hormones such as testosterone) and to lower prostate specific antigen (PSA) levels.[29]

Likewise, a study of 241 women having invasive breast cancer without metastasis compared to 88 women with benign breast conditions found that the women with the highest DHA levels in their breast tissue had the lowest incidence of breast cancer—an incredible 69 percent lower.[30]

The omega-3 fats have also been shown to significantly suppress tumor angiogenesis, which, as we have seen, is critical to tumor growth and spread. The DHA component of the omega-3 oils appears to play the greatest role in this beneficial effect. The omega-6 oils promote angiogenesis by increasing the production of stimulators such as COX-2, 12-hydroxyeicosatetraneoic acid (12-HETE), and 15-hydroxyeicosatetraneoic acid (15-HETE), factors that DHA lowers.[31]

DHA has also been shown to suppress cancer cell stimulation by estrogen.[32] The higher the intake of DHA, the greater the suppression is of the tumor growth. Interestingly, DHA can suppress tumor growth even when the omega-6 fat intake is high, even though it works much better when the intake of the omega-6 fats is reduced. In one study, rats fed a diet containing 8 percent omega-6 fats had very aggressive tumors that frequently metastasized throughout the animals' bodies. By adding 4 percent omega-3 fats to the rats' diet, tumor growth was dramatically reduced. Increasing the percentage of the omega-3 fats even higher produced a more powerful tumor-suppressing effect.

Recent studies have shown that diets high in DHA oils enhance the effectiveness of chemotherapy by suppressing cancer cell reproduction and by increasing apoptosis, a major mechanism utilized by chemotherapy drugs.[33]

Important Points to Remember

Of particular importance is the fact that the type of fat consumed is more important than the percentage of fats in the diet. For example, a diet containing 35 percent fat calories mainly as omega-3 fats is better than a diet of 25 percent fat calories composed mainly of omega-6 fats.

Also important to remember is that the omega-3 fats are easily oxidized—that is, they easily become rancid. Once rancid, these fats are harmful. Omega-3 fats should be kept in the refrigerator, and you should take at least 1,000 international units of natural vitamin E or vitamin E succinate daily. It is not necessary to take the vitamin E and omega-3 oils at the same time. Most of the anticancer effects of the omega-3 oils are accounted for by the DHA component and not the eicosapentaenoic acid (EPA) component. DHA is extracted from algae.

Flaxseed and Flaxseed Oil

Flaxseed contains several anticancer components, including the omega-3 oils and special precursor substances. One study of chemically induced breast cancers in mice found that the animals fed various concentrations of flaxseed oil in their diets had smaller tumors and fewer tumors than did the control mice.[34] We now know a lot more about why and how flaxseed works to inhibit cancer development and growth.

Flaxseed contains extremely high levels of a phytochemical called lignan, which is composed of powerful anticancer chemicals called seoisoloriciresinol diglycoside and matairesinol, which are converted by the friendly bacteria in the colon into two anticancer chemicals, enterolactone and enterodiol. These two chemicals have shown powerful suppressing effects on prostate, colon, and breast cancer.

Lignans have antioxidant, antiproliferative, antiestrogen, and antiangiogenesis properties, all of which suppress the development, growth, and spread of several types of cancer.[35]

Normally, estrogens are secreted into the colon, where they are metabolized in the presence of the friendly bacteria into either a 2-hydroxyestrone metabolite, which has been shown to powerfully suppress cancers, or the 4-hydroxyestrone and 16-alpha hydroxyestrone products, which strongly stimulate the growth of several types of cancer, especially prostate and breast cancer.[36]

In the Finnish Kuopio Breast Cancer Study, in which 194 women with breast cancer were compared to 208 controls, it was found that the women with the highest blood levels of enterolactone had significantly lower breast cancer risk than the women with low levels.[37] This was true for both premenopausal and postmenopausal women.

Of particular importance is the finding that the ratio of the forms of the estrogen metabolites—2-hydroxyestrone and 16-alpha hydroxyestrone—is what determines the risk for breast cancer.[38] The women with the highest ratio had the lowest incidence of breast cancer, and the women with the lowest ration had the highest incidence of breast cancer. The importance of these estrogen metabolites has been confirmed in studies of breast biopsies, in which women with the highest 16-alpha hydroxyestrone levels had the highest incidence of breast cancer.

A woman can increase her 2-hydroxyestrone levels by eating a diet low in the omega-6 fats, exercising regularly, and taking special nutritional supplements. Unfortunately, the 16-alpha hydroxyestrone levels respond very little to these same changes in behavior. A higher intake of the omega-3 oils can lower the harmful 16-alpha hydroxyestrone levels and increase the beneficial 2-hydroxyestrone levels. This can be done by eating 10 grams of flaxseed a day.

Studies have also shown that a high-protein diet lowers the ratio of 2-hydroxy to 16-alpha hydroxyestrone, thereby greatly increasing cancer risk. People wishing to lose weight through the use of a high-protein diet should remember this finding. In addition, this ratio of estrogen products is linked to several other types of cancer as well, such as cervical, endometrial, prostate, and even head and neck cancers.[39,40]

One study found that animals having higher 16-alpha hydroxyestrone levels were more likely to develop breast cancers when exposed to the murine mammary tumor virus than were mice exposed to the virus alone.[41] Some cancer specialists feel that many human breast cancers are linked to a virus.

Lignan has been shown to inhibit the conversion of testosterone to estradiol in the fat cells by blocking the enzyme aromatase.[42] This enzyme is suspected of playing a major role in breast, prostate, and colon cancer. Extra virgin olive oil (but not plain or lite olive oil) contains significant amounts of lignan.[43]

Recent studies have shown that a diet containing 5 percent flaxseed caused a significant fall in the tumor growth promoter insulin-like growth factor-1 (IGF-1).[44] Numerous studies have shown a direct correlation between IGF-1 levels and the risk of developing uncontrollable cancer growth.

One study found that women who frequently take antibiotics are significantly more likely to develop breast cancer than women who take antibiotics less frequently, but only if they are premenopausal.[45] The longer they were followed, the greater was their risk. It was hypothesized that the antibiotics kill the friendly bacteria needed to metabolize the estrogen in the colon.

Special Cancer-Fighting Fats

Several special fats have been shown to significantly inhibit cancer formation, growth, and spread. Fortunately, these oils are readily available as supplements. Some of these oils also improve weight gain in the cancer patient and provide a ready source of concentrated energy without fat gain.

Gamma Linolenic Acid

Gamma linolenic acid (GLA) is a special oil commonly extracted from evening primrose oil and borage oil. Borage oil has the highest levels of GLA. Like the omega-3 oils, GLA is polyunsaturated, making it easy to oxidize. GLA oil has been shown to have a number of antitumor properties. Its ability to kill cancer cells has been demonstrated on many types of cancer.

Recently, GLA was found to readily kill leukemia cells isolated from patients with alpha-cell chronic lymphocytic leukemia.[46] The leukemia cells seemed to be affected the most, with the normal cells spared. In the presence of GLA, 42 percent of the leukemia cells underwent apoptosis, whereas only 20 percent of the cancer cells died when GLA was not present. When dexamethazone (cortisone) was added to the GLA, 86 percent of the cancer cells were killed. While this study was done in a culture dish, it indicated a potential usefulness for GLA oil in leukemia treatment.

Another study, using human tumors, demonstrated that injecting GLA directly into a brain tumor (glioma) caused the tumor to regress.[47] There is significant evidence that GLA kills many cancer cells by dramatically increasing the free radical and lipid peroxidation products within the cancer cells selectively—that is, it affects only cancer cells, not normal cells. When testing GLA in a culture dish, adding antioxidants has been shown to block the killing effect. This would give some credence to the fear that antioxidants might interfere with cancer treatments. Later I will explain the problem with this notion.

Studies using animals with carcinogen-induced tumors or implanted human tumors also demonstrated the ability of GLA to suppress tumor growth.[48] Other studies did not find a beneficial effect with GLA.

It appears that GLA's effectiveness depends heavily on oxidation-induced apoptosis of cancer cells. It may be that smaller amounts of GLA are effective, whereas larger amounts may be detrimental, since GLA can induce inflammatory reactions. As stated previously, anything that increases inflammation also increases tumor formation, growth, and spread.

Because of this narrow window of effectiveness, I would not recommend taking more than 2,000 milligrams of GLA a day as a supplement.

Conjugated Linoleic Acid

Conjugated linoleic acid (CLA) is a special fatty acid that is chemically related to the cancer-promoting linolenic acid, but instead has been shown to have significant anticancer effects in experimental animal studies. In fact, CLA is effective at concentrations of 1 percent or less of total fat intake, which is a very small amount.[49] Unlike some fats, CLA's anticancer activity is not reduced by increasing the concentration of the bad fats in the diet.

The anticancer effect of conjugated linoleic acid has been demonstrated against several types of cancer.[50] Of particular interest is its effect against breast cancer and colon cancer. For example, in one recent study using a powerful chemical to induce precancerous colon changes in rats, it was found that the rats fed CLA had a dramatic reduction in the number of lesions in their colon.[51] These precancerous lesions, called abberant crypt foci, develop in human colon cancer as well. It appears that the CLA caused these precancerous cells to commit suicide while having no effect on the normal cells.

Both animal and human studies have found a decreased incidence of breast cancer in females whose diet contained at least 1 percent CLA oil.[52] Because the amount of this oil needed to suppress breast cancer development is so low, it is considered to have a direct effect on the cancer cells.

It may be that CLA oil acts to prevent cancer by inhibiting the formation of arachidonic acid (one of the cancer fertilizers) from linolenic acid (the major fatty acid in corn, safflower, peanut, and sunflower oils).[53] Further confirmation comes from a study that showed a diet higher in CLA oils reduced the amount of tumor-associated eicosanoid, PGE2, induced by a cancer-causing chemical called phorbol ester.[54] This would explain why CLA oils are especially effective against breast, colon, and prostate cancers, since all of these cancers produce high levels of PGE2 eicosanoids. CLA oils are found primarily in meats and milk products. Because of the adverse effects of both of these sources in terms of cancer development, it is better to obtain CLA from supplements.[55]

Because CLA oil is effective at levels of 1 percent or less of the total dietary fat inake, taking 1,000 to 2,000 milligrams a day of the supplement is adequate.

Medium-Chain Triglycerides

The medium-chain triglycerides (MCTs) are special fats that are made of links of fatty acids that are shorter than those composing the omega-3 or omega-6 fats. In addition, they are metabolized by the body more like carbohydrates than fats—that is, they are rapidly broken down to provide considerable energy without affecting the insulin levels. This is important because excess insulin can powerfully stimulate tumor growth and spread. In addition, earlier studies have shown that the MCT oils can inhibit tumor growth and prevent cancer-related weight loss.

Several studies have shown that the MCT oils have an antitumor effect on several types of cancer. In fact, one study found that the oils increased the death of cancer cells, but had no harmful effect on normal cells.[56] Of special importance is the fact that the MCT oils have shown no negative effects on immunity. They may even enhance the immunity against tumors.

The MCT oils have been shown to reduce inflammation by 50 percent in animal tests using a powerful inflammatory chemical.[57] Again I emphasize that anything that reduces inflammation also reduces cancer growth and spread. A recent double blind, controlled trial utilizing MCT oils found that the oils produced a significant degree of fat loss, especially of subcutaneous fat, and at the same time increased muscle building.[58] This is very important for the cancer patient.

Note that you should not take the MCT oils, either as a liquid or in capsule form, on an empty stomach because they can cause considerable stomach pain and cramping. The MCT oils are always best taken immediately after a meal. I would also limit intake of the MCT oils to three or four tablespoonsful a day. The oils can be mixed with extra virgin olive oil in equal volumes to reduce their gastric-irritating effects. The advantage of the MCT oils over the other oils is that they are metabolized very rapidly to yield high levels of energy. As we have seen, cancer patients need significant amounts of energy, but we cannot use glucose or other simple sugars because they enhance cancer cell growth. The MCT oils solve this problem.

Perillyl Alcohol

Perillyl alcohol is an extract containing the omega-3 oils taken from the plant *Perilla futescens*. Its advantage over the fish oils is that it does not cause stomach upset, has no bad fishy taste, and has anti-inflammatory and cancer-inhibiting effects equal in effectiveness to these other omega-3 oils.

Recent tests using tumor models found that perillyl oil inhibited cancer growth and increased apoptosis in several types of cancer, including colon, breast, and liver cancer.[59] Studies are now being conducted using human cancer patients to see if it will have the same effectiveness. Thus far, it looks promising.

Chemically, perillyl alcohol is a monoterpene. This class of cancer-inhibiting chemicals also includes limonene, a phytochemical found in lemons. Recent studies have shown that perillyl alcohol inhibits cancer development in part by stimulating the production of both the phase one and phase two detoxification enzymes in the liver. The destruction of cancer cells when exposed to perillyl alcohol occurs by several mechanisms, including activation of cancer suicide genes, inhibition of inflammation, and reduction of cancer cell spread. One of the real advantages of this supplement is that it has very low toxicity.

SPECIAL OILS AND CHEMOTHERAPY

An obvious question arises when we consider the significant effect of these special oils on cancer growth and spread: Do they enhance the effectiveness of cancer chemotherapy or do they possibly interfere with its effectiveness? Several studies have shown that some of the oils can significantly enhance the effectiveness of the treatment.

For example, one of the major problems when using chemotherapy drugs is that the cell cycle of the cancer (the time required for cell reproduction) is longer than the half-life of the drug (the time needed for half of the drug to be cleared from the blood). Most of the chemotherapy drugs must be present during the cycling (cell division) of the cancer cells in order to be effective. Since the drug is gone before the cancer cells have completed their division, the cancer cells escape the drug's killing effects.

In one recent study, researchers found that when DHA oil was combined with the anticancer drug paclitaxel, it not only increased the effectiveness of the drug against the cancer, but it removed much of the toxicity normally seen when the paclitaxel is used alone.[60]

The study demonstrated that when combined with DHA oil, paclitaxel is active against cancer sixty-one times longer than when it is used alone. In addition, adding the DHA oil appeared to help aim the drug directly at the tumor. In one part of the study using mice having tumors, the combination was shown to cure all ten animals that received it, whereas the paclitaxal used alone cured none of the animals.

In a phase one study done at Johns Hopkins Hospital using patients having solid tumors (tumors other than blood cell cancers, such as leukemia), researchers found that they were able to give the DHA-paclitaxel combination in a dose 4.6 times higher than the previously approved maximum dose of the chemotherapy agent when used alone. None of the patients lost their hair or suffered from nausea, vomiting, or neuropathy (nerve damage). Their bone marrow depression was significantly reduced as well. In addition, most of the patients reported a significant improvement in their quality of life.

Other special oils have also been shown to enhance the effectiveness of certain chemotherapy agents.[61] For example, GLA, the omega-3 fatty acids, and EPA, in decreasing order of effectiveness, have been effective against breast cancer cells in culture. When GLA was given at the same time as paclitaxel, there was a moderate synergism. If it was given following treatment with the chemotherapy agent, the enhancement was additive only. An additive effect of GLA oil against estrogen-sensitive breast cancer cells has also been shown when GLA oil was added to tamoxifen.[62]

When they combined a low-fat diet with the GLA and tamoxifen, the researchers saw a significantly slower growth of implanted human breast cancers. In addition, they saw a remarkably lower level of estrogen receptor expression. This means that the tumor cells had fewer estrogen receptors and therefore were less susceptible to growth stimulation by estrogens.

Another recent study showed a similarly enhanced effectiveness in the case of alpha-cell chronic leukemia when GLA oil was combined with dexamethasone, a common chemotherapy agent used in this form of leukemia.[63] Normally, 20 percent of leukemia cells spontaneously undergo apoptosis. However, when GLA was added to the culture medium, 42 percent died by apoptosis. And when GLA was added to the dexamethosone, 86 percent of the cancer cells died. The increase in apoptosis was significantly less in normal blood cells.

This is an important finding because one of the primary goals of cancer therapy is to increase the apoptosis of cancer cells without significantly increasing the apoptosis in the normal cells. These studies clearly demonstrated that the fear expressed by oncologists—that is, that nutritional treatments will interfere with the traditional cancer treatments—is totally unfounded. In fact, these studies show that just the opposite effect occurs.

Some oncologists will counter that these oils cause cancer cell death by increasing the free radical and lipid peroxidation in the cancer cells and that antioxidant vitamins would block this effect. In the case of GLA, vitamin E was not able to completely block the enhanced apoptosis. Some studies have shown that DHA's dramatic stimulation of cancer cell apoptosis can be blocked by a powerful nonvitamin antioxidant, butylated hydroxytoluene (BHT). However, there is no evidence that naturally occurring antioxidants can block its effectiveness.[64] This is especially so because many of the nutrient antioxidants, as we shall see, actually have anticancer effects separate from their antioxidant effects.

Proteins, Amino Acids, and Cancer Growth

One of the major problems seen with patients having advanced cancers is a loss of muscle protein, also called cachexia. In an effort to avoid this, or to correct it, doctors and research scientists have utilized high-protein concoctions, amino acid combinations, and single amino acids. Unfortunately, most of the early efforts failed. As our knowledge has increased concerning muscle building and proteins, we have developed better combinations of amino acids. For example, we now know that in order for amino acids to enter and remain in muscle tissue, they must be administered along with carbohydrates or other sources of energy. In addition, we know that certain amino acids play a larger role than others in muscle building. For example, the branch-chained amino acids (leucine, isoleucine, and valine) and glutamine are more important than the other amino acids.

Since rapidly dividing cells have an increased demand for certain amino acids, doctors have worried about the wisdom of giving these amino acids in larger amounts. Would it make the cancer grow faster? This fear is not completely unwarranted. Several studies have shown that the amino acids methionine and arginine can increase the growth of certain types of tumors and may increase the risk of metastasis as well.

Methionine

The strongest evidence concerning the connection between tumor growth and the amino acids is found with L-methionine. Most of the evidence stems from the use of diets depleted of methionine. For example, giving patients with advanced gastric cancer intravenous nutritional supplementation using mixtures containing no methionine significantly slowed the growth of their tumors and made the tumors much more susceptible to chemotherapy. An analysis of the tumors showed that the methionine-deficient diet slowed cell division, freezing the cancer cells in the synthesis phase (S-phase) of reproduction, the phase in which the cell makes a copy of each of its chromosomes in preparation for cell division.[65] This allowed the chemotherapy drug more time to kill more cancer cells.

Similar reductions in tumor growth have been seen in prostate cancer when methionine was restricted in the diet.[66] It appears that at least one mechanism by which removing L-methionine accomplishes this is stimulation of the gene signal c-Jun N-terminal kinase-1 (JNK-1), a primary anibody that triggers spontaneous cancer cell death.

While methionine can increase the growth of existing cancers, in the normal individual it appears to play a vital role in the prevention of cancer development.[67] Methionine's major role in preventing cancer development is based on the fact that it is the primary methyl donor in cells. Biochemically, L-methionine is converted to S-adenosylmethionine (SAMe), which then donates methyl groups for DNA regulation and repair. When there is a deficiency of methyl groups, cancer risk is greatly enhanced. In rare instances, overmethylation of the DNA can lead to cancer. This is why the supplement SAMe should not be taken by cancer patients or by people with a strong family history of cancer.

There is one instance in which too much L-methionine in the diet can increase the risk of cancer. Using a model of human familial polyposis, a disorder in which numerous precancerous polyps develop in the colon early in life, animals were fed a diet rich in L-methionine soon after birth.[68] The researchers found that these animals did not develop more polyps, but that the polyps in the small bowel were larger and more likely to become malignant.

With the rather dramatic results being shown with methionine-deficient diets, we must ask: Will such a diet damage normal cells? As yet, we do not know the answer to this question. As I have mentioned, a low-methionine diet does increase cancer risk. However, one study in which both gastric cancer cells and normal stomach lining (gastric mucosa) cells were exposed to a methionine-deficient medium found that the cancer cells experienced significantly suppressed growth, but the normal cells of the stomach showed no effect.[69]

The major sources of methionine are meats (especially pork), beans, fish, nuts, and brewer's yeast. The highest plant source is the Brazil nut, followed closely by the soybean. Ironically, these methionine sources are also major sources of glutamic acid and aspartate, which are suspected of promoting cancer invasion, especially with brain cancers, as well. Following is a list of foods that are high in methionine:

- Brazil nuts
- Brie cheese
- Chedder cheese
- Crayfish
- Dried eggs
- Dried milk
- Halibut
- Meats (beef, chicken, fish, and pork)

- Parmesan cheese
- Salmon
- Soybeans
- Sunflower seeds
- Whole eggs

Note that beef, chicken, and fish all have about the same levels of methionine—approximately 450 to 650 milligrams per 100 grams of meat—with pork containing somewhat less.

Arginine

L-arginine's story is still being worked out, but we have learned many interesting things about this unique amino acid. Some reports indicate that it can play a powerful role in preventing cancer metastasis, while others indicate that it has a powerful stimulatory role in cancer growth and invasion.[70,71]

One advantage of arginine is its immune-stimulating properties. Some studies in patients have indicated that these properties may suppress tumor growth. Other studies have found that arginine increases the production of nitric oxide by the cells and that this might reduce metastasis. A few studies have found just the opposite.

Because of the question regarding L-arginine's stimulation of cancer growth, I would caution against using high doses of this amino acid at this time. I feel that with more study, we will find L-arginine is a useful adjunct in cancer treatment, but that at the present time, the risk is too great.

Glutamate

Another amino acid of concern is glutamic acid, or glutamate. This amino acid is one of the most abundant neurotransmitters in the brain, but its concentration outside the brain cells needs to be very carefully controlled because of its toxicity. There is substantial evidence that excess glutamate plays a major role in numerous neurological conditions, such as Alzheimer's disease, Parkinson's disease, Lou Gehrig's disease, stroke, brain and spinal cord trauma, encephalitis, and brain infections.[72] Now there is evidence that glutamate also plays a substantial role in certain brain tumors, called gliomas.

Unfortunately, the most common primary brain tumor, called a glioblastoma multiforme, is also the most malignant one. A recent study found that glutamate may play a major role in the invasiveness and aggressiveness of this terrible tumor.[73] It was shown in the study that human glioma tumors secrete excess glutamate, even when the tumors are implanted in other animals.[74] It was also found that gliomas that secrete excess glutamate are much more aggressive and grow faster than tumors that are free of glutamate. The sizes of the tumors were directly related to the amounts of glutamate present.

In the study, the rats with glutamate-secreting tumors died earlier than the animals with non-glutamate-secreting tumors of the same malignant type. Moreover, by using special drugs that block glutamate, the researchers demonstrated shrinking of the tumors. The level of increase in the glutamate did not have to be very high, only fourfold. In cases of head injury and stroke, the levels can reach from 100- to 200-fold higher. Interestingly, the trauma of surgical removal of a tumor can also increase the glutamate levels around the site of the tumor removal for several weeks afterward. This might contribute to recurrence of the tumor, which frequently occurs.

Of major concern is the high level of glutamate in processed foods in the guise of MSG and its other forms. In addition, certain foods are naturally high in glutamate levels. For example, meats, beans (especially soybeans), certain cheeses (Parmesan, Gouda, Brie), sunflower seeds, and peanuts are all relatively high in glutamate.

Normally, the blood-brain barrier works to prevent excess glutamate from entering the brain. The barrier is ineffective when the blood levels of glutamate are excessively high, and it may completely break down when tumors of the brain develop. This means that diets high in glutamate act as strong stimulants for the growth of malignant brain tumors.

Most food processors add glutamate products to their foods to enhance the taste. Unfortunately, these same additives enhance brain cell injury, seizures, and brain tumor invasion and growth.

It may be that glutamate enhances the growth of tumors outside the brain as well. Thus far, no one has looked for such a link. However, we do know that glutamate, in the form of MSG, can alter gene function and increase free radical generation. In fact, there is a strong correlation between glutamate damage to the neurons and free radical generation. Since many cells in the body, such as the endothelial cells, cardiac nerves, pancreatic cells, and ovarian cells, have been shown to contain glutamate receptors, they, too, would be susceptible to glutamate toxicity and free radical generation.

The strong connection between glutamate and the aggressiveness of brain tumors leads to a major concern. Many nutritionists advocate glutamine as a way to enhance gut repair and to prevent the muscle loss common with malignancies.[75] There is little question that glutamine has some very beneficial effects, including improvement of lymphocyte function, reduced permeability of the intestine during radiotherapy, and improvement of muscle bulk. The problem lies in the fact that glutamine is the precusor of glutamate—that is, the cells manufacture glutamate from glutamine. A high intake of glutamine will increase the brain levels of glutamate, potentially increasing the danger imposed by the glutamate stimulation of glioma growth and aggressiveness. This danger was considered by Dr. Jeffery Rothstein and Dr. Henry Brem of Johns Hopkins University when this research was first reported.[76]

So, what about taking glutamine supplements for cancers other than brain tumors? Is it safe? While the jury is still out, it appears that it is safe and that in certain situations it may increase the effectiveness of the chemotherapy. We do know that glutamine added to the diet can dramatically reduce the complications associated with abdominal radiotherapy and chemotherapy, especially as related to gastrointestinal function and lymphocyte function.

As we have seen previously, the intestinal cells use a lot of glutamine. When deficient in glutamine, the intestinal wall begins to leak, allowing bacteria and undigested food particles to enter the bloodstream. This greatly increases the risk of deterioration and even death. In addition, glutamine is a major building block for muscle tissue. Depletion of glutamine, which commonly occurs with cancer, causes muscle loss. This loss can be averted by a diet high in glutamine.

Cancer cells soak up glutamine like a sponge. In fact, they steal glutamine from the liver, muscles, and gastrointestinal tract.[77] Some fast-growing cancers consume glutamine five to ten times faster than normal cells. While glucose is the major fuel for cancer cells, glutamine is also essential. Experimentally, removing all glutamine from a cancer cell results in its death. But will adding glutamine make a cancer grow faster? In experiments using rats with tumors, glutamine given orally did not increase the growth of the tumors, as determined by careful measurements.[78] Nor did the rats experience increased metastasis. There are also no reports of increased tumor growth or metastasis occurring in people receiving glutamine during cancer treatment.[79]

Of great interest is the finding that animals provided a diet high in glutamine while receiving the chemotherapy drug methotrexate had improved antitumor responses to the methotrexate over the animals given the drug alone. In addition, the animals fed the high-glutamine diet had far fewer toxic side effects from the drug.[80]

Another beneficial effect of an increased intake of glutamine is improved immune function. This is because the primary cancer-fighting immune cell, the lymphocyte, requires a lot of glutamine to function properly. With the dramatic loss of glutamine from the blood with cancer growth, the supply to the lymphocytes falls dangerously low, impairing their function. Studies have shown that supplementing the diet with extra glutamine improves immune function.[81]

The benefits of short-term glutamine supplementation probably exceed any of the negative effects. Improved gut function and gut immunity, improved lymphocyte function, enhanced effectiveness of chemotherapy, reduction in treatment complications, and prevention of muscle loss are major gains for the cancer patient.

DO ANTIOXIDANT SUPPLEMENTS INCREASE CANCER GROWTH?

While nutrition has been cleared of any role in stimulating cancer growth, what about nutritional supplements? This is one of the greatest fears of oncologists. This fear is mostly based on the idea that chemotherapy and radiation work by increasing the generation of free radicals within the cancer cells, and that blocking this generation of free radicals will neutralize the cancer treatment.

As we saw in Chapter 2, most chemotherapy drugs inhibit cancer growth and kill cancer cells by mechanisms that have nothing to do with free radicals. In fact, one recent study clearly demonstrated that the chemotherapy drugs oral etopodise (VP-16) and cisplatin kill malignant cells completely independent of free radical damage.[82] In addition, powerful antioxidants did not diminish the killing effectiveness of either of these drugs.

Let us explore this subject by looking at some news stories that caused a real uproar among the public.

Beta-Carotene and Lung Cancer

In 1994, the results of the Alpha-Tocopherol Beta-Carotene Study (ATBC) were announced in the *New England Journal of Medicine*. The results, which then passed through the filter of the general media, supposedly indicated that beta-carotene causes lung cancer.[83] This transformation of meaning, unfortunately, is not uncommon when complicated medical reports are interpreted by the lay media.

In fact, the ATBC, as well as numerous other studies, both in animals and in humans, demonstrated that increased beta-carotene intake reduces the incidence of several types of cancer, including oral, esophageal, ovarian, and cervical cancers. In the study, cancer of the lung was increased only in the men who smoked at least a pack of cigarettes a day and/or consumed excessive alcohol. The Physicians' Health Study, which included 22,071 physicians taking 50 milligrams of beta-carotene every other day over a twelve-year period, did not find an increase in any cancer.[84]

Subsequent studies have indicated that the ATBC study was flawed for several reasons. One of the major criticisms, which was even admitted in the original paper, was that because the subjects were longtime smokers and drinkers, several may already have had small cancers present at the time the study began. This is a valid observation.

It has also been noted that the form of beta-carotene used in the study was a synthetic form of the vitamin, which differs significantly from the form found in fruits and vegetables. Other studies have shown that the synthetic forms of beta-carotene can cause a drastic reduction in the liver stores of the other carotenoids.[85] Some of the other carotenoids are more important in cancer prevention and control than beta-carotene. In addition, high intakes of beta-carotene alone can lower lutein absorption. This effect is not seen with the natural forms of beta-carotene. Lutein has been shown to play a major role in the prevention of lung cancer. A high intake of beta-carotene alone is also known to lower the blood and liver levels of vitamin E.

Another problem is that beta-carotene works best in tissues with a low oxygen content.[86] The lungs have a very high oxygen content, making it more likely that the beta carotene, especially in high concentrations, will oxidize. When beta-carotene or any other antioxidant vitamin oxidizes, it becomes an oxidant—that is, it can damage cells and possibly lead to the development of cancer.

Using any antioxidant alone in high concentrations is hazardous because of this phenomenon. In all biological systems, the antioxidants work together, preventing any one of the antioxidants from oxidizing excessively. For example, vitamin E will convert oxidized vitamin C and beta-carotene back to their reduced, antioxidant forms.[87]

In addition, no scientific evidence exists that taking even large doses of synthetic beta-carotene can increase the lung cancer risk in nonsmokers.

Beta-carotene has been shown consistently to have a very high profile of safety, even in pregnant women, infants, and small children. Despite this, I always advise obtaining the carotenoids from one of two sources: plants (fruits and vegetables) or a supplement containing all of the major forms of the carotenoids, such as the algae *Dunaliella bardawil* or *Dunaliella salina*.

In summary, the problems with the study linking beta-carotene with lung cancer are common to many such human studies: A form of synthetic vitamin known to disrupt the biochemical balance was used, and the vitamin was given in isolation. I would never advocate taking large doses of any single vitamin or mineral, including vitamin C, beta-carotene, and vitamin E. These nutrients work in conjunction with each other and can be harmful if used alone.

Vitamin C and DNA Damage

Another alarming news report was that studies had found that taking higher doses of vitamin C could cause DNA damage. This is another case of using a double standard in science. The typical orthodox physician would never accept as final proof studies that had been done in isolation (in vitro)—that is, that were done in a culture medium using methods that in no way represent the conditions in a person's body. Such studies may hint at a potential problem, but they are not definitive and they certainly cannot be used to formulate health policy or treatment protocols.

The scare stories concerning vitamin C and DNA damage originated with a study using isolated cells in a culture medium exposed to large concentrations of vitamin C in the presence of iron. Under such circumstances, two things can happen. First, the vitamin C may oxidize, becoming dehydroascorbic acid, a weak oxidant, or free radical. Second, the vitamin C may convert the iron to a form that triggers the creation of hydrogen peroxide, which in turn can break down into a powerful free radical called a hydroxyl radical. The bottom line is that the conditions of the study did not represent a natural situation for ascorbate in the body.

In the body, other antioxidants (vitamins, minerals, and flavonoids, as well as antioxidant enzymes and glutathione) prevent vitamin C from oxidizing. In addition, the antioxidant enzymes glutathione peroxidase and catalase prevent hydrogen peroxide from breaking down into powerful hydroxyl radicals.

There is some evidence that should you significantly increase your iron intake at the same time you increase your vitamin C intake, you can elevate your free radical production. Yet, with normal iron intake, the iron is protected from oxidizing by a special set of binding proteins called transferrin and ferritin.

Other studies have shown that vitamin C may, in fact, have a special function in protecting the DNA from free radical damage. This is because ascorbate is water soluble and thereby prevents the membrane surrounding the nucleus of the cell from undergoing lipid peroxidation. This is very important, since lipid peroxidation produces especially caustic substances that can severely damage the DNA.

There is one instance in which higher intakes of vitamin C were shown to be detrimental to certain cancer patients. In this study, it was shown that a small percentage of leukemia patients experienced worsening of their disease when given vitamin C in concentrations higher than 100 milligrams a day.[88] Dr. Chan Park, director of the Cancer Center at the Samsung Medical Center in Seoul, Korea, presented the data to this effect at the Fifteenth International Conference of Human Functioning held in Wichita, Kansas, in September 2000. The responses of the leukemia patients to the higher doses of vitamin C were not always the same, since increasing the dose of vitamin C to very high levels (given intravenously) destroyed the same leukemia cells.

In summary, there is no evidence that taking even high doses of ascorbate (buffered vitamin C) damages the DNA, but there is abundant evidence that it protects the DNA and reduces cancer incidence for several types of cancer.

Conclusion

What we have learned is that nutrition, for the most part, is very beneficial to the cancer patient, but at times it can be a two-edged sword. Because cancer cells are different from normal cells in terms of their biochemical makeup, physiology, and metabolism, they are more dependent on certain nutrients than normal cells. For example, cancer cells have a voracious appetite for glutamine, methionine, glucose, and iron, and under certain conditions, and with specific cancers, you may want to avoid these nutrients.

In addition, we have seen that most of the oncologists' fears concerning nutrition stimulating the growth of cancers are totally unfounded. In fact, the nutrition being promoted by oncologists and many oncology dietitians is infinitely more dangerous in terms of stimulating cancer growth. It is truly frightening to see what is being suggested for cancer patients in terms of dietary choices.

We have also learned that a properly designed nutrition program can improve cancer patients' sense of well-being, increase their energy levels, reduce their treatment complications and side effects, and even enhance the effectiveness of the treatments themselves.

Many patients are forced to stop their treatments because of complications associated with the treatments. And it is known that interruption of the treatments can significantly lower their chance of being successful. Patients on well-designed nutritional programs rarely have to interrupt their treatments.

Because of their improved mood and energy level, cancer patients on a proper nutrition program feel less depressed and more hopeful. We know that depression, especially when severe and unrelieved, can suppress immunity and reduce the chances of a favorable outcome.

6

Nutrition and Cancer Treatments

Most of my patients tell me the same story about what happened when they informed their oncologist that they were going to see someone about a nutrition program. The oncologist screwed up his or her face, looked very grim, and remarked, "That's fine. Just don't let him put you on any antioxidants. Antioxidants will interfere with the treatments." This myth is so firmly ingrained in the oncology world that it is difficult to remove.

One of my patients, being treated at the university oncology center, asked his panicked oncologist what scientific evidence he had to show that antioxidant supplements interfered with cancer treatments. The oncologist thought for a long time and then said, "It's soft evidence, but there is some evidence that they can interfere with the treatments." This is the usual response.

Dr. Jerome Block, professor of medicine at the University of California at Los Angeles (UCLA) School of Medicine and former chief of medical oncology at the Harbor-UCLA Medical Center, concluded, in a recent review of this debate:

> The hypotheses that antioxidants' inhibition of free-radical activity may negate cytotoxic properties of some cancer therapies have been dependent on naïve and inaccurate assumptions.[1]

In an article in the *Journal of the American Nutraceutical Association* in 2000, I reviewed the available evidence on both sides of the issue and also concluded that the bulk of the evidence falls on the side of antioxidants being a tremendous benefit to the cancer patient.[2]

It is ironic that oncologists rarely object to a diet high in vegetables or even to juicing vegetables. It is ironic because these vegetables contain antioxidant combinations that are infinitely more powerful and versatile than any of the antioxidant supplements to which oncologists object so vehemently. The reason oncologists don't object to the foods is that they are not aware of this fact.

THE EVIDENCE AGAINST SUPPLEMENTS

For the most part, there is little support for the idea that nutritional supplementation interferes with the traditional cancer treatments. Most of the fears are based on the extrapolation of the effects of the nutritional supplements on normal cells to their possible effects on cancer cells. For instance, we know that antioxidants can completely protect normal cells from the free radical damage caused by chemotherapy drugs and radiotherapy.[3]

We also know that low doses of vitamins, when used alone, can cause some tumors to grow faster. This has been shown with vitamin C and leukemia and cancers of the parotid gland.[4] It has also been demonstrated when low doses of beta-carotene were given to animals having melanomas.[5] I emphasize "low doses" and "when used alone." High doses of vitamins, when used in combinations, have the opposite effect, as we shall see.

I have known many people who took only a single vitamin, such as vitamin C or E, thinking this was all they needed to do, since the chosen vitamin was the latest hot item on the news. This is very hazardous, not just in terms of cancer, but also regarding all degenerative diseases.

When vitamins are taken alone, they are subject to becoming oxidized—that is, they can become free radicals. Vitamin C will become dehydroascorbate, a weak free radical. The same is true for vitamin E and the carotenoids. Vitamins, as well as the other cellular antioxidants, were meant to be used together.

One study found that giving animals vitamin C as ascorbic acid increased the number of chemically induced bladder cancers.[6] Once again, we see that the form of the vitamin is critical, since the ascorbate form of vitamin C does not increase bladder cancer.

Finally, in the case of human lung cancers transplanted to mice, vitamin B_6 in high doses did stimulate tumor growth.[7] Vitamin B_6 inhibits tumors of other types. In essence, the only scientific studies demonstrating increased tumor growth or interference with chemotherapy effectiveness occurred when the antioxidant vitamins were used alone.

THE EVIDENCE FOR SUPPLEMENTS

The majority of studies examining the effects of nutritional supplementation have demonstrated a reduction in cancer risk, a reduction in the growth of established cancers, and even a reduction in the invasion and metastasis of certain cancers. So why do individual vitamins, especially in lower doses, increase the growth of cancers? To fully understand this, we need to go back to the stages of cancer development.

The initiation stage of cancer development involves DNA injuries by free radicals that accumulate in a specific sequence. It may take many years or even decades for these injuries to produce the genetic cellular growth stimulation needed to start the process. These random mutations are speeded up when the DNA repair enzymes are defective or in short supply. This can be due either to heredity, damage from toxins (such as mercury, fluoride, or arsenic), a deficiency of antioxidant protection, or a deficiency in the vitamins and amino acids used in DNA repair.

During the initiation stage, mutations also occur among the genes responsible for making the cells mature. When a cell reverts to a more immature state, it is more prone to become immortal—that is, malignant. As the mutations accumulate, the cells may form a precancerous lesion, such as a colon polyp or sun-damaged skin. These abnormal collections of cells contain numerous DNA mutations.

Dr. Kedar Prasad, working at the Center for Vitamins and Cancer Research at the Colorado Health Sciences Center in Denver, Colorado, notes that these precancerous lesions contain cells with varying types of gene damage, which explains why it has been so difficult to ascribe one type of gene injury to cancer development.

The final stage of cancer development, according to Dr. Prasad, is of critical importance in understanding the value of antioxidant vitamins in cancer treatment. Even after a cancer has formed, further free radical damage can make the cancer much more aggressive.[8] By inhibiting further free radical damage to the cell's DNA, advancement of the aggressiveness can, at least potentially, be blocked. The exact mechanism by which this can be accomplished has not been worked out as yet. Experimentally, antioxidants have been shown to prevent cancer progression at all of the stages and to enhance the conversion of immature cells to more mature cells.

As the cancer develops and spreads, the number of free radicals increases progressively. This causes the cancer to become more aggressive over time. Patients receiving chemotherapy also have high rates of free radical generation throughout their body. Logically, this should increase the aggressiveness of the cancer, causing it to be more difficult to control later in the course of the disease. This would suggest that chemotherapy that does not successfully kill or control a cancer may actually make it incurable.

We know that once a chemotherapy program fails, further attempts at control of the cancer are extremely difficult, if not impossible—that is, the cancer becomes resistant. Cancer resistance has been explained by assuming there are two basic populations of cancer cells mixed together within a tumor. One type of cancer cell is very susceptible to chemotherapy and is easily killed off. The second type of cancer cell is extremely resistant to chemotherapy, even from the very beginning of treatment. This explains why tumors may shrink early in the course of treatment and then suddenly start to grow very rapidly. In time, the tumor is composed solely of the resistant type of cancer cell, which grows very rapidly and frequently metastasizes.

It has now been determined that the resistant cancer cells differ from the susceptible cancer cells in that they have a special mechanism to expel the chemotherapy drug from the cell as fast as it can enter. The most successful ways to block this resistance have involved using special nutrients, many of which have been antioxidant vitamins.

The contention by oncologists that free radicals are responsible for the effectiveness of chemotherapy is easily disproved, since if this were true, anything that increases free radical generation would work as well as any anticancer drug. We know that the omega-6 fats increase free radical formation, yet they also increase cancer growth and spread. In addition, they make cancers more aggressive. The same is true for substances that increase inflammation. As we have seen, the food additive carrageenan causes intense inflammation when it is injected into tissues, and this intense inflammation can generate an enormous number of free radicals in the area of the injection. Yet injecting carrageenan near a tumor will cause that tumor to grow at a significantly faster rate and to metastasize widely. In fact, the number of free radicals formed usually exceeds the amount produced by most chemotherapy drugs. If free radicals were how chemotherapy killed cancer cells, then carrageenan would be one of the best anticancer drugs known. Instead, the opposite is true: Carrageenan stimulates cancer growth and spread.

It should also be noted that in the leukemia study mentioned previously, vitamin C increased cancer cell growth only when it was used alone and in smaller concentrations. When it was used in higher concentrations, it caused the cancer cells to begin to die. This gives some credence to the theories of Linus Pauling concerning very high dose vitamin C and cancer suppression.

Of more importance have been the observations of Dr. Prasad and his associates that a mixture of vitamins can suppress the growth of certain cancers, when no effect is seen when the vitamins are used individually. For example, these researchers found that a mixture of vitamin A (as 13-cis-retinoic acid), sodium ascorbate, d-alpha-tocopheryl succinate (vitamin E), and polar carotenoids (with no beta-carotene) significantly reduced the growth of human melanoma cells in culture, whereas the individual vitamins, in the same concentrations, had no effect.[9] Similar results were found when the vitamin mixture was used on human parotid carcinoma cells. Of particular interest was the finding that doubling the dose of one of the vitamins in the mixture further reduced the growth of the tumors.

Butyric acid, a fatty product (a short-chain fatty acid) produced during the fermentation of soluble fiber in the colon, has been shown to have significant anticancer properties by itself. In addition, it is a major energy fuel for the cells lining the gastrointestinal tract, keeping them healthy and functioning at peak activity. When vitamin E, in the form of alpha-tocopheryl succinate, is added to butyric acid, the combination dramatically enhances the inhibition of cancer growth by the butyric acid.[10]

It is quite evident from these studies that when vitamins are used together, they can act powerfully to inhibit cancer formation, and in the case of existing cancers, they can inhibit their growth, invasion, and metastasis. In none of these studies was there evidence that the vitamins stimulated cancer growth when used in this manner.

It has been shown that the most important factors in determining the effectiveness of a nutrient combination against a cancer are its dose, the form of the vitamins used, and how long the mixture is used. For example, when two antioxidant vitamins are used together in the presence of cancer cells and one is used in a high dose and the other in a low dose, the anticancer effect is no better than when the high-dose vitamin is used alone.[11] Yet, when both the vitamins are given in high doses, we see a synergistic killing or suppression of the cancer cells.

What about studies using people? Unfortunately, relatively few careful studies have been done in people receiving chemotherapy. As I stated at the beginning of this book, in over twenty-four years of combining antioxidants with traditional treatments, I have never seen the antioxidants interfere with the chemotherapy drugs, and I know of no one else, including oncologists, who has seen this either. But I have seen significant improvement in the effectiveness of cancer treatments when they are combined with the proper nutritional supplementation.

Dr. Jerome Block has noted that antioxidants have been used extensively in patients in an effort to reduce the toxicity of such chemotherapy agents as amifostine combined with cisplatin, dextrazazone combined with adriamycin, and mesna combined with ifosphomide.[12] With none of these have the antioxidants been reported to reduce the effectiveness of the treatments.

In three separate studies, the powerful antioxidant glutathione was shown not to interfere with the chemotherapy drug's effectiveness, and in fact, it enhanced the drug's antitumor effectiveness.

Why Cancer Cells Act Differently Than Normal Cells

In all of the studies using vitamin mixtures, the inhibition of cell growth occurred only with cancer cells and not with normal cells. This is important, especially in the treatment of childhood cancers, since you do not want to interfere with the normal growth of the children. Even in adults, you do not want to inhibit the reproduction of the cells that normally divide very rapidly and frequently, such as those lining the gastrointestinal tract, located in the bone marrow, and found in the hair follicles.

So why does this selective toxic effect occur only in cancer cells? It appears that cancer cells, at least in certain instances, take up these antioxidant vitamins in much higher concentrations than do normal cells.[13] There is growing evidence that these vitamins kill cancer cells, or at least inhibit their growth, by a number of mechanisms, many of which have nothing to do with their antioxidant effect.

These nutrients also selectively enhance the detoxification systems used to neutralize the cancer-causing chemicals obtained either in the diet or from the environment. As we shall see later, some of these dietary chemicals are quite potent in this regard.

On a cellular level, several of the vitamins can block DNA reproduction, induce apoptosis, inhibit critical cancer growth signals, and block essential enzymes needed for tumor growth, invasion, and angiogenesis. In addition, several flavonoids, vitamins, and special fats can powerfully block the eicosanoid pathways, which trigger inflammation, suppress immunity, and directly stimulate tumor growth and metastasis. It is these effects of which oncologists are unaware and that lead them to hypothesize that nutrients will interfere with their treatments. Because cancer cells concentrate these nutrients in much higher strengths than normal cells, the effectiveness of this inhibition is even greater.

The important thing to remember is that these nutrients not only increase the killing of cancer cells by the conventional treatments, but also protect normal cells from these powerful cell toxins.

SPECIAL WAYS NUTRIENTS FIGHT CANCER

In Chapter 2, I said that from the very beginning, doctors have been searching for a way to kill cancer cells without harming the body's normal cells, something referred to as selective toxicity or targeted therapy. Unfortunately, this goal has remained elusive for the pharmacological manufacturers and hence for oncologists.

Throughout this book, I have shown that many nutrients and nutritional supplements do act with great selectivity. Many not only spare the normal cell from treatment toxicity, but also enhance the normal cell's health. This is important, not only in terms of the immediate protection from toxicity, but also in preventing the occurrences of secondary cancers—that is, cancers caused by the treatments themselves.

Now let us look at the specific ways in which nutrients help us attain these goals.

Nutrients Improve Cell Communication

We saw in Chapter 1 that normal cells are constantly in communication with each other, in a process called gap junction intercellular communication (GJIC). This line of communication is necessary in order to prevent the cells from getting anarchistic notions about going out on their own and defying all the rules. Because all of our organs and tissues are made of groups of specialized cells, for normal function to occur, these cells must remain orderly and must carefully follow instructions. They help each other to stay in line by this system of communication.

It is thought that one of the earliest changes in carcinogenesis is the loss of this cell-to-cell communication. The phone lines that keep this communication link are based on chemical messages. One of the primary links is through a chemical called connexin 43. We know that early on in the cancer process, this chemical messenger is lost or significantly decreased.

The good news is that several nutrients found in foods can significantly increase this chemical messenger. Unfortunately, this works only before the cell becomes fully cancerous. For this reason, nutrition is most helpful in the prevention of cancer, which would make it particularly important in the prevention of secondary cancers.

In one study, it was found that certain flavonoids, called apigenin and tangeretin, can significantly increase connexin 43.[14] Apigenin is found in higher concentrations in celery and parsley, and tangeretin is found in tangerine oil. In addition, these flavonoids also prevented the suppression of connexin 43 caused by powerful tumor-promoting chemicals. Three carotenoids found in many fruits and colorful vegetables—beta-carotene, lycopene, and canthaxanthin—were also found to increase the production of this chemical messenger in the cells. Lycopene is the carotenoid that gives tomatoes, watermelons, and pink grapefruit their red color. Many of the carotenoids, some forty in the human diet, are broken down into numerous metabolic products, several of which have their own anticancer effects.

Nutrients Turn Off Cancer Genes

The prevailing theory of cancer causation involves the occurrence of repeated, accumulative damage to a cell's DNA, which changes the cell from a mortal cell to an immortal cell. Despite the body's powerful DNA repair mechanisms, DNA damage is fairly common in normal cells, but much more common in tumor cells.[15] With aging, these DNA injuries accumulate. Smoking, a very powerful free radical generator, dramatically increases this cumulative damage.

While many prevention studies have shown that several of the antioxidant vitamins and other nutrients can prevent cancer from developing even in the presence of powerful carcinogens, in some cases they had little effect. The reason for this may be that some of the damaging free radicals and lipid peroxidation products created during cellular oxidation are not neutralized by the more common antioxidants, such as vitamin C, vitamin E, and the carotenoids. However, other antioxidants, such as the flavonoids and glutathione, can efficiently neutralize these harmful radicals. This again emphasizes the importance of including all of the antioxidant vitamins, minerals, and flavonoids in your diet and supplement program.

Certain of the vitamins have shown the remarkable ability to inhibit the conversion of normal cells to cancer cells by oncogenic viruses. For example, tocotrienol, a vitamin E product found in high concentrations in palm oil, has been shown to inhibit the Epstein-Barr virus from inducing cancer.[16] The Epstein-Barr virus has been associated with lymphomas in humans. It is the gamma and delta fractions of tocotrienol that have the most powerful protective effects.

The carotenoids and vitamin A (retinoids) have also shown a strong ability to inhibit cancer induction, not only by viruses, but by chemicals and radiation as well. At least part of the effect is from these nutrients acting directly on the genes.[17]

Plant flavonoids have also been found to strongly prevent cells from becoming cancerous in the face of powerful carcinogens. What makes them special is that they can have numerous effects on the cells, both on normal cells and cancer cells. In normal cells, they provide powerful protection against a large number of free radicals. Also, they enhance the protection offered by the vitamins. With cancer cells, they behave differently. They can strongly inhibit cancer cell growth and may even cause apoptosis.

Apigenin (found in celery and parsley), kaempferol (found in fruits and ginkgo biloba), and geinstein (found in soybeans) have been found to be significantly effective in preventing cancer formation. A substance extracted from green tea called epigallocatechin gallate has been shown to significantly protect the DNA from damage caused by peroxinitrite, a free radical that is not neutralized by most of the antioxidant vitamins.[18] Other studies have shown that green and black tea, both caffeinated and decaffeinated, strongly inhibit damage to the DNA caused by powerful mutagens.[19] Green tea has also been shown to significantly inhibit leukemia cell growth.[20] When green and black tea are mixed together, they form a much more powerful protective combination.

Some people don't care for the taste of green tea, especially when it is served as iced tea, as is common in the South. Mixing black and green tea will kill the unpleasant taste for those few people, while boosting the tea's anticancer effectiveness. Actually, green and black tea are the same tea. Green tea is in the raw state. Black tea is what most people think of as "tea."

Quercetin, one of the most commonly found flavonoids in fruits and vegetables, demonstrates a special ability to protect the DNA in cells.[21] Analysis indicates that quercetin collects around the nucleus of cells, offering this highly sensitive structure powerful antioxidant protection. Quercetin is one of the most commonly found flavonoids in fruits and vegetables, especially in onions, teas, apples, and cranberries. Ginkgo biloba also contains large amounts of quercetin.

The protective ability of these phytochemicals was recently demonstrated in a study of seven flavonoids and vitamin C using a high-tech method to measure DNA damage called the comet assay.[22] Of the flavonoids tested, the three most powerful in terms of DNA protection were luteolin (found in celery), myricetin (found in black currants), and quercetin (found in teas, apples, and onions). Vitamin C alone offered the least DNA protection, but when it was added to quercetin, its protection was significantly boosted.

In the case of prostate cancer, another plant extract called silymarin holds much promise by affecting gene activation. Studies have shown silymarin to also be effective against other types of cancer, including breast cancer, skin cancers, and other carcinomas.[23] Silymarin is an extract found in the herb milk thistle. As we have seen, this extract is also important in protecting the liver, which is vital during chemotherapy.

Thus far, I have discussed plant extracts, vitamins, and other individual nutrients. What about whole plants, such as a tomato or broccoli? In fact, whole plants have been tested. Overall, it was found that of the approximately twenty-four fruits and thirty-four vegetables examined, 68 percent demonstrated at least some antimutagenic effects—that is, they protected the DNA from damage. Among the fruits, the strongest activity was in blackberries, sweet and sour cherries, black currants, pineapples, and watermelon. Moderate activity was seen in kiwis, mangoes, honeydew melons, and plums.

If we look at the vegetables, we see that the cruciferous vegetables (such as broccoli, Brussels sprouts, kale, and cauliflower) as well as beets, chives, horseradish, onions, rubarb, and spinach have very strong antimutagenic activity, whereas green beans and tomatoes have only moderate activity.

When apples, apricots, kiwis, pineapples, beets, cabbage, cauliflower, cucumbers, onions, radishes, and rubarb were heated (cooked), they lost most of their protective effect. Blackberries, blueberries, sweet and sour cherries, honeydew melons, plums, Brussels sprouts, eggplant, pumpkin, and spinach retained their antimutagenic activity when cooked.

So, we see that many fruits and vegetables can significantly protect the DNA in normal cells from damage by mutagens such as chemotherapy.

Nutrients Interfere with Cancer Cell Reproduction

In order for most of the chemotherapy drugs to work, they must be in the tumor in high concentrations during the time the cancer cells are dividing. Unfortunately, the cells do not all divide at the same time. This means that some cells will be killed and others will escape as the concentration of the drug falls. In the minds of scientists, there are two answers to this problem: Either force all the cells to divide at the same time or give the drug over a very long time period in high doses.

Several drugs were tested to see if they could make the cancer cells start dividing at the same time, but the results in patients were disappointing. Therefore, the second of the two options was settled upon. Today, chemotherapy drugs are given in long cycles, lasting from weeks to months. In some instances, they are given over several years.

For some tumors, special pumps were implanted in the body that continuously infused the tumor with very high concentrations of the drug. While this method did show some initial success, eventually the tumors became resistant and continued to grow, usually at a faster pace.

The problem with extending treatment this way is that it also increases the likelihood of complications, especially with prolonged immune suppression. Malnutritious patients and/or patients with advanced cancers are more likely to suffer from complications during their treatments.

Many phytochemicals, such as apigenin, genistein, curcumin, green tea extract, and indole-3-carbinol, have been shown to prevent cancer cells from dividing, but have no effect on normal cells. This not only slows the growth of the tumor, but allows the chemotherapy drugs more time to kill the cancer cells.

Vitamin E succinate has also been shown to stop the reproduction of cancer cells, with no effect on the reproduction of normal cells. Combinations of vitamin E succinate and beta-carotene have been shown to have the same effect on melanoma, prostate, oral, lung, and breast cancer cells in culture.

Nutrients Cause Apoptosis

When God designed us, He placed in all our cells special genes that would protect us against abnormal cell function. Should free radical damage reach a level that endangers the cell, two options become available: Either the cell will slow its growth to allow more time for DNA repair, or should the damage be too extensive, a built-in suicide gene will be activated to kill the cell.

In general, once enough DNA damage is done to result in the transformation of the cell to a cancer, the cell will opt for suicide. Fortunately, this keeps us from developing cancer at a much higher rate than we do already. The problem is that the same process that damages the DNA leading to activation of the cancer genes (oncogenes) also frequently damages the suicide genes as well. This shuts down our protection. Two of the major suicide genes are labeled protein 53 (p53) and protein 21 (p21), but more are being found.

Experts believe that turning these suicide genes back on might allow us to rid ourselves of cancer cells without further intervention. In fact, many of the cancer chemotherapy drugs, as well as radiation treatments, also depend on increasing cancer cell suicide. Several nutrient extracts have been shown to have a powerful ability to turn on these helpful suicide genes as well.

One study found that green tea extract (catechin and epigallocatechin gallate) and persimmon extract caused human lymphoid leukemia cells to undergo increased spontaneous death just like what is seen when using the chemotherapy drugs.[24] The difference was that the extracts did not cause normal cells to die. In essence, the extracts reactivated the suicide gene. Curcumin was shown to have the same effect on breast cancer cells. The higher the dose of curcumin used, the greater was the killing effect. Once again, the flavonoid had no effect on normal cells.

Apigenin, luteolin, and quercetin, all flavonoids found in many fruits and vegetables, have been shown to restore the suicide gene. The herb Panax gensing has also been shown to activate the p53 and p21 suicide genes in cancer cells. Vitamin E succinate has demonstrated a similar effect.

Resveratrol, extracted from the skin of grapes, potently kills cancer cells by activating the apoptosis gene. In addition, it inhibits the growth of prostate cancer by blocking the activation of DNA by androgens. Some nutrient combinations are even more effective. For example, vitamin E succinate combined with retinoic acid (vitamin A) efficiently killed human B lymphoma cells in culture, but protected normal lymphocytes.

Vitamin E succinate was shown to enhance the effectiveness of the chemotherapeutic drug adriamycin against prostate cancer cells in culture. It also enhanced the effectiveness of tamoxifen, cisplatin, DTIC, interferon-alpha2b, 5-FU, and cyclophosphamide against cancer cells.

Quercetin was shown to increase the effectiveness of cisplatin as well as that of other agents in cancer cell cultures in animal studies. It also reduced the chemotherapy toxicity to normal cells. In one study, quercetin significantly increased the effectiveness of adriamycin in breast cancers resistant to numerous chemotherapy drugs (multidrug resistance). The omega-3 fat component DHA also enhanced the apoptosis of cancer cells while protecting normal cells.

Nutrients Inhibit Cancer-Dependent Enzymes

Once cancer cells develop, they begin to produce important growth-related enzymes within the cells, one of which is called ornithine decarboxylase. This enzyme is responsible for the production of a cell growth protein called polyamine. It has been shown that the activity of ornithine decarboxylase determines the speed with which certain cancers progress—that is, how aggressive they become. High enzyme activity was associated with rapidly growing tumors, and low enzyme activity was associated with slowly growing tumors.

Several flavonoids and plant extracts have been shown to powerfully inhibit this cancer growth enzyme. These flavonoids and plant extracts include green tea extract (epigallocatechin galate), apigenin, retinoids, curcumin, genistein, and isothiocyanates (found in broccoli). In fact, several even inhibited the enzyme when powerful cancer-promoting chemicals were used.

Experts believe that this explains, in part, how a diet high in fruits and vegetables not only can prevent cancer from occurring, but can also interfere with the growth of cancers that already exist. As we will see, there is now a lot of science behind the idea that fruit and vegetable extracts can be used to treat cancer and not just prevent it.

Another pivotal enzyme is tyrosine kinase, which is responsible for the production of a powerful substance called epidermal growth factor. When activated, epidermal growth factor increases the ability of cancer cells to invade the surrounding normal tissues. Numerous nutritional supplements are able to suppress this enzyme and reduce the growth of tumors.

Many such enzymes, such as protein kinase C, phospholipase A2, and the ones mentioned above, play a pivotal role in cancer growth and spread, and have become a target for cancer treatment. Many nutrients powerfully suppress these cancer-dependent enzymes.

For example, in one study of eight different natural products, the plant flavonoids quercetin and luteolin were found to be the most potent in inhibiting this enzyme.[25] Other studies found apigenin, genistein, and kaempferol to be very effective.[26] Apigenin not only suppressed tyrosine kinase, but inhibited another enzyme, topoisomerase, a target for some anticancer drugs.[27] This would suggest a mechanism by which the mixtures of plant flavonoids and vitamins enhance the effectiveness of the chemotherapy drugs. A high density of these powerful anticancer flavonoids is what is found in blenderized vegetables.

Most of these flavonoids are found in fruits and vegetables, but as I have indicated, certain ones are present in higher concentrations in particular fruits or vegetables. This is why it is important to eat a wide variety of fruits and vegetables and not just your favorite ones. Some herbs also contain some of these flavonoids in higher concentrations. For example, ginkgo biloba contains several of the very powerful anticancer flavonoids, including quercetin, kaempferol, and apigenin.

Another key enzyme for cancer cell growth is protein kinase C. Much attention is being given to ways this enzyme can be inhibited, since it is so critical in controlling the growth of cancers. The flavonoids fisetin, quercetin, apigenin, myricetin, and luteolin all powerfully inhibit this enzyme.[28] Again, all of these flavonoids are commonly found in fruits and vegetables. Epigallocatechin gallate, epicatechin, galagin, and kaempferol are all moderately active in suppressing protein kinase C.

In one study in which fifteen flavonoids were tested against chemically promoted cancer cells, curcumin, apigenin, kaempferol, and genistein were found to significantly inhibit protein kinase C and to change cells from cancerous to more mature—that is, to less cancerous.[29] This explains the observation that people who have cancer and switch to a diet higher in fruits and vegetables, especially vegetables, have tumors that are less aggressive and less likely to metastasize than people who eat diet composed mostly of meats, "bad" oils, and carbohydrates.

Vitamin E has also been shown to powerfully inhibit protein kinase C.[30] The d-alpha-tocopheryl succinate form of vitamin E has the greatest potency in inhibiting this growth-promoting enzyme.[31] This again emphasizes the importance of using the right form of a vitamin. Vitamin E acetate, commonly sold in pharmacies and discount outlets, has very little effect on this tumor growth–promoting enzyme.

In addition, taking the flavonoids (as vegetables or supplements), vitamins, and other phytonutrients together dramatically increases their anticancer effectiveness. It is suspected that the effect of combining all of these nutrients is synergistic rather than just additive.

Nutrients Inhibit Inflammation

The national media announced not long ago the new finding that women who took an aspirin daily had a lung cancer rate half that of women who did not take aspirin. Similar results had previously been found in the cases of breast cancer and colon cancer. So, what accounts for this almost miraculous effect?

When cells become cancerous, they stimulate the production of certain types of eicosanoids, in particular PGE2. These eicosanoids are known to suppress the immune system and activate inflammation, both of which increase the growth of cancer cells. The biochemical reaction responsible for the eventual production of these cancer-stimulating products is quite complicated, but basically it involves the release of a special fatty acid, called arachidonic acid (one of the cancer fertilizers), from the membrane of the cancer cell. It is the enzyme protein kinase C that brings this about. To complete the dietary connection, all of these harmful compounds are made from the omega-6 fats.

Once the arachidonic acid is released into the cell, two other enzymes act on it to generate all of the various types of eicosanoids, especially the PGE2. These enzymes, called cyclooxygenase (COX) and lipoxygenase (LOX) enzymes, are key players in this process. A growing list of cancers, including prostate, colon, endometrial, cervical, lung, glioma, and breast cancer, are known to have significantly elevated levels of these enzymes. Experimental studies have shown that inhibiting these enzymes can make some of these cancers either stop growing altogether or grow significantly more slowly. It is these enzymes, especially the COX enzymes, that are the targets of aspirin and the arthritis medications called nonsteroidal anti-inflammatory drugs.

The drugs that block the COX enzymes have been shown to be especially effective in colon cancer patients. Numerous experimental studies have also demonstrated the value of blocking the COX enzymes not only for cancer prevention, but for the inhibition of cancer growth as well. There are at least two forms of the COX enzyme, designated COX-1 and COX-2. It is the COX-2 enzyme that seems to play the most important role in cancer growth.

Stimulation of the COX-2 enzyme has been shown to greatly accelerate cancer growth in experimental animals. In one recent study in mice, it was shown that injecting even a very dilute concentration of the powerful inflammatory seaweed extract carrageenan could dramatically increase the malignancy of an implanted carcinoma.[32] Carrageenan powerfully activates the COX-2 enzyme.

This seems to indicate a close correlation between the presence of inflammation in the body and the likelihood that a cancer will spread widely in the body, as we have seen previously. Therefore, high levels of inflammatory chemicals (arachidonic acid, the omega-6 fats, COX-2, LOX, and PGE2) in the body carry a poorer prognosis than when the levels are low.

Given less attention than the COX-2 enzyme is the enzyme lipoxygenase, or LOX, which plays the key role in the production of an inflammatory substance called leukotriene. There is some evidence that LOX also plays a role in the development of some types of cancer. A Japanese study found that treatment with a drug that blocks the LOX enzyme selectively could significantly inhibit the development of mammary cancer in rats exposed to a powerful breast cancer carcinogen.[33] The importance of this finding is that most of the drugs used to prevent inflammation do not block the LOX enzyme. Blocking this enzyme as well as the COX-2 enzyme may improve the reduction in cancer growth even more. While aspirin and the other arthritis drugs do not suppress the LOX enzyme, the flavonoids can suppress this enzyme. Especially powerful is the flavonoid quercetin, which has shown significant cancer-inhibiting properties.

There are several plant flavonoids known to be rather powerful blockers of these enzymes. They include the following:

- Amentoflavone—inhibits the COX enzyme
- Apigenin—powerfully inhibits both the LOX and COX enzymes
- Curcumin—very powerfully inhibits the COX enzyme

- Kaempferol—inhibits both the LOX and COX enzymes
- Quercetin—inhibits primarily the LOX enzyme

Some breast cancers are known to generate large quantities of PGE2, produced by the COX-2 enzyme. An analysis of these cancers found that estrogen-sensitive breast cancer cells had high levels of the COX-1-type enzyme and very low levels of the COX-2 type, while non-estrogen-sensitive cancers had high levels of the COX-2 enzyme but very low levels of the COX-1-type enzyme.[34] This is important because the non-estrogen-sensitive breast cancers—that is, the breast cancers that do not need estrogen to grow—are much more aggressive than the estrogen-sensitive breast cancers.

Animal studies using a highly metastatic type of breast cancer disclosed that inhibiting the COX-2 enzyme reduced tumor invasiveness, migration, and angiogenesis.[35] Since many of the vegetable and fruit flavonoids can powerfully inhibit the COX-2 enzyme, as well as the LOX exzyme, this may explain their powerful anticancer effects. None of the chemotherapy drugs inhibit this cancer-promoting enzyme.

Prostate cancer cells also produce large amounts of the COX-2 enzyme. An examination of prostate cancers removed from patients demonstrated that the tumors had been secreting abnormal levels of only the COX-2 enzyme and not the COX-1 enzyme.[36] This means that inhibiting the COX-2 enzyme not only can treat existing prostate cancer, but may also prevent the cancer from developing in the first place. We know that even an inflamed prostate gland has higher levels of the COX-2 enzyme.

One of the ways increased activation of the COX-2 enzyme boosts the malignancy of cancers is by strongly stimulating angiogenesis—that is, the production of tumor blood vessels.[37] This has been shown in prostate cancer as well as in other cancers. As we saw in Chapter 2, inhibiting angiogenesis is a very powerful anticancer tool.

Individuals who have inherited the gene for familial polyposis have a much higher incidence of colon cancer because they produce so many colon polyps. Several clinical studies as well as animal studies have shown that drugs that inhibit the COX-2 enzyme can significantly reduce the development of these precancerous polyps, plus reduce the incidence of colorectal cancer.[38]

Normally, the cells lining the colon do not have high levels of COX-2 enzyme activation. People with chronic inflammatory bowel diseases such as ulcerative colitis usually have high COX-2 enzyme activation and also have a significantly higher incidence of colorectal cancer. The COX-2 enzyme therefore increases in the face of inflammation, and as we have seen, chronic inflammation is a common cause of cancer of various types.[39]

The presence of COX-2 enzyme elevation in ovarian cancers, according to a study of some 117 patients with epithelial ovarian cancer, appears to indicate a poor prognosis, especially in women under the age of sixty.[40]

While the COX-2 enzyme has been getting most of the attention, there is evidence that in at least two types of cervical cancer, squamous and adenocarcinoma, the COX-1 enzyme appears to run the show.[41] Careful studies indicate that it is the COX-1 enzyme that is highest in these cervical cancers and that, if the enzyme is blocked, the cancer either does not develop or grows much slower. The flavonoids inhibit both the COX-1 and the COX-2 enzymes.

As a neurosurgeon, I was particularly interested in COX-2 enzyme expression in brain tumors, especially in the glioma type of brain tumor. Indeed, the COX-2 enzyme is increased in gliomas, and in fact, the more malignant a tumor is, the greater is its level of the COX-2 enzyme.[42] Glioblastoma multiforme is verification of this, since the level of the COX-2 enzyme is very high in this form of glioma. Furthermore, the higher the percentage of COX-2-enzyme-activated cells in the tumor, the worse the prognosis. There is evidence that the inhibitors of the COX-2 enzyme slow the growth of malignant gliomas.[43] An added advantage to using nutrients to suppress these enzymes is that, unlike the arthritis medications and aspirin, they do not damage the liver or kidneys, or cause the stomach to bleed.

A component of the herb ginkgo biloba called amentoflavone was found to be as potent as indomethacin, a powerful nonsteroidal anti-inflammatory drug, in inhibiting the COX enzymes.[44] Curcumin has also been shown to be a very powerful inhibitor of the COX enzymes, which in part explains its potent anticancer effects.

Another study found that the plant flavonoids apigenin, genistein, and kaempferol were very powerful inhibitors of the activation of the COX-2 enzyme.[45] Of these three flavonoids, apigenin was the most potent. Apigenin is found in many vegetables, but is present in higher concentrations in celery. Combining these flavonoids gives you special advantages over using them alone. For example, by combining curcumin and quercetin, you can get maximal inhibition of both the COX and the LOX enzymes. This appears to be especially important in some breast and cervical cancers.

All of this tells us that there is a good scientific explanation for the dramatic reduction in cancer risk in people who eat a diet high in fruits and vegetables, low in the omega-6 fats, and high in the omega-3 fats.

Nutrients Inhibit Tumor Invasion

In Chapter 2, we learned that in order for tumors to invade surrounding tissues, special eroding enzymes called matrix metalloproteinase-2 (MMP-2) and matrix metalloproteinase-9 (MMP-9) are necessary. Under intensive study, these enzymes appear to play a major role in the cancer patient's outcome. Experimental studies have shown that by suppressing these enzymes, we can halt cancer invasion and spread.

Several natural products can reduce the levels of MMP-2 and MMP-9. One of the easiest ways to reduce these invasion enzymes is to eat less of the bad fats. Studies have shown that diets high in linolenic acid increase the amount of MMP-2 in the more aggressive types of breast cancer (estrogen-receptor-negative cancers).[46] The same is true of prostate cancers. Increasing the omega-3 fatty acids in the diet removes the stimulus for producing the proteinases and helps to control the cancer.

Another powerful inhibitor of the proteinase enzymes is curcumin. Tests using curcumin against a human cancer showing a very powerful ability to invade surrounding tissues demonstrated significant inhibition of MMP-9 and, as a result, a dramatic reduction in tumor invasion.[47] An additional advantage of curcumin is that it enhances the healing of normal tissues, which is important if you will be undergoing surgery.[48] The plant flavonoids luteolin and quercetin have also demonstrated an ability to powerfully inhibit MMP-2 and MMP-9.[49] Luteolin is found in high concentrations in celery and artichoke extracts.

Nutrients Block Angiogenesis

Even though I touched on angiogenesis (the growing of new tumor blood vessels) briefly, I will go a little deeper into how nutrition can play a profound role in the process. On some occasions, cancer cells invade normal blood vessels. The stronger the basement wall around a blood vessel, the more difficult it will be for cancer cells to enter the vessel and the less likely will be a successful metastasis. A flavonoid called catechin, found in grape seed extract and Pycnogenol, significantly increases the basement membrane's resistance to tumor invasion.[50] By strengthening this barrier, you lessen the chance that your cancer will spread. You should begin strengthening these vessels right away.

You should also avoid the things that we know increase angiogenesis. A recent study found that nicotine strongly stimulated angiogenesis, even in animals with implanted tumors.[51] The animals receiving nicotine had tumors significantly larger than the animals free of nicotine. It appears that nicotine stimulates all of the growth factors needed to produce new blood vessels. This means that smoking is especially dangerous for a person with even a very small tumor. Even using the nicotine patches intended to help people quit smoking can promote tumor growth.

While the exact mechanism of angiogenesis has not been fully worked out, we know that the eicosanoid system plays a major role. The eicosanoid system is the fatty acid–altering system involving the COX and LOX enzymes. We know that three major products from this system, PGE2 and 12- and 15-HETE, play major roles in the process. These hormonelike (paracrine) chemicals promote the growth of infant blood vessels.

There is good evidence that the suppression of the eicosanoids is one of the principle ways in which the omega-3 oil product DHA inhibits angiogenesis.[52] It also explains, in part, why a diet high in the omega-6 fats powerfully promotes cancer growth and spread, since this fat dramatically increases the production of PGE2 and 12- and 15-HETE.

The flavonoids from edible plants can also inhibit angiogenesis. One of the early findings was that genistein, extracted from soybeans, significantly suppresses angiogenesis. This led to the widespread promotion of soybean products as inhibitors of cancer growth. What was less well known was the fact that six other flavonoids are actually much more powerful as angiogenesis inhibitors and do not have the serious negative effects of genistein.[53] More common among these are apigenin and luteolin, both of which occur in higher concentrations in celery.

Doing two things will significantly reduce tumor angiogenesis: correcting your dietary ratio of the omega-6 and omega-3 fats and increasing your intake of vegetables. While there are additional supplements that can help, these are the basics.

Nutrients Exert Antihormone Effects

Hormones are known to have a growth stimulating effect on certain cancers, most obviously breast cancer and prostate cancer. In addition, they may have effects on other cancers as well. For example, there is evidence that estrogen plays a role in the development and progression of colorectal cancer. In this case, an enzyme called aromatase increases the production of estrone, one of the three major forms of estrogen, in colon adenocarcinoma. It does this by converting testosterone to estrogen compounds within the cells themselves. Aromatase is also thought to play a major role in breast and prostate cancer.

A study of four compounds found that three—quercetin (a flavonoid), tamoxifen (a chemotherapy drug), and raloxifene (a drug used to prevent postmenopausal osteoporosis)—significantly inhibited the activity of aromatase. This is consistent with the findings of tumor inhibition by quercetin in colon and breast cancer.

A surprising finding was that genistein actually increased the activity of the aromatase enzyme. This should increase tumor growth and spread, and there is evidence that it does just that. A recent study by Dr. Clinton Allred and his coworkers at the Department of Food Sciences and Human Nutrition, University of Illinois, demonstrated that genistein extracted from soybeans can significantly enhance the growth and development of breast cancers in mice.[54] This is one of the reasons I caution women, as well as men, against using soy products.

In addition, the breast biopsies of women who eat large amounts of soy products have also shown increased growth of breast ductal tissue, the source of most breast cancers.[55]

The relationship between the aromatase levels in breast cancers and tumor growth is so strong that this enzyme has become a major target of oncology researchers. A Russian study from the Petrov Research Institute of Oncology in which fifty women having breast tumors were studied found that there was a direct correlation among the concentration of the aromatase enzyme, the size of the tumor, and the degree of the cell differentiation of the tumor—that is, how active the aromatase enzyme is determines the aggressiveness of the tumor.[56]

What makes these aromotase findings so important is that the estrogen levels in the blood can be normal or even low, but if high levels of estrogen are being produced in the breast tissue itself, cancer is much more likely to develop. And when it does, it is more likely to grow aggressively and to spread. Scientists working at the Department of Medicine at the University of Virginia demonstrated that normal breast tissue can, when stimulated by hormones, increase the aromatase levels up to 10,000 times higher than normal.[57] This can lead to a very high level of estrogen in the breast itself.

This finding is important because most doctors test only the blood levels of estrogen. Finding normal blood levels of estrogen may give the doctor, and subsequently the patient, a false sense of security. Unfortunately, there are no available tests for the breast levels of this enzyme or for the hormone it produces.

The estrogen concentration in the breast ductal fluid is normally forty times higher than it is in the blood plasma.[58] The good news is that many plant flavonoids are rather powerful aromatase inhibitors. The flavonoids apigenin and coumestrol have also shown an ability to inhibit both breast cancer cells and prostate cancer cells. Another study tested breast and prostate cancer cells that were very sensitive to stimulation by androgens, progestins, and steroids, and found that apigenin, naringenin, and eleven other flavonoids showed blocking effects on these hormone-stimulated cancer cells.[59] What that means is that quite a few plant flavonoids can block the stimulation of cancer growth by the female hormones.

Some flavonoids, such as quercetin, naringenin, and kaempferol, have been shown to inhibit the binding of estrogen to its receptor.[60] This blocks the growth-stimulating effect of estrogen on breast cancer, at least in tissue cultures. Whether it will do the same in people with breast cancer has not been proven, but it may, in part, explain why a diet high in fruits and vegetables is associated with a lower incidence of hormone-sensitive cancers. Again, the difference between genistein and quercetin is that even though both are weak stimulators of the estrogen receptors, genistein stimulates aromatase production whereas quercetin, the same as kaempferol, inhibits aromatase production.

Using aromatase-producing tissues from both animal and human sources, researchers found that, compared to a standard aromatase enzyme inhibitor, apigenin was 8.7 times more potent and quercetin was 1.5 times more potent in inhibiting the enzyme.[61]

Thus far, such powerful aromatase-inhibiting flavonoids as apigenin and kaempferol have not been available as supplement extracts. This means that we must resort to juicing or blending our vegetables, since vegetables contain these flavonoids in high concentrations. Good vegetables to use include kale, turnip greens, and broccoli for kaempferol; grapefruit for naringenin; and celery and parsley for apigenin.

Nutrients Act as Chelating Agents

As we have already discussed, iron is a powerful stimulus for cancer growth, invasion, and metastasis. This is because iron is critical for the function of the enzyme ribonucleotide reductase, which synthesizes DNA. A study done in 1992 using rats exposed to a carcinogenic agent demonstrated that the rats deficient in iron had a significantly lower incidence of breast cancer development than the rats with even normal levels of iron.[62]

A number of flavonoids and plant components are known to remove iron from the tissues and to prevent its absorption. The most potent include:

- Curcumin
- Green and especially black tea
- Hesperidin
- Naringenin
- Inositol phosphate-6 (IP-6)
- Quercetin

Controlling the iron levels can be done purely through nutrition. One of the best ways to remove excess iron from your body is to increase the phytates in your diet. The phytates are natural substances found in grains, potatoes, and many other foods. These compounds bind tightly with iron in a process called chelation, preventing the iron from doing harm.

An especially good supplement to use is inositol phosphate-6 (IP-6), which combines the phytates and inositol. Inositol has been known for some time to inhibit the growth of cancer. When you take this combination supplement with your meals, it will bind and remove the iron from your food, preventing it from being absorbed. When you take the supplement on an empty stomach, it will be absorbed and will bind the iron from your blood and tissues, particularly from any cancerous tissue. The main effect of this supplement is that it will strongly stimulate your natural killer cells and T-helper cells, which the immune system uses to kill cancer cells. Therefore, you will get a combined beneficial effect. The iron-binding effect of this combination supplement is so powerful that it is used to treat hemochromatosis.

Some time ago, researchers discovered that certain women with iron deficiency anemia did not improve their iron status, even when they were given iron supplements. The researchers then discovered that these women were heavy tea drinkers. Most iron supplements are given with meals. It turned out that tea contains compounds (catechins) that firmly bind iron, thus preventing it from being absorbed.

Since this early discovery, it has been shown that many flavonoids can chelate iron. The most powerful iron-binding flavonoids are rutin, hesperidin, quercetin, and naringenin. All of these flavonoids can be purchased as individual supplements. Other flavonoids that have demonstrated good iron-chelating effects include apigenin, fisetin, taxifolin, and diosmin. These are all found in common fruits and vegetables.[63]

It may be the iron-binding properties of the flavonoids found in vegetables that account for the observation that eating vegetables with a high-red-meat diet reduces the incidence of cancer associated with such a diet. The flavonoids in the vegetables bind the iron in the red meat, preventing it from being absorbed.

Once absorbed, the flavonoids also bind any free iron that may exist in the tissues. Normally, when a cancer begins to grow, the body will quickly bind any excess iron to ferritin in an attempt to deny iron to the cancer cells. The flavonoids assist in this effort.

The question then arises: Can eating too many vegetables lead to iron-deficiency anemia? Carefully done studies have shown that the flavonoids in foods allow just enough iron to be absorbed to prevent anemia. In general, the iron stores have to be severely depleted to lead to clinically significant anemia. The flavonoids in tea are the exception, since they can produce anemia if they are consumed with every meal.

Nutrients Improve Detoxification

In Chapter 2, I demonstrated the importance of the liver's detoxification systems not only in preventing cancer, but also in removing the toxic waste products generated during conventional cancer treatments. Because chemotherapy drugs are so powerful, they can damage the liver cells as well as other cells in the body. While all the cells contain detoxification systems, it is the liver that shoulders most of the work.

One mistake many doctors make is assuming that because the conventional liver tests come out normal, the liver's detoxification systems are working well. This is just not true. The liver's detoxification system is a very complex biochemical factory that has many parts, and each part must work at optimal activity to protect you against drug and environmental toxicity.

The liver's detoxification system, as discussed earlier, is divided into two major systems, referred to as phase one and phase two. These two systems must work in tandem in order to protect you fully. If phase one is working well, but part or all of phase two is working below par, toxins can build up in your system. Both systems can be enhanced by supplementing with nutrients such as the carotenoids, indole-3-carbinol, and curcumin, and eating a diet high in the cruciferous vegetables.

Sometimes, the inhibition of portions of the phase one system can actually reduce cancer risk. This is because the enzymes in this detoxification system will convert a totally benign chemical into a dangerous carcinogen in an attempt to detoxify it. Of particular importance when this happens is the phase two detoxification system. Phase two's main goal is to convert the toxins either passed down to it from phase one or directly presented to it into water-soluble chemicals. This makes the substances easier to remove from the body. Fat-soluble chemicals tend to stay in the fat stores of the body for a very long time, as we learned in our discussion of pesticides and herbicides in Chapter 2.

The phase one detoxification system includes several biochemical pathways, including ones that use glutathione, sulfate, glycine, and glucuronide. Each of these pathways has a specific function in detoxification. For example, the glycine pathway is used mainly to rid the body of salicylates (such as aspirin) and benzoates. Benzoates are frequently used as food preservatives. Acetaminophen, neurotransmitters, steroid hormones, and certain prescription drugs use the sulfation pathway.

All of the body's detoxification systems, both in the liver and in the individual cells, depend upon nutrition. For example, a low intake of sulfates in the diet can seriously impair a vital part of the phase two system. In addition, not only can the detoxification systems be improved by supplying their required nutrients in the diet, but consuming specific other nutrients can enhance or inhibit certain parts of the detoxification process. For example, several of the phytochemicals, such as resveratrol, quercetin, apigenin, chrysin, ferulic acid, chlorogenic acid, isothiocyanates, and indole-3-carbinol, can inhibit various of the protein 450 (p450) enzymes of phase one detoxification.[64] This is beneficial in preventing carcinogen production.

Of special importance are the phytochemicals from edible plants that can stimulate phase two detoxification, since this phase plays the most important part in neutralizing toxins of all types. Indole-3-carbinol and isothiocyanates from cruciferous vegetables are potent stimulants of phase two detoxification. Broccoli sprouts have up to a hundred times more isothiocyanates than mature broccoli flowers, making them especially potent.

Tangeretin extracted from tangerines has been shown to increase some of the phase one enzymes, while curcumin, astaxanthin, and canthaxanthin increase both phase one and two detoxification enzymes.[65] The latter two, astaxanthin and canthaxanthan, are carotenoids found in most fruits and vegetables.

Especially potent in inhibiting the phase one enzymes is naringenin extracted from grapefruit. In fact, people who eat grapefruit or drink grapefruit juice in large amounts generally find that their caffeine high is exaggerated and prolonged, since the flavonoid inhibits detoxification of caffeine. This may explain, in part, the anticancer effect of grapefruit. As strange as this seems at first glance, by inhibiting the phase one detoxification enzymes, naringenin prevents the conversion of otherwise harmless environmental chemicals and even weak carcinogens into powerful carcinogens.

Some people are born with an impaired ability to detoxify drugs and toxins. This has been shown to lead to an increased risk of cancer.[66] These are the people who are very sensitive to many drugs, often requiring doses much lower than normal. It is vital in these people to enhance the effectiveness of the detoxification pathways not so affected.

During chemotherapy or radiation treatments, the toxic load caused by cell injury can be so high that it endangers life. This is why it is critical to maintain your detoxification systems at peak activity.

As I said earlier in this chapter, the ducts of the breasts contain cells that can generate very high levels of estrogen (estradiol) while the blood levels of estrogen remain normal. In such a case, a well-functioning liver detoxification system would be of little help, since the toxic levels of the estrogen are localized in the breast and not in the blood. By using nutritional methods to enhance detoxification both in the liver and in the cells, you can increase detoxification.

Also playing a big role in detoxification is the gastrointestinal tract, which has been estimated to process more than twenty-five tons of food in a lifetime.[67] It also processes massive amounts of environmental toxins, drugs, and toxins generated in the colon. All of this material has to be detoxified by the liver.

Normally, the intestine contains its own powerful detoxification enzymes within the cells lining the lumen of the gut. But during chemotherapy and abdominal radiation treatments, these cells can be severely damaged. This not only dramatically reduces gut detoxification, but also increases the load of toxins flooding the liver, since the normal barriers in the intestine are severely injured.

It is for this reason that protection and repair of the intestinal cells is critical during conventional treatments, as outlined in Chapter 3. A flood of toxins from the intestines can also overload the phase one and phase two enzymes, leading to severely impaired liver detoxification.

In addition, the conventional cancer treatments, as well as the use of antibiotics or steroids, can severely disrupt the normal colon bacteria, leading to an overgrowth of pathogenic organisms. These organisms often release powerful toxins into the circulation, again taxing the liver's detoxification system. Once again, this is why it is crucial for cancer patients to consume a healthy, balanced diet.

CONCLUSION

We have seen in this chapter that the evidence justifying the oncologist's fear of nutrition stimulating tumor growth and interfering with the conventional cancer therapies stands, at best, on shaky ground. The vast majority of studies have demonstrated an enhancement of tumor growth only when single vitamins were used in low doses. Even these cases have been inconsistent. For example, studies have shown the inhibition of cancer even when synthetic beta-carotene was used. There have been no studies showing the stimulation of cancer growth when natural beta-carotene was used, especially in combination with other antioxidants. The same is true for vitamin E.

As we have seen, when synthetic beta-carotene is used, other, more powerful carotenoids, such as lutein and canthaxanthin, can become depleted in vital tissues. A similar effect is seen with a high intake of synthetic beta-carotene alone, which can depress the tissue and plasma levels of vitamin E.[68] In addition, the testing of commercially available synthetic beta-carotene supplements has shown that several brands contain no intact beta-carotene at all.

So, why is synthetic beta-carotene used in virtually all cancer prevention and treatment experiments? Incredibly, because it is cheap and often donated to the researchers by the companies that manufacture the supplement. This is despite the fact that it is widely known that the synthetic product is much less effective against cancer than the natural form.[69] The use of the synthetic vitamin makes all of these experiments and studies invalid.

We have also known for a long time that antioxidant vitamins can become oxidized when they are used in isolated forms, especially in conditions that promote high rates of free radical generation and lipid peroxidation, such as when the subjects are smokers or alcohol abusers. When these vitamins are oxidized, they become free radicals themselves. If they are allowed to accumulate, they can damage the cells just like any other free radical.

The oxidation of antioxidant vitamins is of special concern in the case of ascorbic acid, or ascorbate, since vitamin C can potentially trigger the production of iron-activated free radicals. This is how an excess of iron in the body leads to an increased risk of cancer, as well as of other degenerative diseases. Of major importance is the concentration of vitamin C in the diet. For instance, animal studies have shown that the subjects on diets including marginal amounts of vitamin C developed high rates of lipid peroxidation in the presence of even small amounts of iron. When the animals were given high doses of ascorbate, the lipid peroxidation was significantly reduced.

This indicates that we should keep our vitamin C levels high in order to prevent the damaging effects of iron. We need to remember that vitamin C increases the absorption of iron from the gut, and that in the hereditary condition hemochromatosis, iron absorption is excessive, leading to very high tissue levels of the mineral. In this case, the ability of iron to produce free radicals exceeds the ability of vitamin C to neutralize the radicals. A combination of antioxidants including vitamins C and E would help solve the problem, since the nutrients would prevent each other from remaining oxidized—that is, the vitamin E would help restore the vitamin C, and the vitamin C would help restore the alpha-tocopherol.

The effectiveness of a nutritional mixture in combating cancer does not rely solely on its antioxidant effects, however; as we have seen, it relies also on a number of critical biochemical processes essential to cancer cell growth. This explains the dose-related effectiveness of the nutritional combinations. In addition, each nutrient in a combination appears to affect a different set of biochemical processes in the cancer cell, so that by mixing the vitamins and flavonoids together, we see a greater inhibition of the cancer. As we will see in the remaining chapters of this book, the effectiveness of nutritional therapy against cancer depends not only on suppressing or killing cancer cells, but also on causing them to return to a more normal function—that is, to once again become normal (differentiated) cells.

Finally, we have seen that our nutritional choices can play a major role in the effectiveness of our immune system, especially in the portion that plays the primary role in the fight against cancer. Biochemicals found in plants, such as the flavonoids, can directly interfere with a cancer's growth and spread, but have no negative effects on normal cells. Of even greater importance is the finding that many of the components found in plant foods can greatly enhance the effectiveness of the conventional cancer treatments while significantly reducing their associated complications. Good nutritional choices can mean the difference between success and failure in cancer treatment.

7

Nutrition, Cancer, and Immunity

If I had to pick the one thing, and only one thing, that is most important to defeating cancer, it would be immunity. We know that people who have immune deficiency diseases, such as AIDS, also have a significantly higher incidence of cancer. The same is true for transplant patients, since they have to take special drugs to suppress their immunity.

For many years, the prevailing thought was that the immune system has a finite ability to rid the body of cancer cells, able to sweep away usually no more than a few million cells, which would just about cover your thumbnail. However, a case reported in the *New England Journal of Medicine* a little more than twenty years ago seemed to indicate that the immune system's power had been grossly underestimated.

It was during the early years of kidney transplant surgery, before the organs for transplant were as carefully scrutinized for disease as they are today, that the following incident occurred. It seems a young man received a kidney that, unknown to his doctors, contained cancer cells. The transplant surgery went well, and there were no signs of organ rejection. Within a few weeks, the patient began to complain of severe shortness of breath. A chest X-ray was taken, and much to the doctors' surprise, it showed that both of the young man's lungs were filled with tumors. A further workup determined that the tumors had spread throughout his body. Not knowing what else to do, the young man's doctors stopped his immune-suppressing drugs and removed the kidney. To their relief, within a very short period of time, all of the tumors disappeared.

Not only had the young man's newly restored immune system cleared the tumors in his lungs, but it had killed all of the cancer cells throughout his body. The total volume of tumor destroyed by his immune system far exceeded what was thought possible.

A very interesting book of collected cases of the spontaneous disappearance of cancer appeared in the fifties, collected by a surgeon from North Carolina named Dr. Emerson Cole. These were cases in which far-advanced cancers just suddenly disappeared for no known reason. A second look at the cases found that most could be explained by sudden immune activation against the cancers.

One case I clearly remember involved a farmer with extensively metastasized malignant melanoma sent home by his doctors to die. For some reason, the farmer received a vaccination for smallpox. Shortly afterwards, all of his tumors disappeared. Other patients had their cancers disappear following an infection. Numerous other cases also indicated immune stimulation as the cause for the sudden cure.

What these cases demonstrate is that even extensive cancers can be cured if the immune system is stimulated and working properly. The question is: Why doesn't this occur more often? While we have some of the answers to this critical question, many more lie ahead.

The importance of immunity in cancer control is emphasized by the close correlation between immune response to the tumor and survival. In one study, 40 percent of women with breast cancers were found to have immune reactions to their tumors.[1] The women who did not show immunity to their tumors generally had a worse outcome.

In another study, twenty-one of seventy-seven women with breast cancer showed an immune reaction to their tumors, and of these twenty-one, 95 percent remained disease-free for up to twelve years after their initial treatment.[2] Of the fifty-six patients who showed no immune reaction, 41 percent had their cancer return, resulting in their death. The researchers found no correlation between a tumor's size, the presence of lymph node involvement, and the degree of malignancy on microscopic examination. In other words, the state of the immune reaction was far more important than any of the other factors.

IMMUNE SURVEILLANCE: SEARCHING OUT THE ENEMY

It was hypothesized many years ago that normal cells continuously undergo malignant transformation, but that they are destroyed as fast as they can transform. So, what is killing them?

The theory goes, and there is good evidence to support it, that the immune system has special cells called natural killer cells whose job it is to seek out and kill these budding cancers before they can fully develop. To do so, these natural killer cells must roam throughout the body checking each cell.

As we have seen, in fact, there are numerous safeguards against wayward cells taking root in the body, including the suicide genes. It is believed that millions of cells constantly undergo malignant transformation at any one time, but that most of them are killed by one of these mechanisms.

The reason we develop cancer in the first place, or so the theory goes, is that some part of the mechanism breaks down; in this case, it is the immune surveillance system. We know, for instance, that the two peak times for lymphoma and leukemia to develop overlap the very periods when immune strength is at its lowest—early childhood and middle age. Likewise, the cancer rates dramatically increase with the onset of age-related loss of immune power and continue to increase progressively thereafter.

Studies have also shown that the greatest risk for developing cancer is when cellular immunity falls, especially when the portion known to play the biggest role in fighting cancer takes a dip. Previously, I stated that having a chronic illness significantly increases the risk for developing a cancer later. This is true for two reasons: One, chronic illness is associated with excessive free radical production, and two, it is also associated with immune suppression, especially of cellular immunity.

LATENT CANCERS: MALIGNANT CELLS IN HIDING

We know that after the age of fifty, about 40 percent of men have cancer cells in their prostate gland. Yet, only a fraction of these men develop full-blown prostate cancer. After the age of seventy, the incidence of prostate cancer goes up to almost 70 percent. The same appears to be true for breast cancers. After the age of fifty, about 40 percent of women have some cancer cells in their breast. Again, however, most will never develop full-blown breast cancer.

So, it appears that our immune surveillance is not foolproof. Apparently, some cancer cells can just lie dormant waiting for their time to strike. The question again is: Why do so few cancer cells ever do this? Part of the answer is that the immune system apparently can keep cancer cells dormant without actually killing them. Certain nutrients can do the same thing.

For example, it was shown in animals that high doses of beta-carotene could keep a cancer from growing, but if the supplement was stopped, after a lag period, the cancer would suddenly start growing very rapidly.[3] However, as long as the animals' beta-carotene levels were kept high, the tumors never grew. The same was shown for vitamin A.

It may be that many cancers are not cured, but rather controlled. This would explain the extremely long latent period between the apparent cure of some tumors and their dramatic reappearance many years later. This again emphasizes the importance of keeping your defenses, especially your immune system, in perfect working order.

It is not enough to just keep your defenses in good health; you must also avoid the foods that are known to promote cancer growth. For example, a diet high in the omega-6 fats and low in the omega-3 fats would strongly stimulate dormant cancer cells to start growing again.

CANCER VACCINES

The idea of using vaccines to treat cancer had its beginning with Dr. William B. Coley in 1893, long before the science of cancer immunology existed. Basically, Dr. Coley's methods consisted of using various bacterial products and toxins to stimulate the body's immune cells to attack and kill the cancer cells. A review of the cases he treated shows that his results were, in fact, quite impressive. For example, of thirty patients with inoperable cancer that he treated with his vaccines, twenty survived for more than twenty years. Overall, some 270 cancer patients that he treated with his Coley's toxin underwent a complete remission of their disease.

Ironically, Dr. Coley's methods were not adequately studied until recently to see if they had any merit as cancer treatments. In fact, a review of his data published in 1966 by the American Cancer Society under the title "Unproven Methods of Cancer Treatment" concluded that there was little objective basis to believe the treatments altered the course of the disease in any significant way. I'm sure the American Cancer Society wishes no one would read that ridiculous statement today, since Dr. Coley's work laid the foundation for modern immunotherapy.

Vaccinations, in modern times, have been used to treat primarily colon cancers, melanomas, and breast cancers. The results have been varied. The most impressive results have been with melanomas, for which vaccines have now even become a standard treatment.

One of the problems with treating cancer using immunotherapy is that the cancer can alter the body's immunity, preventing the immune cells from recognizing the vaccine. Cancers can also secrete special proteins, which bind antibodies and form immune-blocking complexes. When this happens, even with a very powerful immune system, the cancer will remain hidden.

Some evidence exists that one way to bypass this problem is to break up the immune complexes using proteolytic enzymes. Proteolytic enzymes are protein-dissolving enzymes available from nutrition companies and health food stores. Proteolytic enzymes must be taken on an empty stomach in order to be effective. The idea is to have the enzyme enter the bloodstream and eventually the tumors. If taken with food, they will be used up digesting the food. Once the immune complexes are broken down, the immune cells can seek out and kill the cancer cells.

Two other enzymes of possible use are bromelain and trypsin.

Bromelain is a proteolytic enzyme found in pineapples, and trypsin is a digestive enzyme found in many digestive enzyme preparations. Again, these should be taken on an empty stomach. In addition, do not eat for at least one hour after taking the enzymes. If you have an ulcer or gastritis, take the enzymes only under the supervision of your doctor, since the enzymes can make these conditions flare up.

Some vitamins, such as vitamin E, can increase the antigenicity of cancer cells. This means that they will make the cancer cells more susceptible to immune attack.

One of the problems with most studies using cancer immunotherapy is that they never use nutritional immune support and stimulation in conjunction with the therapy. It has been my experience that when cancer immunotherapy is combined with a proper nutritional program and proteolytic enzymes, the results are greatly improved.

CONVENTIONAL TREATMENTS AND IMMUNITY

While most oncologists are aware that chemotherapy and radiation treatments can severely damage the immune system, most are not aware that the damage can be reversed by nutritional therapy. Before I discuss the specifics of how to protect and enhance your immune function, let us take a look at the true impact of chemotherapy and radiation damage.

In an evaluation of 142 patients before and after chemotherapy treatments, it was shown that 58 percent of the patients demonstrated impaired T-lymphocyte responses before treatment and 80 percent demonstrated impaired responses two to four weeks after completion of their treatments.[4] This represents a 22 percent increase in immune suppression caused by the chemotherapy itself.

A big surprise in the study was that 20 percent of the patients actually had an increase in their immune responses—that is, the chemotherapy made their immune systems work better. While no one knows why this occurred, it may be that the cancer cells killed by the chemotherapy released their tumor antigens into the tissues and blood, resulting in autoimmune stimulation.

One of the most common effects of the exposure to radiation is the suppression of immunity, especially of cellular immunity. In fact, a severe sunburn can significantly suppress the immunity not only of the skin, but also of the entire body. For patients who receive radiation treatments, the greatest dangers involve the axial skeleton (spine and pelvis), spleen, abdomen (gastrointestinal tract), thymus gland, and long bones of the arms and legs. These are the sites of the major immune centers.

In general, the immune cells in these sites will recover rapidly, as long as the patient is provided good nutrition. One of the mistakes the early researchers made was to look only at the number of immune cells when measuring immune competence. For example, a normal lymphocyte count was considered to be a sign of adequate immune function.

We now know that the immune cells not only have to be present, but also have to be working. To measure this, we now expose the lymphocytes to various substances known to elicit strong immune reactions. By doing this, we know that the immune cells not only are present in sufficient numbers, but also are working at peak activity.

Surgery and Immunity

Most cancer treatments begin with the surgical removal of the cancer. This can be either a simple office procedure or an extensive, prolonged surgical operation lasting many hours. We know that immune suppression is common during prolonged surgical procedures and may last for several weeks afterwards.

While the stress of surgery accounts for some of the immune suppression that cancer patients experience, it appears that most of it is due to the anesthesia. Procedures lasting less than an hour are much less likely to cause significant immune suppression than longer operations. Blood transfusions—even of just a single unit of blood—are also known to cause severe immune suppression. Multiple transfusions are especially hazardous.

Like chemotherapy-related immune suppression, surgical immune suppression can be prevented and/or reversed using nutritional treatments. We will discuss this more later.

STRESS AND IMMUNITY

There is little in life that is more stressful than having cancer. This is not only because of the fear generated by the diagnosis, but also because of the prolonged, often physically taxing treatments and their complications. When you have cancer, your life is completely disrupted, totally wrapped around your disease. It is as if you become a slave to your cancer.

If all this weren't enough, your sleep is often disrupted. You feel tired and exhausted, which frustrates you. And you find that you cannot do many of the things you previously enjoyed. All of this adds to your stress.

We know from experimental studies that stress is much more than psychologcial; it can have profound physical effects that can be quite harmful. For example, animals put under chronic, unrelieved stress have been found to have severe depression of their immune system, especially of their cellular immune cells. This immune depression can persist for a very long time. In addition, chronic stress can dramatically increase the formation of free radicals.

This combination of increased free radical generation and immune suppression increases the likelihood not only that your tumor will recur, but also that you will develop a secondary cancer. So, you may be thinking about now, how can nutrition help with stress?

Actually, nutrition can help in many ways. Melatonin can help you to sleep better, and recent studies have indicated that it may also have anticancer effects of its own. In addition, it protects the brain against stress-related free radical damage.

In addition, by improving your general nutrition, you will have a lot more energy, greater endurance, and far fewer complications associated with your treatments. Most patients feel a greater sense of well-being once they establish better eating habits. In addition, they begin to feel that they, not their cancer, are in control.

REPAIRING AND STIMULATING THE IMMUNE SYSTEM

As we have seen, there are many things that can weaken the immune system in the cancer patient. Fortunately, all of them can be reversed using nutrition. Interestingly, most antioxidants can also improve immune function. When a large number of free radicals are being produced, as we see with chemotherapy and any chronic disease such as cancer, the immune cells work less efficiently.

This is true even though the immune cells generate their own free radicals to kill the foreign invaders or cancer cells. Normally, the immune cells protect themselves from their own free radicals by maintaining a much higher level of antioxidants than most of the other cells. In cases of severe nutritional deficiency, as we see with chemotherapy, these immune cells lose much of their antioxidant defense, causing them to die off in large numbers.

Because the immune cells have such a high metabolic rate, they also have a high demand for the water-soluble vitamins. Stress, chemotherapy, and many medications are known to deplete these critical vitamins very quickly. The water-soluble vitamins, such as the B vitamins and vitamin C, are not stored in the body. The fat-soluble vitamins, such as vitamins A, D, and K and the carotenoids, are much more difficult to deplete.

In addition, when the body is attacked, either by infection or cancer, the immune system must produce billions of white blood cells very quickly. This requires an adequate supply of the nutrients necessary for cell reproduction, especially niacinamide, vitamin B_6, folate, and vitamin B_{12}. All of these vitamins can be quickly depleted with the stress of conventional cancer treatment.

We also know that immunity is very dependent on several of the minerals, including zinc, magnesium, and selenium. This is especially true for cell-mediated immunity. In addition, of critical importance is the balance of the omega-6 fatty acids and omega-3 fatty acids. An excess of the omega-6 fats can significantly suppress the immune system, whereas the omega-3 fats can powerfully enhance immunity. Several studies have shown that diets high in the omega-3 fats can prevent anesthesia-induced immune suppression. The same is true for immune suppression caused by chemotherapy.

Of particular importance in the protection and restoration of the immune system are the carotenoids, especially lutein, astaxanthin, beta-carotene, and canthaxanthen. All of these can be found in mixed carotenoid supplements derived from the algae *D. salina*. The carotenoids have been shown to be very effective at restoring age-related immune loss.

WHEN TO BEGIN YOUR NUTRITION PROGRAM

You should begin your nutrition program as soon as possible. This will allow the nutritional factors time to stimulate cell repair, strengthen the normal cells (especially of the DNA), increase protein synthesis in the muscles, and build up the immune system.

With the immune system working at peak activity, tumor reduction can begin before the chemotherapy or radiotherapy is started. In addition, the immune system can begin the process of killing off the cancer cells that have already escaped into the bloodstream and lymphatic system. Of special importance, the nutrients can begin to interfere with the metabolism of the cancer cells, causing them to be much more vulnerable to the conventional treatments.

The beauty of nutritional treatment is that it still works, though less efficiently, even after you have started your other treatments. The longer you continue your nutrition program, the better it will work. Many of the nutrient building blocks, especially the omega-3 fats, will be slowly incorporated into the membranes of your cells. This replacement process will continue throughout your life.

Some of my patients asked me if they should delay their chemotherapy or radiation treatments a few weeks to allow their nutrition program to take effect. In most cases, I said yes. Improving the body's protection, especially its immune protection, exceeds the value of immediately starting the chemotherapy or radiotherapy treatments. There are no studies demonstrating that delaying these treatments by two to three weeks will significantly affect their outcome.

You must also consider the fact that the chemotherapy, and possibly the radiotherapy, will damage your intestinal cells, significantly impairing your nutrient absorption, even when your diet is filled with all the correct nutrients. By starting your diet before the treatments, you will protect these delicate intestinal cells.

Another thing most doctors never consider is that any manipulation of the tumor may spread cancer cells into the system, increasing the likelihood of future metastasis. This includes mammograms (during which the breast is literally crushed), palpation of the tumor by the doctor or patient, and surgical manipulation of the tumor during its removal. Most patients, even before they have gone to the doctor, will have pushed, probed, and felt the tumor many times, just to be sure it is really there.

The bottom line is that you want to have your immune system ready to deal with this flood of escaping cancer cells. With the profound immune suppression caused by anesthesia during surgery, many of these cancers will successfully metastasize, later to grow rapidly. By stimulating your immune system before surgery, the immune suppression will be either minimal and short lived or will not occur at all.

The Most Important Part of the Nutrition Program

Many people think that the nutritional treatment of cancer involves only nutritional supplementation, such as with vitamins or isolated phytochemicals. While important, of even more importance is the basic diet, both in terms of what you eat and of what you avoid.

As we have seen throughout this book, many things in the diet can actually promote the growth and spread of cancer and make it much less likely that you will have a successful outcome for your disease. This is especially true concerning the omega-6 fats, which can powerfully stimulate cancer growth and spread.

In addition, a high-calorie diet can also promote cancer growth, especially when those excess calories come from sugar.

We have also seen that certain amino acids, especially methionine, can promote cancer growth. Some foods, such as dried milk, cheese, egg yolks, and dried egg, contain more methionine than others. Based on these studies, perhaps we should avoid these high-methionine-containing foods.

On the flip side of the coin, there are some foods we should increase in our diet, such as vegetables, some fruits, special protein sources, and whole grains. Of special importance are the vegetables, since they contain the flavonoids and other anticancer phytochemicals. The way to get the greatest benefits from these plants is to blenderize them, which greatly improves their absorption.

Without a good basic diet, the supplements you take will be much less effective. This is why so many reports in the medical literature claim that selected nutrients have little or no effectiveness against cancers. Whatever beneficial effects a supplement offers are often neutralized by foods in the diet that promote cancer.

SPECIAL SUPPLEMENTS TO ENHANCE IMMUNITY

When we talk about enhancing immunity, we need to be more specific. The immune system is an enormously complex system involving numerous types of cells, special proteins called antibodies and complements, and a vast array of immune chemicals known as cytokines. While each of these plays a role in combating cancer, of particular importance is their balance.

The immune system is divided into the cellular immune system, composed mainly of T-lymphocytes (T-cells) and macrophages, and the humoral immune system, composed of antibodies. The antibodies are manufactured by B-lymphocytes (B-cells). It is now thought that the main defense against cancers comes from the cellular immune system. In fact, antibodies may actually help protect the cancer cells from cellular immune attack.

The cancer cells have to be recognized before the immune

cells can seek them out and kill them. Cancer cells have special recognition sites on their surfaces called tumor antigens that act somewhat like beacon lights. Some cancers have very strong antigens and some have very weak ones. The stronger the tumor antigen, the easier it is for the immune system to control the cancer. Malignant melanomas, choriocarcinomas, testicular cancers, and renal cell cancers all have rather powerful tumor antigens.

We also know that cancers can change their antigens over time, making it more difficult for the immune system to find them. In addition, when a cancer spreads, the metastasis will often have a different set of antigens than the main tumor. This explains why it is so difficult for the immune system to eradicate cancers.

If all this weren't enough, cancers can also secrete proteins that bind up the antibodies into large molecules (immune complexes) that block cellular immunity.

All of this has to be considered when attempting to use your immune system to kill your cancer. It is not just a matter of boosting immunity, which in most cases is fairly easy to do. The aim in cancer immunotherapy is to boost cellular immunity without boosting humoral immunity—or at least, to keep the cellular immunity way ahead of the antibody production.

Some nutrients boost both cellular immunity and humoral immunity. These are less desirable than nutrients that boost predominantly cellular immunity. When immunity is boosted, the immune cells begin to secrete chemicals called cytokines (biological response modifiers). Some of these cytokines help fight cancer, and some can actually make it grow faster.

The use of cytokines to fight cancer is an area of very intense research. Unfortunately, when used alone in high concentrations, cytokines can cause some very bad complications. Recent studies have shown that several types of cytokines not only work better when combined with nutrients, but are less toxic to the body.[5] Nutrients can also control cytokine release.

Now, let us look at some of the more useful immune-enhancing agents, presented, more or less, in their order of importance.

Beta-Glucans

The beta-glucans are powerful immune modulators that come from the outer cell wall of several types of bacteria, yeast, and mushrooms. Chemically, they are polysaccharides that include beta-1,3-glucan and beta-1,6-glucan. Early experiments with crude extracts of baker's yeast found that the beta-glucans could powerfully stimulate the immune system. Unfortunately, they were associated with some bad complications as well. These complications disappeared once the product used was purified.

The beta-glucans have been found to possess the ability to stimulate the immune system of a wide variety of animals. These animals include earthworms, shrimp, fish, chickens, rats, rabbits, pigs, sheep, and humans.[6]

The major sources of the beta-glucans are baker's yeast (*Saccharomyces cerevisiae*) and mushrooms (shiitake, maitaki, and reishi). Most of the research has been done on the product derived from baker's yeast. Basically, the beta-glucans work by stimulating a special immune cell called a macrophage. This cell is sort of the brains of the whole immunity operation. Its job is to evaluate the situation and issue the orders to the other immune cells regarding exactly how to defeat the cancer.

Clinical tests on patients have clearly demonstrated that the beta-glucans dramatically protected them from infections. Tests utilizing cancer patients have been impressive as well. In fact, for some types of cancer, the use of these immune stimulants has become standard.[7]

Because beta-glucans supplements work by interacting with receptors on the macrophage cell, the dose is critical. There is a specific dose range for effectiveness that must be followed. If you take too low a dose, you will experience very little effect. If you take too high a dose, you may actually depress your immunity.

This latter effect may explain how yeast overgrowth in cancer patients causes immune suppression. All yeast organisms, including *Candida albicans*, have beta-glucans in their cell walls. When yeast overgrows and invades the bloodstream and tissues, as more and more of the organisms die, they release their beta-glucans in great numbers, which can eventually paralyze the macrophages. This is why it is important to identify and treat a yeast infection early.

While beta-1,3-glucan is considered the most potent of the glucans, the beta-1,6-glucan form appears to enhance the effectiveness of the other form. Try to find a product that combines the two. For the added benefit of iron chelation and further boosting of the cellular immunity, look for a product that combines these two forms of beta-glucans with inositol phosphate-6, or IP-6.

Another advantage of beta-1,3-glucan is that it can cause minimal stimulation of the humoral immunity. This reduces the risk of the immune promotion of cancer growth, which, on rare occasions, can occur.

For most cancer patients, I recommend 15 milligrams of beta-1,3-glucan combined with beta-1,6-glucan three times a day on an empty stomach. Do not eat for one hour after taking the product. I often recommend also taking IP-6 as a separate supplement to take full advantage of its iron-binding effect. (For a complete discussion of IP-6, see page 214.)

Thymus Protein Extract

The thymus gland, a small triangular mass of tissue located in the chest, is the site of the production of our cellular immunity, mainly the T-lymphocytes. The thymus gland manufactures several hormones that stimulate immune stem cells to mature into the various cell types, including T-helper cells, that play a major role in the destruction of cancer cells.

As we age, our thymus gland begins to shrink, until sometime after the age of forty, it becomes almost invisible to the naked eye. It has been shown that the thymus gland is dependent on vitamin A and the carotenoids, which may explain in part why these vitamins can improve our immunity and resistance to cancer.

Terry Beardsley, Ph.D., an immunologist at Baylor College of Medicine, Texas, isolated a particular thymic protein that seems to play the major role in how the thymus gland assigns immune functions to the T-lymphocytes. He calls it thymic protein A.

Earlier in this chapter, I discussed the role played by immune complexes in stimulating cancers to grow out of control. There is growing evidence that immune complexes are more likely to form if the cellular immune system is not working properly. Thymic protein A has been shown to stimulate the production of active cellular immunity and to inhibit the creation of immune complexes by the humoral immunity.

Of even greater interest is the finding that when tested in the presence of cancer cells, this thymic factor powerfully inhibits cancer cell growth, especially in the cases of leukemia and lymphomas. It appears to inhibit these cancers by two mechanisms: one, by increasing the activated cellular immunity, and two, by directly inducing cancer cells to commit suicide. By also inhibiting the production of immune complexes, this thymic factor shows great promise in cancer control and eradication.

Mushrooms

By mushrooms, I mean medicinal mushrooms, not wild mushrooms or the so-called magic mushrooms. Three particular species of medicinal mushrooms have received the most attention: maitake, shiitake, and reishi. The active ingredients in medicinal mushrooms for immune stimulation are the beta-glucans, which are a type of polysaccharide (sugar). The shiitake and reishi mushroom extracts are effective only if given by injection. The maitake mushroom extract is effective when taken orally. Two other mushooms that have shown anticancer effects are the kawaratake (*Coriolus versicolor*) and suehirotake (*Schizophyllum commune*).

The maitake mushroom (*Grifola frondosa*) appears to be the most effective against cancer from among the mushroom products. The name *maitake* in Japanese means dancing mushroom. While the active ingredients in all of these mushrooms are beta-glucans, it is the form in the maitake species that is the most potent.

A Japanese mycologist by the name of Hiroaki Nanba, Ph.D., was the first person to isolate the active component, named the D-fraction, a protein composed of beta-1,3-glucan and beta-1,6-glucan linked to a very large protein molecule.[8]

What makes it different from the form found in the other glucans is its chemical configuration—specifically, its side branches.

Dr. Nanba found that the D-fraction is even more potent at stimulating the immune system than the whole mushroom extract. Since his initial discovery, he has further refined the D-fraction to what is now known as the MD-fraction, which is even more potent.

Tests have demonstrated that the D- and MD-fractions strongly stimulate the body's natural killer cells, cytotoxic T-cells, interleukin-1, interleukin-2, and lymphokines, all of which are critical to fighting cancer. Animals exposed to powerful carcinogens were found to be much more resistant to tumor growth when fed maitake D- and MD-fractions. In one test, of the animals fed the maitake D-fraction only, 30.7 percent developed tumors, whereas 93.2 percent of the control animals developed tumors. In addition, the maitake D-fraction appeared to prevent metastasis. In another test, less than 10 percent of the animals given the maitake D-fraction developed metastasis, whereas 100 percent of the animals not given the extract developed metastasis.

Tests using cancer patients also showed that the maitake D-fraction improved the results of the conventional treatments, even in those patients with advanced cancers. In one study of thirty-six patients having stage two to stage four cancer, the people in which the maitake D-fraction was used either alone or in combination with chemotherapy showed better improvement than the patients given chemotherapy alone.[9] The combination appeared to work best for breast, lung, and liver cancers and was less effective for bone and stomach cancers and leukemia.

Cancer regression or significant symptom improvement was seen in eleven of sixteen breast cancer patients, seven of twelve liver cancer patients, and five of eight lung cancer patients. In one patient having a liver cancer called hepatocellular carcinoma, the tumor completely disappeared while the patient was using MD-fraction and maitake powder as the only treatment.

An additional benefit of the maitake D-fraction was that it dramatically reduced the side effects of chemotherapy, including nausea and vomiting, hair loss, and a fall in white blood cells (leukopenia). Pain was significantly reduced in 83 percent of the patients receiving the extract. It also appeared to improve diabetes as well.

A recent study using an animal model implanted with a lung cancer called Lewis lung carcinoma found that the animals treated with the chemotherapy agent cyclophosphamide alone had a 57 percent reduction in tumor growth, but the animals treated with the drug combined with beta-1,3-glucan had a 94 percent reduction.[10]

As I have already discussed, cancer patients often have yeast infections. By using the maitake D- or MD-fraction, you also benefit from a reduction in these infections. In addition, the immune stimulation afforded by these mushroom extracts reduces the risk of postoperative infections and pneumonia.

Finally, one recent study found that white button mushrooms (*Araricus busporus*) suppressed aromatase, the enzyme that is responsible for estrogen production in fat tissue.[11] As you will recall, suppressing aromatase inhibits the occurrence of breast cancer and slows its growth and spread.

The dose of maitake mushroom extract taken by the cancer patients in these studies varied from 40 to 100 milligrams of the D- or MD-fraction. Some of the patients took 5 to 6 grams of the whole maitake tablets.

Herbal Combinations

While not many clinical tests have been done using herbal combinations in cancer patients, the results that are available, when combined with the results of animal studies, are quite impressive. In one study of 112 patients having non-Hodgkin's lymphoma, the patients receiving Chinese herbs combined with conventional chemotherapy showed a statistically significant improvement in their three-year survival as compared to the patients who received only chemotherapy.[12]

The study found that the patients receiving the Chinese herbs had a significant improvement in their immune function and better blood flow than the control patients. In addition, the patients taking the herbs had fewer and milder side effects.

An additional impressive study, this time using animals, found that a combination of eight Chinese herbs dramatically reduced the incidence of a bladder cancer induced by a powerful carcinogen.[13] The herbal combination was shown to significantly increase the ability of the immune cells to kill cancer cells.

Mushroom combination products have shown some impressive results in a number of immune disorders, including cancer. Some of these products add herbs such as aloe vera and cat's claw to the mix to enhance the immune-stimulating and -modulating properties.

One study found that a combination of four Chinese herbal extracts could significantly inhibit the growth of both drug-resistant and drug-sensitive small-cell lung cancers.[14] The extract combinations included *Glycorrhiza glabra*, *Olenandria diffusa*, SPES (a combination of fifteen Chinese herbs), and PC-SPES (a combination of eight Chinese herbs). The study demonstrated that these herbal combinations were as effective as the conventional chemotherapetic drugs, but were more selective and had fewer side effects. (For a complete discussion of PC-SPES, see page 218).

Another study demonstrated the unique ability of herbal combinations not only to stimulate immunity, but also to directly inhibit HIV viral replication.[15] The product used, labeled XQ-9302, was a combination of twenty Chinese herbs precisely purified and balanced. What made the study especially exciting was that the herbal combination increased immunity in the HIV-infected patients and dramatically lowered their viral load, all without side effects.

Several studies have shown that it is the combination of the herbs that is critical, since individually, herbs have much less effectiveness.

Lactoferrin

Lactoferrin is a glycoprotein (a sugar combined with a protein) found originally in milk secretions. It is now known that lactoferrin is secreted by the cells lining the gastrointestinal tract, lungs, nasal passages, and all other mucous membranes. Its importance lies in its ability to powerfully stimulate the immune system, bind iron, inhibit the growth of cancer cells, increase phagocytosis (the killing of bacteria by phagocytes, or white blood cells), and prevent autoimmunity. Despite the fact that lactoferrin is not absorbed from the intestines, it is able to stimulate the immune cells for the entire body. This is because it stimulates the immune cells in the gut. As you will recall, the gut contains more than 50 percent of the body's immune cells.

One remarkable property of lactoferrin is its ability to prevent cancers from metastasizing.[16] Several studies on animals have shown that it dramatically inhibits cancer metastasis even for some of the more aggressive cancers. In part, this is because of its unusual ability to stimulate the production of interferon-gamma, an immune cytokine. It also stimulates the natural killer cells, T-cell cytotoxicity, and macrophages.

Another important property for the cancer patient is that lactoferrin inhibits inflammation.[17] You will recall that inflammation increases the growth and spread of cancers. In addition, lactoferrin is a powerful chelator of iron, making it beneficial in preventing cancer growth and spread. This property makes it a powerful antibacterial and antifungal substance as well.

There are several supplements that supply lactoferrin, including colostrum and whey protein. Colostrum is the early excretion of milk, which contains a highly concentrated form of powerful immune factors. Whey protein is a special protein found in milk products. (For complete discussions of colostrum and whey protein, see pages 215 and 216, respectively.) Lactoferrin can also be purchased as a pure product. The dose is six capsules a day on an empty stomach.

Inositol Phosphate-6

Inositol phosphate-6, or IP-6 for short, is found in many plants and cereal grains, usually in low concentrations. For some time, we have known that inositol inhibits the growth of cancer. An IP-6 combination developed by a cancer researcher at the University of Maryland School of Medicine contains additional inositol, resulting in a supplement with potent iron-binding ability. This product can also powerfully stimulate cellular immunity and chelate heavy metals such as lead and mercury.

If you use IP-6 with additional inositol, you must carefully monitor your iron levels to avoid lowering them too far.

Extremely low iron levels can impair immune function. If your iron levels are high based on your blood iron studies, you should take 500 milligrams with each meal. This will bind the iron so as to prevent absorption. Another way to accomplish this goal is to take 200 milligrams of decaffeinated green tea extract with each meal.

To get the best immune stimulation, take 1,000 milligrams of IP-6 with additional inositol between meals. Do not eat for one hour afterward. This will allow the IP-6 to enter your bloodstream and tissues, and exert maximum cellular immune stimulation and iron chelation.

IP-6 can be found in certain combination products, although the dose is usually too low for cancer treatment. IP-6 can also be purchased in a pure form.

MGN-3

MGN-3 is a biological response modifier composed of a combination of powerful immune-stimulating extracts, including arabinoxylane, a polysaccharide obtained from modified rice bran and hydrolyzed using the enzymes from several types of mushrooms, including the shiitake, kawaratake, and suehirotake species. Studies have shown that MGN-3 boosts several cancer-fighting parts of the immune system. For example, it enhances the activity of the natural killer cells and increases the production of interferon-gamma, tumor necrosis factor-alpha, and interleukin-2.

The usual dose of MGN-3 is 3 grams a day, divided. Take the MGN-3 on an empty stomach.

Colostrum

The first secretions of breast milk contain the highest concentrations of colostrum. This is so infants can have immune protection while their own immune systems finish developing. Colostrum contains lactoferrin; immunoglobulins; proline-rich polypeptides, which promote thymus gland function; and a special growth factor called transforming growth factor beta (TGF-B), which improves intestinal health.

Because the colostrum in supplements is derived from cows,

it is very important to use only products certified to come from cows that are free of bovine spongiform encephalopathy (BSE), also called mad cow disease, as well as antibiotics, pesticides, and herbicides. Look for a product that is standardized to contain 40-percent immunoglobulin G (IgG). Each capsule should contain 450 milligrams of colostrum. The dose is five to seven capsules a day on an empty stomach.

Whey Protein

Whey protein is a special protein found in milk products. Because of its unique abilities to enhance immunity as well as increase muscle building, it has undergone a tremendous amount of research study. However, one of the downsides of whey protein is that it has a rather high content of glutamate, making it unsuitable for patients with brain cancers, especially gliomas.

A fairly recent study found an important property of whey protein. We know that part of the reason cancer cells can become resistant to chemotherapy is that they increase the amount of glutathione inside the cells. In fact, some oncologists have proposed cellular glutathione levels as a way to predict multidrug resistance.

This is where whey protein comes in. It has the ability to increase the levels of glutathione in normal cells but to decrease it in cancer cells. This makes the cancer cell more vulnerable to sudden death, as well as to death cause by conventional treatments. In addition, whey protein appears to prevent multidrug resistance.

Astragalus

Astragalus is an herb that is also known as Mongolian milk, milk vetch, and beg kei. Astragalus has been shown to stimulate immunity against cancer as well as viruses, fungi, and bacteria. In fact, it has broad-spectrum antibacterial activity, much like prescription antibiotics. It has also been shown to increase the blood flow through the coronary arteries and to improve the symptoms of congestive heart failure.

One fascinating property of astragalus when it is combined with the herb *Ligustrum lucidum* is that it increases the survival of individuals treated with radiation therapy or chemotherapy for various cancers.

Astragalus also stimulates the bone marrow stem cells, allowing them to recover more quickly from chemotherapy-induced bone marrow suppression. The immune effects of the herb appear to be a combination of the effects of the more than forty saponins, astragaloside, several flavonoids, and coumarins found in the extract. The flavonoids act as powerful antioxidants.

As for the beta-glucans, the dose of astragalus is critical. The dose should not exceed 28 grams per day, since higher doses have been shown to actually suppress the immune system.

Moducare

Moducare has been a very important addition to the variety of plant-derived immune stimulants and immune modulators available for use by cancer patients. As we have seen, stimulating the wrong part of the immune system can sometimes actually cause cancers to grow faster. In general, it is the humoral system (antibody-making cells) that causes the problem.

The sterols and sterolins found in Moducare have been shown to inhibit the humoral immune system when it is overactive and to stimulate the cancer-fighting cellular immune system. This allows you to benefit from immune stimulation should you also have an autoimmune disorder, such as rheumatoid arthritis or lupus.

I recommend taking the extract in increasing doses. Start with one capsule a day for three days, then increase to two capsules a day for three more days. Do not take more than two capsules three times a day. Moducare must be taken on an empty stomach and only with water. Do not eat for one hour after taking the supplement.

Mistletoe Extract

Mistletoe extract has been used as a healing herb for centuries. However, it was not until 1989 that components of the extract were shown to have anticancer effects. One component, a glycoprotein called lectin-1, has been shown to induce the death of cancer cells in culture. Another component, lectin-2, has been shown to increase the binding of T-lymphocytes to receptors on the cancer cells, thereby increasing the ability of the immune cells to kill cancer cells.

Animal studies indicate that mistletoe extract possesses potent anticancer effects against several types of tumors, especially sarcomas. Studies in cancer patients have indicated that it indeed increases the number of immune cells and, by increasing the brain production of endorphins, also produces a sense of well-being. The only major side effects of mistletoe extract include an occasional increase in blood pressure and increased heart rate.

OTHER SPECIAL ANTICANCER SUPPLEMENTS

There are several other anticancer supplements that do not fall into any particular category but deserve attention. Here are some of the nutrients that hold the most promise.

PC-SPES

PC-SPES is a combination of eight highly concentrated Chinese herbs that has been found to be very effective against both androgen-dependent and androgen-independent prostate cancers. Its mechanism of action involves the inhibition of several of the systems used by the cancer cells for their growth and survival. It has been shown to inhibit cancer cell reproduction, suppress growth factors that contribute to the tumor growth, stimulate the p53 gene, and induce apoptosis in the cancer cells. It also has some weak estrogenic properties.

PC-SPES contains chrysanthemum, dyers woad, licorice, reishi, san-qi ginseng, rabdosia, saw palmetto, and baikal skullcap. In one study of the ability of this herbal combination to suppress PSA, it was found that all the men taking PC-SPES experienced a lowering of their previously elevated PSA levels.[18] Of this group, the PSA levels of 88 percent continued to stay low, and in only 12 percent, the PSA returned to the previous levels. When examined up to four years later, 93 percent of the men who had initially responded to the PC-SPES continued to have low PSA levels. In some cases, the PSA had fallen to an undetectable level.

Several clinical trials using PC-SPES have shown the herbal combination to be a valuable option for patients with prostate cancer.[19] One suggested a major side effect, but did not prove it. In this study, a patient receiving PC-SPES developed a pulmonary embolus (blood clot to the lungs) and a blood clot in the deep femoral vein, the major vein of the leg. The problem with the study was that the patient was recovering from radical prostate surgery at the time. Pulmonary embolism is a recognized complication of major surgery, as well as of cancer itself. Other studies have found no significant complications with the use of PC-SPES. Despite this, its use has been banned by the FDA.

One question that immediately pops up is this: Are all of the herbs in PC-SPES really necessary or does one in particular account for the effectiveness of the extract? A recent study looked into this question and found that while some of the individual herbs do have anticancer effects, only the entire combination produces the full effect.[20]

Another combination showing impressive results is called Equi guard, which contains nine herbs: *Herba epimedium brevicornum Maxum, Radix morindae offinialis, Fructus rosa laevigatae michx, Rubus chingii Hu, Schisandra chinesis Baill, Ligustrum lucidum Ait, Cuscuta chinensis Lam, Psoralea coryifola L,* and *Astragalus membranaceus*. In culture tests using prostate cancer cells from both androgen-sensitive and androgen-insensitive tumors, the combination significantly reduced cancer cell growth, induced apoptosis, and inhibited the production of androgen receptor (AR) and prostate specific antigen (PSA).[21]

Olive Leaf Extract

While not strictly an immune stimulant, olive leaf extract has been shown to increase phagocytosis of the white blood cells used to kill and remove cancer cells. Its real value lies in its ability to kill a large number of microorganisms, including viruses, rickettsia, fungi, and mycoplasma. These are all organisms that commonly infect cancer patients and, in some cases, are suspected of causing cancer themselves.

The beauty of olive leaf extract is that it is virtually nontoxic and mostly free of side effects. In addition, viruses, rickettsia, fungi, and mycoplasma do not appear to be able to develop resistance to olive oil's antimicrobial action, which they commonly do to pharmaceutical drugs.

Olive leaf extract is especially useful in combating fungal infections such as Candida and aspergillus. The active component in the extract is oleuropein. Fungal infections, especially in immune-compromised patients, can be fatal. Conventional treatments can have toxic effects on the liver, kidneys, and bone marrow. Combining conventional drugs and olive leaf extract can dramatically increase the effectiveness of the drugs and reduce their complications.

In addition to its antibacterial activity, olive leaf extract has been shown to increase the blood flow to the coronary arteries, lower blood sugar, and prevent the oxidation of cholesterol.

If you suspect you have an infection, I recommend starting with 500 milligrams of olive leaf extract twice a day, which is the maintenance dose. If you are sure you have an infection, increase the dose to 1,000 milligrams three times a day.

The only real side effect of olive leaf extract is what is called the Herxheimer reaction, or "die-off " response. This reaction occurs because the body is flooded with dead organisms, resulting in the production of immune complexes and in toxin release from the mycelia of the fungi. In most cases, the reaction lasts for only a few days to a few weeks, depending on the severity of the infection and the patient's ability to clear the dead organisms out of his or her system.

For most people, the Herxheimer reaction is confined to feeling "bad," while some people may experience chills and fever, muscle aches, headache, and a feeling of having the flu. In the case of a heavy yeast overgrowth in the colon, the Herxheimer reaction can be reduced by taking several colon-cleansing enemas. The enemas will remove the dead and dying organisms. Drinking a lot of water will also help.

We know that Candida organisms can induce powerful free

radical reactions. This again emphasizes the importance of taking antioxidant supplements and eating a diet high in antioxidants of various types.

Panax Ginseng

Panax ginseng holds great promise in the fight against cancer. Numerous culture studies, animal studies, and clinical studies have shown it to be of tremendous benefit.

The ginseng species of plants have been shown to contain thirty-five different ginsenosides, most of which are saponins. Of the various species of ginseng, the most impressive is red ginseng. A recent review of cancer prevention associated with long-term consumption of ginseng products found that, overall, the people who regularly consumed ginseng had a cancer rate 60 percent lower than a matched population of people.[22] Most impressive was the finding that none of the people taking the red ginseng developed cancer. The study included more than 4,000 people. Protection was seen for all types of cancer.

Studies of ginseng have shown that the herb has multiple effects against cancer, including the stimulation of natural killer cell function,[23] the prevention of tumor invasion,[24] the inhibition of angiogenesis,[25] the inhibition of cell cycling,[26] the activation of the apoptosis genes (p53 and p21),[27] and even the promotion of cancer cell differentation[28]—that is, the stimulation of cancer cells to become normal cells. Red ginseng has also been shown to inhibit the metastasis of tumors such as malignant melanomas.[29] As if this were not enough, red ginseng has also been shown to enhance memory and to protect the brain cells that are responsible for memory (hippocampal neurons).[30]

Before purchasing your ginseng product, you need to know several things. First, only plants that are five or six years old have the anticarcinogenic effects.[31] Second, a recent analysis of twenty-five products found that the amount of the anticancer ginsenosides varied by fifteenfold among capsules to thirty-six-fold among the various brands of liquids.[32]

The best way to assure you are getting a good product is to buy only from a manufacturer that specializes in herbs and to buy herbs that are standardized. To make sure you are getting a standardized product, check the label, which should tell you the percentage of the active ingredient within the preparation.

The only two problems I have found with taking ginseng products are insomnia, which is secondary to its stimulating effects, and hypoglycemia. Cerebral excitation is directly related to the dose. It is best to take the herb in the morning and to start at a lower dose, gradually increasing it to your level of tolerance.

The hypoglycemic effects of the herb are a benefit to diabetic patients, but a problem for people with reactive hypoglycemia. If you are hypoglycemic, avoid sugar, which will allow you to better tolerate the herb. The higher the dose, the greater will be the hypoglycemic effect.

THE BRAIN HAS ITS OWN IMMUNE SYSTEM

In the 1970s, the prevailing thought was that the brain existed as an isolated organ beyond the body's immune system—that is, the immune system was believed to be unable to defend the brain against bacterial invasion or cancer. In fact, the brain is partially isolated from the rest of the body. However, we now know that the immune system can reach into the brain to at least help during a time of need.

The brain is unique in that it does have its own immune system, consisting primarily of special cells called microglia. These cells, when activated, not only can produce immune cytokines and antibodies, and engulf bacteria and cancer cells, but can also migrate throughout the brain to seek out these unwanted invaders.

What is remarkable is that these special immune cells can be activated by stimulating immune cells anywhere in the body, including in the gastrointestinal tract. This is one mechanism that explains how the use of live viruses for vaccination can produce the brain damage of autism. It also explains what we know as "sick behavior"—that is, a sense of feeling sick.

When the immune system is activated, it secretes special cytokines that stimulate special areas in the brain that cause us to feel sick. This slows us down so that the immune system can do its job. Overactivity of this system can make us feel really bad, as when we have the flu.

The advantage of being able to increase the brain's immune activity at a distance is that this can help to protect the brain against metastatic invasion by cancers. This means that all of the immune stimulants and modulators that we have so far discussed can improve the brain's immune defenses as well.

CONCLUSION

In this chapter, we have seen that building our immune defenses is vital in our war against cancer. This includes not only utilizing special immune stimulants, but also improving our general nutrition to properly maintain all of the trillions of immune cells that we will need.

Chemotherapy, surgery, and radiotherapy are all very powerful immune inhibitors that allow cancer cells to grow rapidly, invade surrounding tissues, and eventually metastasize widely throughout the body. We now know that much of this immune suppression can be either avoided or reversed by adhering to certain nutritional principles.

These nutritional principles include eating a diet rich in flavonoids, vitamins, and minerals—that is, a diet high in fruits and vegetables, especially vegetables. Of equal importance is eating a diet devoid of the known immune-suppressing foods, such as the omega-6 fats and sugar, as well as cancer-stimulating nutrients such as methionine, iron, and copper.

Because we want our immune system working at peak activity, we must also use a carefully designed combination of the immune-stimulating supplements. In addition, we need to be careful not to exceed the recommended doses because, for some of the immune stimulators, an excessive dose can have the opposite effect that we want—that is, immune suppression.

8

Fighting the Special Problems of Cancer Therapy

In this chapter, I will discuss some of the special problems facing the cancer patient and how these problems can be improved or corrected using nutrition. In addition, I will tie together all of the information presented in this book so that you will have a better idea of how to proceed.

FATIGUE

One of the big complaints of cancer patients is that when they attempt to tell their oncologist about a specific problem, the oncologist does not seem to listen. This is especially a problem with complaints about fatigue. For example, in one study, it was found that while 75 percent of the cancer patients complained that fatigue was adversely affecting their life, only 32 percent of the oncologists recognized it as a problem in their patients.[1]

Fatigue is more often seen in patients with metastatic disease, especially in cases of ovarian or lung cancer. The causes of fatigue are many and include poor appetite, recurrent vomiting, anemia, particular types of chemotherapy drugs, and deficient nutrient intake. Of these, deficient nutrient intake is the most important.

I have found that most patients undergoing chemotherapy or radiotherapy experience a dramatic improvement in their energy level and a sense of well-being merely by taking a good multiple vitamin. Most patients are severely deficient in the water-soluble vitamins, which include the B vitamins and ascorbate. All of these vitamins play a major role in energy production.

In addition, most chemotherapy drugs damage the mitochondria, the energy factories of the cells. This can cause major decreases in cellular energy production, leading to feelings of intense fatigue. Fortunately, there are many ways to increase mitochondrial energy production.

Acetyl-L-carnitine, a natural substance found in all cells, plays a major role in cellular energy production. In addition, it protects the brain, chelates free iron, improves cell membrane function, regulates fatty acid metabolism, improves heart function, and improves DNA repair in normal cells.

Alpha lipoic acid also plays a significant role in cellular energy production. In addition, it plays a major role in cellular glutathione generation, is a powerful antioxidant, restores the other antioxidant vitamins, chelates some heavy metals, and prevents excitotoxic damage to the brain.

One product, called Propax with NT Factor, combines many of these cellular energy components into a supplement. It is one of the few products that have been tested in cancer patients undergoing chemotherapy treatments. The study involved thirty-six patients in a double-blind, placebo-controlled, randomized study and twenty-two other cancer patients in an open-label (where they knew they were receiving the supplement) study.

Interestingly, the open-label and double-blind studies showed similar results, indicating that bias and placebo effect played no significant role in the outcome. The results of the supplementation with the Propax with NT Factor were scored both by the patients themselves and by the nurses. At the end of the open-label, 75 percent of the nurses reported an improvement in the patients' quality-of-life scores. In the same study, 81 percent of the patients reported a reduction in their fatigue and their chemotherapy side effects.

The reason the nurses were chosen to score the patients is that it is the nurse, not the doctor, who most often recognizes a patients' complaints, as we have seen. In many practices, the oncology nurse is the one who follows the patients during most of their return visits and is certainly the one who listens most closely to the patients.

Tests using NT Factor alone have shown that it increases mitochondrial energy production significantly. It does this by improving the functioning of the membrane surrounding the mitochondria, which is vital for the energy reactions.

Another study, done by Dr. David Newburg, director of the Program in Glycobiology at the Shriver Center for Mental Retardation and a biochemist at Harvard University, found that the phosphoglycolipid in NT Factor contains very high concentrations of a special form of the product called lysolecithin, which increases cancer cell death. The amount of this lysolecithin in the supplement can destroy cancer cells without harming normal cells.

An additional advantage of NT Factor is that it has also been shown to be very protective of the brain, especially in preventing the effects of aging. It can be taken either as a separate supplement or as part of the multivitamin-and-mineral, antioxidant, and omega-3 fatty acid supplement Propax.

WEIGHT LOSS

The medical term for the severe weight loss seen in some cancer patients is cachexia. The cause of this loss of fat and muscle has only recently been discovered. Not long ago, it was thought that cancer patients lose weight because they eat poorly, secondary to their nausea and gastrointestinal upset. However, careful studies have demonstrated that even with adequate caloric and protein intakes, their weight loss proceeds unabated. Some researchers have proposed that cancer somehow interferes with nutrient absorption. More often, these researchers believe, the cancer treatments damage the absorptive cells of the gastrointestinal tract. But still, this does not explain the weight loss in most advanced cancer patients.

Recently, it was found that immune cytokines (immune helper chemicals), especially tumor necrosis factor alpha (TNF-alpha), play a pivotal role in this syndrome. In fact, this explains weight loss in many conditions, including autoimmune diseases, chronic infections, and even age-related muscle loss. A central event in all these conditions is inflammation, which causes the release of TNF-alpha.

Several nutrients have been shown to reduce the level of this cytokine, including vitamin E, plant flavonoids, curcumin, quercetin, hesperidin, grape seed extract, Pycnogenol, and lactoferrin. One recent report found that combining vitamin E with aspirin significantly lowered TNF-alpha levels. Another study found that muscle loss could be reversed in the elderly by lowering their TNF-alpha levels using anti-inflammatory supplements.

Whey protein has also been shown to increase muscle building in patients with cachexia. The only problem I have with whey protein is that it is relatively high in glutamate, an excitotoxin. As you will recall, high levels of glutamate can stimulate the rapid growth of brain cancers. For this reason, I would not recommend whey protein for patients with brain tumors. A safer protein source is egg white protein, which has a perfect balance of the amino acids, without high levels of the excitotoxic amino acids.

Another product that has shown great promise in preventing weight loss in cancer patients is MCT oil. Several studies have shown that MCT oil promotes significant muscle building and is not stored as fat—that is, it will not make you fat. In fact, MCT oil is used by the body much like carbohydrates, except that it does not stimulate insulin release.

MCT oil can be purchased as capsules or a liquid. I prefer the liquid, since it allows you to avoid the gelatin of the capsules. The dose is one tablespoonful three times a day. Do not take MCT oil on an empty stomach, since it can cause stomach cramping. It is best taken after a meal. Another way to take MCT oil is to mix it with an equal amount of extra virgin olive oil. You can also mix in all of your oil-soluble supplements, such as curcumin and CoQ_{10}. You should keep the prepared oil in the refrigerator.

In general, you can increase your intake of complex carbohydrates should weight loss become a problem. Choose carbohydrates that do not significantly stimulate insulin release.

Unfortunately, many oncologists tell their patients that it is important simply to gain weight, no matter what they eat. Far too many suggest eating such things as cakes, pies, energy bars, and commercial liquid diets. Most canned liquid meals contain cancer growth–promoting fats, high-calorie sugars, and the ineffective acetate form of vitamin E. Many contain several forms of excitotoxins as well.

What to Eat

"What can I eat?" is by far the most common question I am asked by patients after I complete my dietary discussion with them. Most of us are so accustomed to eating only what we like that the idea of eating for health comes as a shock. I have had some patients who just could not do it. These few were food addicts in the same way that some people are hopelessly addicted to cigarettes.

I have had some patients tell me that they would starve if they followed the diet. The problem is not the quantity of food, but that all the foods of intense taste or excessive sugar, oil, or salt are avoided or consumed in reduced quantities. You can eat all the vegetables you wish. You can even consume all the extra virgin olive oil you wish. You can have some bread, limited fruits, and some meat.

Following the anticancer diet means that you will have to give up seared meats, barbeque, smoked meats, processed meats, beef and pork, milk and milk products, seafood, commercially prepared foods, and sweets. In addition, you will replace coffee with tea, stop smoking, and avoid alcohol.

After you begin following the diet, you will notice that you have much more energy than ever before, your mind is clearer, your aches and pains are improved or gone, and your bowel movements are much more regular and normal in appearance.

Patients with cancer-related pain notice that their pain level is significantly reduced. I had one patient who came to my office barely able to walk with a cane, suffering from terrible back and hip pains secondary to metastatic bone disease. After two weeks on her diet, she had no further pain and could walk normally. Her energy level was so high, I had to make her slow down.

The benefits of switching to a healthy diet are numerous. It is easier if the entire family switches to the diet. We know that healthy diets work best if started early in life, so get the kids involved as well. If bad, junk foods are nowhere in the house, staying with the anticancer diet is much easier.

So what about eating out? This is a real problem and not one easily solved. Unfortunately, the vast majority of restaurants serve foods that promote poor health. After all, the whole idea is to make the customers enjoy their meal. This means lots of fats, sugar, salt, gravies, MSG, and MSG-containing additives. The only solution is to avoid eating out. If that is impossible, then eat only bland foods without sauces or gravies. Shun the appetizers, and forgo the desserts.

The anticancer diet has to be adhered to very stringently. Even seemingly minor deviations can cause disaster. You have to keep in mind that you have a potentially fatal disease and that any sacrifice is worth preserving the life you have been given.

Proteins

Proteins make up most of the solid structure of the body, including the cells, connective tissue, and even components in the tissue fluid and blood. They do much more than provide structure for the body. Many form very complex molecules that allow the cells to function properly. Low protein levels can impair the immune system.

As we saw in the section on cachexia, loss of muscle protein is a major problem in the cancer patient. Unfortunately, a lot more is involved than supplying a lot of protein in the diet. High-protein diets have several disadvantages. For one, they cause acidosis (a buildup of acid in the body). Most of the enzymes in the body operate within a narrow range of pH (acid-alkaline balance). Acidosis will cause some of the more sensitive enzymes to function at less than an optimal level.

As a result, the body has an elaborate buffering system to prevent acidosis. With prolonged acidosis, however, this buffering system can be taxed. When this happens, one of the body's more powerful buffering systems takes over. Special cells in the bones called osteoclasts are activated and begin dissolving the minerals from the bone, releasing the calcium in an effort to buffer the acid. This loss of calcium from the bone, if extensive and prolonged, can lead to osteoporosis.

In addition, as we saw earlier, certain of the amino acids in proteins can strongly stimulate the growth of cancers. Arginine and methionine are the main culprits. The strongest evidence is with methionine.

Most important, you should avoid eating red meats, especially beef, pork, and lamb. All of these meats are high in iron content, and the iron is highly absorbable. In addition, they all contain high levels of a special fat called arachidonic acid, which, as I explained earlier, is a powerful cancer fertilizer that plays a vital role in the COX-2 enzyme pathway.

This leaves chicken and turkey. However, you still need to be choosy. First, you should avoid processed meats as much as possible. Organic chicken and turkey are best, but can be expensive. The next best option is minimally processed poultry. It should be free of injections of broth, MSG, hydrolyzed proteins, and other additives.

Most chickens are washed in chlorine at the processing plant to prevent salmonellosis. This means that you must wash the chicken thoroughly before preparing it for cooking. Remove most of the skin and excess fat as well. Bake or broil the meat, but try to avoid searing it. Barbequing over a grill is the most carcinogenic way to prepare the meat.

How much meat are you allowed to eat? In general, you should limit your meat intake to six ounces per meal. This is an amount that will fit in the palm of your hand, a trick used by Dr. Barry Sears, author of *The Zone* series of diet books.

So what about seafood? A recent study found that the healthiest diet is a vegetarian diet plus fish. This is basically the Japanese diet. Unfortunately, most seafood is now polluted with mercury, as well as with other heavy metals and industrial toxins. Even much farm-raised fish is contaminated because of the use of pesticides and herbicides on nearby land.

It is the omega-3 fatty acids that make seafood so nutritionally useful. Unfortunately, many of the previous sources of these fats, such as salmon, are now farm raised. Farm-raised fish have little or no omega-3 fats in their tissues since they are grain fed.

One of the most hazardous sources of the omega-3 fats are the bottom-dwelling sea creatures, such as shrimp, oysters, crabs, and lobsters, especially those harvested from the Gulf of

Mexico. Tons of industrial pollutants pour out of the mouth of the Mississippi River because of the long line of industrial plants scattered along its banks. In fact, this zone has such a high cancer rate that it is referred to as the "cancer belt."

I am often asked about wild meat, such as venison. While it is true that wild meat has a much lower fat content and a higher omega-3 fatty acid content than farmed meat, it also is high in iron and arachidonic acid. There is little question that it is less hazardous for the cancer patient than industrial beef and pork. Nevertheless, you should eat it rarely, if at all.

Carbohydrates

In the past, carbohydrates were called starches. Biochemically, carbohydrates are made from large conglomerations of sugar units joined together. As we have already discussed, cancer cells have a voracious appetite for sugar (glucose), and feeding a cancer patient a high-sugar diet could increase the growth and spread of the cancer.

In part, this is due to feeding the tumor the fuel it needs, but it is also because insulin is a growth-promoting hormone for cancers. When we eat a high-sugar diet, our pancreas releases a large burst of insulin. Insulin can promote tumor growth by several mechanisms, including direct stimulation and promotion of inflammation via the COX-2 enzyme.

In the past, it was thought that all starches had the same effect on insulin release. We now know that the effect is highly variable and depends on the type of starch involved. Based on this new understanding, nutritionists have worked out a table, called the glycemic index, that ranks foods according to the insulin response they trigger. Carbohydrates that are absorbed rapidly can trigger a sudden burst of insulin and are placed high on the list. For example, white bread has a score of 100, which is the same score given to sugar. Many beans are very low on the list.

In general, you want to eat primarily carbohydrates that are below 50 on the glycemic index list. You should eat the items ranked above 50 only in moderation and never alone. For example, you can eat a few strawberries after you have finished your meal, but you should not eat them alone as a snack. This is because when your stomach is full, the sugar from strawberries is absorbed slowly, whereas when your stomach is empty, the sugar from strawberries is absorbed very rapidly.

Fruits are generally discouraged on the anticancer diet, despite the fact that they contain some very powerful anticancer and antioxidant flavonoids. They should especially be avoided by patients already having metastasis. Patients without metastasis can enjoy fruits with a low sugar content, such as strawberries, raspberries, and grapefruit, but only in limited amounts. This means no more than half a cup a day. Raspberries contain very high levels of a cancer-inhibiting flavonoid called ellagic acid.

Pastas are allowable on the anticancer diet in limited amounts—that is, no more than twice a week. One of the problems with pasta is that the federal government, in all its wisdom, passed a law forcing the addition of iron to all breads, cereals, and pastas. Many innovative types of pasta, but also containing iron, can be found in health food stores and fresh markets, including spinach pasta, Jerusalem artichoke pasta, and whole-wheat pasta.

When buying breads and other baked goods, be sure to check the label for carrageenan. If this additive is present, do not buy the product. Also, check the label for the type of oil used. The best alternative is to make your own bread using extra virgin olive oil, fresh ingredients, and stevia for the sweetener, and avoiding all the harmful ingredients we have so far discussed.

Healthy Fats

As we have seen throughout this book, the type of fat you eat can play a major role in the eventual outcome of your disease. An excessive intake of the bad fats—that is, the omega-6 fats—can make your tumor grow faster and increases the likelihood that it will spread. In addition, eating bad fats will suppress your immune system and increase inflammation, which also promotes tumor aggressiveness.

Most commercial foods are prepared with the omega-6 fats, including corn, safflower, peanut, sunflower, soybean, and canola oils. Margarines are made with these same cancer-stimulating fats. In place of margarine, you should use butter, but this does not mean drowning your vegetables or layering your toast with a thick sheen of it. Use only a small amount.

Another common source of the bad fats is salad dressings. All commercial dressings use these oils, even when olive oil is prominently displayed on the label. Read the fine print, and you will see other oils listed. There are two options. First, make your own dressing. Second, pour off the oil in the commercial brand and replace it with extra virgin olive oil. This can be done with oil-based dressings that contain no forms of MSG. Some people may prefer to just squeeze some lemon on their salad or to use herbs and salt. This is perfectly fine.

Extra virgin olive oil is the healthiest oil to use. It is best consumed unheated. You can dip bread in it or even take it by the teaspoon. There are no limits on this oil's use. I generally use extra virgin olive oil for cooking as well. Since it is monounsaturated and contains numerous flavonoids, it is resistant to becoming rancid. To add to its antioxidant effectiveness, you can sprinkle turmeric in it. Turmeric also has antibacterial activity, which allows you to use the oil over and over for cooking. Several spices and herbs have antibacterial activity.

In general, you should avoid animal fat as much as possible. Pesticides and herbicides accumulate mainly in fatty tissues, including the fatty tissues of animals. Mercury also collects in the fatty tissues. Remove all the skin and excess fats when preparing your meats.

Flaxseed oil, as we discussed in Chapter 5, has several cancer-fighting components and is highly recommended. Of the fish oils, however, only a few are suitable for use. Most commercial brands of fish oils contain only 30 percent or less of pure omega-3 oils; the remaining 70 percent or more of the fish oil consists of saturated fats and other unhealthy oils. Another problem with some of these oils is that they have rather low contents of DHA. As you will recall, it is the DHA component that has most of the anticancer effect.

Another alternative, and the one I prefer, is to use pure DHA itself. DHA oil is extracted from algae, the same source from which the fish get their DHA. In our body, about 9 percent of the DHA is converted to EPA. This 9 percent is the normal physiological percentage. In addition, using DHA oil allows pure vegan vegetarians to avoid consuming fish. Because DHA oil is highly unsaturated, it is vulnerable to oxidation. For this reason, it should be kept in the refrigerator. DHA oil should never be used for cooking.

Fiber

Food fiber exists in two basic forms: soluble and insoluble. Both forms have a specific function in maintaining health. Insoluble fiber acts as a scrub brush, cleaning the intestinal walls and absorbing various toxins. A high content of this fiber increases the elimination of stool from the colon, thus removing the toxins from the body. A person should have at least one good bowel movement a day.

Insoluble fiber does even more. In the intestine, it is digested and broken down into various short-chained fatty acids, the most important of which is N-butyrate. N-butyrate is the most important fuel for the cells lining the digestive tract. When supplies of this fatty acid are low, we see a significant increase in bowel diseases such as irritable bowel syndrome and colon cancer. N-butyrate is a powerful anticancer substance. When combined with vitamin E and some of the flavonoids, it becomes even more powerful.

In addition, when soluble fiber is fermented in the colon, the beneficial bacteria (the *Lactobacillus* and *Bifidobacterum* species) are able to grow and proliferate. These bacteria, as we have seen, not only improve the digestive health, but suppress the growth of the bad (pathogenic) bacteria and yeast as well. In addition, they increase the power of the entire immune system, increasing our protection against cancers of all kinds.

When the beneficial bacteria are in good supply, the proper metabolism of the estrogens entering the colon from the bile is enhanced. As you may recall, estrogen in the colon can be metabolized either as a 2-hydroxyestrone product, which is protective against breast cancer, or as the 4-hydroxyestrone and 16-alpha hydroxyestrone products, which strongly promote breast cancer.

So, we can see that having the right balance of fiber in our diet is very important not only for cancer prevention, but for general health as well. The Western diet is very low in both types of fiber; the average American consumes somewhere around 5 to 15 grams of fiber a day. The optimal amount is 30 to 40 grams a day. The high-fiber foods include all the vegetables, most of the fruits, green peas, and cereals. There is some evidence that vegetable fiber is more protective than cereal fiber. Drinking blenderized vegetable juice daily (see Chapter 1) will add a considerable amount of both soluble and insoluble fiber to your diet.

Water

Dr. Lorrane Day, a miraculous survivor of advanced breast cancer, emphasizes drinking a lot of water. In fact, she bases this recommendaton on good scientific reasoning. The way the body rids itself of toxins, including those detoxified by the liver and cells, is by dissolving them in the fluid between the cells, which is derived from the water we drink. Most people are chronically dehydrated, especially after the age of fifty.

So, what do I mean by pure water? Basically, I mean water that is devoid of impurities, especially those that can adversely affect the health. Most municipal water systems are significantly contaminated with pesticides, herbicides, industrial pollutants, heavy metals, and fluoride.

While most water filters, either attached to the faucet, free standing, or under the sink, can filter out the majority of these pollutants, they cannot completely remove fluoride. The only exceptions are the reverse osmosis filter and distillation. Distilling water is a viable option, but you should filter even this water through a free filter system, such as a Pu¯r or Brita pitcher–type filter. These free filter systems will completely remove the volatile chemicals that are carried over in the distilled water.

One reason many people avoid drinking a lot of water is because they get tired of going to the bathroom, especially at night. This becomes a particular problem as we get older. Trips to the bathroom in the middle of the night can severely interrupt sleep. But dehydration is much more dangerous. It not only interferes with the fight against cancer, but also increases the likelihood of stroke and heart attack. To avoid having to run to the bathroom after bedtime, drink most of your water before 6:00 P.M.

In general, drink approximately six to eight 8-ounce glasses of pure water a day. Keep in mind, however, that your real requirements will depend on the time of year it is, the amount of exercise you do, and your propensity to sweat. While thirst is normally a good guide, chemotherapy often causes the thirst receptors to become impaired.

WHAT TO AVOID

One factor often forgotten in designing diets for cancer patients is the effect of certain foods and food additives on cancer growth and spread. We have seen that cancer primarily develops because of accumulated injuries to the cells' DNA. At least two items, food additives and fluoride, have been shown to result in DNA injury. Also detrimental to cancer patients are unhealthy snacks and dairy products.

Food Additives

There are many reasons to avoid food additives. Most food additives are complex chemicals, foreign to the body. They, therefore, must be detoxified. This not only puts a strain on the body's already overburdened detoxification system, but can also interfere with the detoxification of carcinogens.

While the scientists at the FDA try to examine food additives for carcinogenic potential, they do not test them for synergistic or additive carcinogenic potential. More and more, however, we are finding that chemicals, when used together, can act in ways not seen when tested individually.

Of special concern are the excitotoxin food additives, which include glutamate (MSG and hydrolyzed vegetable protein), aspartate (aspartame), and cysteine. These additives can cause the neurons to become overexcited. They can also cause the death of nerve cells, leading to brain damage. In fact, these excitatory amino acids have been closely linked to several of the neurodegenerative diseases.

In addition, excitotoxin food additives have been found to cause damage to the DNA and to affect organs other than the brain. For example, glutamate receptors have been found in the ovaries, pancreas, the cells lining all the blood vessels, and the nerve conduction system of the heart. In several cases, foods high in MSG or hydrolyzed vegetable protein have been shown to cause sudden cardiac death, especially in people with low magnesium levels. Magnesium deficiency is common in people having chronic diseases and especially in cancer patients undergoing chemotherapy treatments.

Of greatest concern is the effect of glutamate on primary brain tumors, such as glioblastiomas and malignant gliomas. As we have seen, recent studies found that glutamate dramatically increases the growth and aggressiveness of glioma-type brain tumors. We know that glutamate from food additives will enter the brain. The defenders of glutamate safety frequently assure consumers that glutamate cannot enter the brain because of the protective blood-brain barrier. This is just not so, however, especially in the face of a brain tumor.

Glutamate food additives also have several other bad effects. For example, experiments have shown that free glutamate (MSG) can precipitate type II diabetes in animals. The widespread use of MSG in processed foods may explain, in part, the tremendous rise in type II diabetes over the past ten years, especially among teenagers.

We now also know that glutamate plays a major role in pain sensation. This is because glutamate is a neurotransmitter. Blocking glutamate has been shown to relieve pain. Avoiding foods containing glutamate will reduce pain levels.

The only way to avoid glutamate is to avoid processed foods. However, very few foods are completely free of MSG or one of its cousins. To ensure the greatest avoidance possible of glutamate, prepare all your foods fresh. Note that portabello mushrooms also contain very high levels of glutamate naturally. When cooked, they release this as free glutamate, which then causes all the problems associated with MSG use. These mushrooms have become very popular, especially in restaurants. The free glutamate greatly enhances the taste of the dish, imparting a steak-like flavor.

Fluoride

As we have already discussed, fluoride is the source of many potential problems both for people with cancer and for people without the disease. These problems include neurological damage, as well as damage to the bones, teeth, and other organs. Of special concern to the cancer patient is fluoride's strong connection to cancer, including lung cancer, head and neck cancers, and cancer of the bone.

Studies have shown that fluoride can boost the potency of carcinogens and increase tumor growth by as much as 25 percent.[2] Because of this startling finding, I recommend that you purify your water if your community fluoridates it. This will require either filtration by reverse osmosis or distillation, as just discussed in the section on water. If you choose to use a reverse osmosis filter, you will need to change the filter every three months because fluoride tends to erode these types of filters. If you use distilled water, you should still filter your water through a separate filter to remove the soluble contaminants that are not removed during the distillation process.

Particularly frightening is the finding that cancer death rates were significantly higher for cities with fluoridated water compared to cities with unfluoridated water. The increased rate was especially high for people over the age of sixty-five years.[3] Cancer of the bone in young men was 50 percent higher in one study of cities with fluoridated water, and in another study, it was six times higher.[4] Fluoride accumulates in the bones, eventually reaching levels that can destroy the bone. This condition is called skeletal fluorosis.

Fluoride, even in very small concentrations, such as the amounts that are currently added to water supplies, can damage the DNA repair enzymes. As you will recall, these repair enzymes are especially important in preventing cancer. Individuals with faulty repair enzymes are known to have very high cancer rates.

At the very least, you should avoid all fluoridated toothpastes, dental fluoride treatments, and fluoride tablets. This is especially important for young children, since they can accumulate large concentrations of fluoride in their bones and brain over a lifetime of exposure.

Ironically, all of the large studies comparing cities with fluoridated water supplies to cities with unflouridated water supplies have found not only that the fluoridated water did not cause any reduction in cavities, but that the fluoridated cities often had higher cavity rates. This is because fluoride weakens and eventually destroys the tooth enamel, a condition called dental fluorosis. Experts believe that the incidence of cavities began to fall before fluoride use became popular because of the better nutrition and public health measures that were instituted.

One of the most frightening aspects of fluoridation is that crops watered with treated water absorb the fluoride. Over time, the concentration of the fluoride becomes significantly increased. Many fruit juices are reconstituted with fluoridated water, with some fruit juices having amounts that exceed the government safety levels. This is another reason to avoid commercially made fruit juices.

Unhealthy Snacks

As I have already mentioned, many oncology dietitians and hospital services encourage cancer patients to snack on high-calorie foods to prevent weight loss. The snacks they recommend often include cheesecake, crackers, cakes, muffins, biscuits, rolls, peanut butter crackers, potato chips, and even Goldfish crackers. This is unbelievable!

These snacks contain mostly procarcinogenic oils and high amounts of sugar, methionine, and food additives. Because these snacks are high on the glycemic index, they increase insulin release, which, as we have seen, promotes cancer growth.

Some chips, such as taco chips and barbeque- and ranch-flavored potato chips, contain high levels of MSG. In addition, almost all are cooked in omega-6 vegetable oils. So, in one snack, you can get a high concentration of cancer-stimulating additives and ingredients.

One of the liquid snacks that have become popular is the

high-calorie milkshake-like drink. There is little doubt that you will gain weight with these canned liquid drinks, but the gain will come mainly from fat weight. In the case of many female cancers and prostate cancer in males, increasing body fat is counterproductive. Breast cancer, as we have seen, is sensitive to body fat, since fat cells can manufacture estrogens. Obesity is one of the factors known to increase the levels of 16-alpha hydroxyestrone, the metabolic product of estrogen breakdown that has been shown to powerfully stimulate the growth and spread of breast cancers.

In general, confine your snacks to vegetables, such as celery. The people who will have a real problem choosing snacks are those who suffer from reactive hypoglycemia. Being very sensitive to anything containing sugar, they are limited in what they can eat. One important step is to avoid all products and drinks that contain caffeine. Caffeine greatly magnifies the symptoms of hypoglycemia, especially the jitteriness, tremulousness, anxious feeling, anger, and weakness.

Note also that many of the flavonoids and herbs, including curcumin, ginseng, hesperidin, and quercetin, can produce hypoglycemia. Because of this, you should always take these supplements near or during a meal. These substances produce hypoglycemia by increasing the effectiveness of insulin at the level of the cell membrane, not by increasing the release of insulin.

Keep in mind that you want to prevent weight loss to protect your body against the damaging effects of a loss of vital nutrients, not to please your dietitian.

Dairy Products

When I refer to dairy products, I mean the products made from cow's milk. Cow's milk contains a very large protein molecule that is responsible for a high incidence of milk allergy. This protein molecule is also responsible for juvenile diabetes, according to several recent studies. Children having a gene for juvenile diabetes will not develop the disease unless they are exposed to an environmental trigger—in this case, cow's milk. It seems that the milk protein closely resembles a protein in the islet cells of the pancreas that is responsible for insulin production. During the immune attack on the milk protein, the islet protein is also attacked in what is called molecular mimicry. MSG also is a trigger.

As we learned in Chapter 7, when you have cancer, you do not want your immune system to do anything but fight the cancer. If your immune factors are tied up interacting with milk protein, they will not be available in sufficient concentrations to defeat the cancer. In addition, this immune attack on the milk proteins will produce a state of chronic inflammation, which will also promote cancer growth.

Also of concern is the fact that cow's milk contains a significant number of cancer viruses, primarily those responsible for leukemia and lymphoma, two of the most common diseases in cattle.[5] In fact, in the United States, approximately 60 percent of the herds examined were infected. This is also another reason you should not eat beef, especially cooked rare—that is, with a pink center. The meat from cows also contains numerous carcinogenic viruses.

Studies have shown a statistically significant increase in the incidence of acute lymphoid leukemia in people living in areas where the cattle have a high incidence of infection. While pasteurization will kill a number of these viruses, a significant number of white blood cells are present in pasteurized milk. The white blood cells are what contain the viruses.

Most of us are familiar with the horrid taste of rancid milk. The reason milk turns rancid so rapidly is that the bacteria already in the milk, after pasteurization, begin to grow rapidly. The contamination is not from your refrigerator. This is a good demonstration of just how many organisms exist in pasteurized milk.

Contaminated milk can also affect babies before birth if the mothers drink it during their pregnancy. This can be especially serious, since a baby's immune system will not react to the virus due to what is called immunological tolerance. As a result, the virus will be allowed to take up residence without the danger of attack by the child's immune system even after birth.

Many of my patients take on a look of intense disappointment at this point in our discussion and want to know what they can use on their cereal. The only safe substitute is ultrapasteurized goat's milk. Ultrapasteurization kills off the viruses and bacteria in milk. Never drink raw goat's milk. Goats also carry a number of viruses that are transmitted into their milk.

Many of my patients also ask me about other alternatives, such as soymilk, rice milk, and almond milk. Most of these beverages are very sweet, especially the last two. Soymilk contains a very high level of free glutamate. In addition, recent studies suggest that the genistein in soymilk may increase the aggressive growth of breast cancers.

Ice cream not only contains milk, but also always contains carrageenan. In addition, it has added sugar. Artificially sweetened ice cream contains aspartame.

Measuring Inflammation

Growing evidence indicates that one of the best ways to follow cancer growth is to keep an eye on the level of C-reactive protein, which is a measure of inflammation.[6] This can be done via a simple, inexpensive blood test that can be performed in most laboratories. The blood level of C-reactive protein has been shown to be a reliable predictor of survival in cases of multiple myeloma, melanoma, and lymphoma, as well as in ovarian, pancreatic, and colon cancers. The higher the level—that is, the greater the inflammation—the worse the prognosis is. Improvement in the level of C-reactive protein is believed to indicate an improving control over the cancer.

Like C-reactive protein, blood ferritin levels are also a good way to follow the progress of your cancer. Very high levels are often seen with advanced cancers, especially cancers that have metastasized. Falling ferritin levels can mean improved control of the cancer. Tests for blood ferritin levels are available in most laboratories and are relatively inexpensive. In some instances, a high blood ferritin level is the first evidence of a malignant disease.

The most common cause for an elevated ferritin level is a disorder called hemochromatosis, a hereditary condition in which far too much iron is absorbed into the blood. In an effort to control the massive amount of iron pouring into the system, the body produces huge amounts of ferritin. Because iron is so destructive, over years the liver is destroyed, often leading to a need for a liver transplant.

People with hemochromatosis have an increased risk of developing liver cancer (hepatoma) as well as other malignancies. One way to effectively lower the iron stores in the body is to give a unit of blood. In fact, this is the primary treatment for people with hemochromatosis. It has also been shown that people without hemochromatosis who give blood regularly have a lowered risk of cancer.

Women, during the years that they menstruate, do not store iron. This lowers their incidence of cancer. Once they reach menopause, however, they begin to store iron very rapidly, which puts them at a significantly higher risk of cancer, as well as of heart disease and stroke. Men begin to store iron rather early in life, putting them at a higher risk for numerous diseases.

Unfortunately, the elderly were told for many years that they needed more iron. In fact, products were designed for the elderly just for this problem. Little did these special consumers know that such products were actually increasing their cancer risk, as well as their risk of all degenerative diseases. If they already had cancer, it caused their cancer to grow faster and spread more rapidly.

In addition, most multivitamin supplements also included a healthy dose of iron for many years. Fortunately, many manufacturers have gotten the message and have removed the iron from their supplements.

HOW TO CHOOSE SUPPLEMENTS

Many doctors and medical authorities repeat the nonsense that we do not need to take vitamins because we get all that we need from our diet. They say this despite the evidence that the vast majority of people eat diets that are severely deficient in the vitamins and minerals. Furthermore, because of depleted soils and nutrient-deficient fertilizers, the foods grown in the Western countries are severely nutrient deficient themselves.

In addition, many of the foods we consume in large amounts are high in the omega-6 fats, additives, artificial sweeteners, and sugar, which deplete the nutrients in our body and interfere with normal metabolism. Recent studies indicate that as we age, our enzymes function less well, but that we can restore these enzymes by taking vitamin supplements in doses much higher than those recommended by the authorities.

For all these reasons, we need to supplement even the best of diets. In addition, at higher doses, some of the vitamins have special effects, such as energy production and lowering of elevated blood pressure. We also know that as we age, free radicals do more damage in the body, even if our antioxidant vitamin levels are normal. This indicates that these vitamins need to be at levels above what is considered normal.

In this section, we will discuss the basic supplements that, when used together, will help you to protect your normal cells against the toxicity of your conventional cancer treatments while enhancing the treatments' effectiveness.

Vitamins

First of all, you need to arm yourself with the basic vitamins. These include vitamins A, B_6, B_{12}, C, D, E, and K, as well as biotin, choline, folic acid, niacinamide, pantothenic acid, riboflavin, thiamine, and tocotrienol.

Vitamin A

Vitamin A, also called retinol, is a fat-soluble vitamin that plays a major role in DNA stability and activation. DNA contains special receptors that are activated by vitamin A. Numerous studies have shown that vitamin A inhibits cancer induction and growth by many mechanisms, including its effects on DNA, immune enhancement, and regulation of cell communication.

Interestingly, vitamin A can be derived from beta-carotene, but the conversion is inefficient in humans. This has the advantage of supplying the body with enough vitamin A, but not so much as to be toxic. In addition, beta-carotene, as well as the other carotenoids, has anticancer activities not seen with vitamin A, including inhibition of cancer growth chemicals and of inflammatory signals. As we have discussed, some of the carotenoids (lutein, alpha-cryptoxanthin, canthaxanthin, and zeaxanthin) are not converted to vitamin A and can have these special anticancer effects.

The human diet contains about fifty types of carotenoids, many of which have anticancer effects. It is best to use a mixture of these carotenoids rather than just taking beta-carotene alone. These mixed carotenoids are available in supplements in which the source of the carotenoids is identified as the algae *Dunaliella salina* (*D. salina*). I usually tell my patients to take a combination of 5,000 international units of retinyl palmitate and 5,000 to 6,000 international units of mixed carotenoids every day.

Vitamin B_6

Vitamin B_6, also called pyridoxine, is a very critical vitamin, especially in the repair of DNA and the protection of the brain against glutamate toxicity. The body uses this vitamin in the form of pyridoxal-5-phosphate. Therefore, I prefer supplementing with the pyridoxal-5-phosphate form of the vitamin. The dose is 34 milligrams a day. Several studies have shown that vitamin B_6 suppresses the formation of malignant melanoma and may aid in preventing it from metastasizing.

Vitamin B_{12}

Vitamin B_{12}, known as cobalamin, also plays a major role in the repair of the DNA. Many cheaper supplements use cyanocobalamin, which cannot be used by the body until the cyanide unit has been removed by enzymes in your tissues. Some people's systems are unable to do this, in which case the vitamin has no value. Therefore, look for vitamin B_{12} in the form of methycobalamin or adenosylcobalamin. The dose is 1,000 to 5,000 micrograms a day, depending on the level of stress you are under.

Vitamin C

Supplemental vitamin C should always be buffered and not in the form of ascorbic acid. The body cannot handle ascorbic acid very well, so this form of vitamin C can cause acidosis. The buffered form is well tolerated and well absorbed, and enters the tissues much better. Use either magnesium ascorbate or calcium ascorbate; do not buy sodium ascorbate. A fat-soluble form of vitamin C called ascorbyl palmitate is also available. The usual dose of vitamin C is 500 to 2,000 milligrams three times a day, depending on your condition. Cancer patients should take the higher of this dose range.

Vitamin D

Vitamin D plays a larger role than just assisting bone metabolism. It also protects the cells and prevents cancer, especially colon cancer. Sometimes you will see it as vitamin D_3. Recently, researchers concluded that the recommendations for vitamin D were too low. It had been thought that taking 400 international units a day was sufficient. Now, most evidence indicates that 1,000 international units a day are better. The only caution is that with some cancers, such as multiple myeloma, an excess of calcium can result, and vitamin D can worsen the condition by boosting the body's absorption of the mineral even further.

Vitamin E

Vitamin E actually consists of eight different forms: four tocopherols and four tocotrienols. Most supplements have one or more of the first four forms. Since alpha-tocopherol is the most abundant form of vitamin E found in the body, most supplements contain only this component. You will see notations such as d-alpha tocopheryl and dl-alpha-tocopheryl used frequently. The only one you want is the d- form.

In addition, alpha-tocopheryl comes in several forms. The most commonly sold is d-alpha tocopheryl acetate. Unfortunately, d-alpha tocopheryl acetate is poorly absorbed, does not enter the brain very well, and has little or no activity against cancer. A better form is d-alpha tocopheryl succinate, now widely available. This form of vitamin E has been shown to be the most active against cancer and is able to enter all tissues, including the brain, in high concentrations. It is also the most powerful antioxidant form of vitamin E. An additional advantage is that it comes as a powder.

The next best form of vitamin E is what is called the mixed tocopherols. This simply means that it contains all four basic forms of vitamin E: the alpha, beta, gamma, and delta forms. This is the form found in nature. We know very little about the remaining four forms of vitamin E except that gamma tocopherol appears to play a more important role than the others in preventing heart attacks and colon cancer.

For cancer patients, I recommend 400 international units of d-alpha tocopheryl succinate three times a day. I prefer this form because of its ability to directly inhibit the cellular components needed by cancer cells, in addition to its antioxidant effects.

To be sure that you are maintaining your levels of the other vitamin E components, I also recommend taking 200 international units of the mixed tocopherols. The mixed tocopherols are also called natural vitamin E.

Vitamin K

While vitamin K plays a major role in blood coagulation, it also has anticancer effects and has been shown to reduce the toxicity of several chemotherapy agents without interfering with their effectiveness. You should not take this vitamin if you are currently taking an anticoagulant medication, such as warfarin, since it will interfere with the drug's effectiveness. The recommended dose of vitamin K is 150 micrograms a day.

Biotin

Biotin plays a major role in the metabolism of fatty acids and, therefore, in energy storage. It also plays a unique role in the brain. Significant deficiencies of biotin are seen with severe prolonged illnesses, such as cancer, especially when chemotherapy is used. Eating raw eggs (specifically, the avitin in the egg whites) can also produce severe deficiencies. Of interest to patients on chemotherapy is the role that biotin plays in hair growth. The daily dose of biotin is 3,000 micrograms a day.

Choline

While not strictly a vitamin, choline is important in maintaining a healthy liver and in the production of acetylcholine, a neurotransmitter in the nervous system. The best form of choline is phosphotidylcholine, found in high concentrations in lecithin and egg yolks. The recommended maintenance dose of choline is 750 milligrams twice a day.

Folic Acid

Folic acid is a critical vitamin in the DNA repair process. People with high levels of folic acid have been found to have a very low risk of several cancers, including cancers of the breast, lung, and colon. In addition, folic acid plays a major role in preventing heart attacks and strokes, as well as neurodegenerative diseases. The recommended dose of folic acid is 800 micrograms a day.

Niacinamide

Niacinamide, also known as vitamin B_3, is the form of niacin that the body uses. Its advantage is that it does not cause itching or flushing. It is also nontoxic to the liver. Niacinamide is a water-soluble vitamin used in many biochemical reactions. Its major function is in DNA repair. It also greatly improves the effectiveness of radiotherapy. For this purpose, it should be taken in a dose of 500 milligrams twice a day throughout the treatment period. The maintenance dose is 100 milligrams a day. Another form of vitamin B_3 is inositol hexanicotinate, which can be used in the same doses.

Pantothenic Acid

Pantothenic acid, or vitamin B_5, is another of the water-soluble vitamins utilized to generate energy. In many supplements, it comes in the form of calcium pantothenate. Its active form in the body is called pantethine, which is commercially available. The dose of pantethine is 50 milligrams a day. If you cannot find pantethine in that dose, take calcium pantothenate in a dose of 50 milligrams a day.

Riboflavin

Riboflavin, called vitamin B_2, is also a water-soluble vitamin. It is involved in numerous biochemical reactions, most of which are concerned with energy production and DNA repair. Riboflavin is the vitamin that makes your urine a bright yellow. This is not harmful in any way. It just tells you that you are getting an adequate amount of the vitamin.

Riboflavin, like thiamine (see below), is stress sensitive. For maintenance, take 10 to 15 milligrams a day. During times of stress, you may want to increase the dose to 50 milligrams a day. The metabolic form of the vitamin is called riboflavin-5-phosphate and can be utilized by the body more efficiently than riboflavin itself.

Thiamine

Thiamine, known as vitamin B_1, plays a major role in energy production. Deficiencies of thiamine can cause severe brain injuries. There is a close link between magnesium, thiamine, and carbohydrate intake. Deficiencies of these nutrients are common in alcoholics, the very ill, starving people, and people on high-sugar diets. People having a low thiamine level in combination with a low magnesium level can experience a sudden, dramatic collapse upon receiving a large dose of glucose or a high-carbohydrate meal. This can quickly lead to coma and death.

This reaction has occurred many times in hospitals. In a typical case, a patient suffering from a severe disease, such as cancer, becomes deficient in the water-soluble vitamins and magnesium, and in an effort to improve the patient's energy loss, the doctor starts an intravenous drip containing dextrose and water (sugar water) but no vitamins or minerals. The patient becomes delirious and combative, and starts to hallucinate. Shortly thereafter, the patient lapses into a deep coma, and if nothing is done to correct the situation, the patient dies.

Adding thiamine and magnesium to the diet can avert this deadly effect. The water-soluble vitamins, primarily the B vitamins and ascorbate, are quickly lost under stressful conditions, such as surgery, chemotherapy, and radiotherapy. Maintaining an adequate intake of thiamine before such a stress occurs can avert disaster.

The recommended maintenance dose of thiamine is 10 to 15 milligrams a day. During periods of intense stress, you should increase the dose to 50 to 100 milligrams a day. Afterward, you can go back to the maintenance dose.

Tocotrienol

Tocotrienol is a part of vitamin E and consists of four separate units designated alpha, beta, gamma, and delta. The gamma and delta units have the strongest anticancer effect. Tocotrienol has been shown to significantly increase the effectiveness of chemotherapy treatments, especially in the case of breast cancer. The recommended dose for maintenance is 50 milligrams a day. The recommended dose during the treatment of an active cancer is 50 milligrams twice a day.

Minerals

In addition to the above vitamins, you also need to take the basic minerals. These include boron, calcium, chromium, magnesium, manganese, molybdenum, selenium, and zinc.

Boron

Boron is an essential mineral that regulates other minerals, especially calcium and magnesium. Human studies indicate that it plays a vital role in brain function and bone metabolism, and regulates steroid hormone function. It appears to play an especially important role in estrogen metabolism. In the male, it plays a role in testosterone metabolism. The recommended dose is 2 milligrams a day.

Calcium

Americans now take calcium supplements by the handfuls in an effort to avoid osteoporosis. However, we need to keep in mind that one of the problems with aging is a loss of calcium homeostasis or control. All the cells of the body carefully regulate calcium entry into their interior. This is because calcium is the trigger for many very destructive reactions. Calcium channel blocking drugs have been shown to inhibit some cancers. No clear proof that these drugs can promote cancer growth has been shown, but few researchers have looked into this question.

The reason calcium inhibits colon cancer is that it binds to fats in the colon, blocking their cancer-stimulating effects. This removes the calcium from the cells as well. Vegetables, especially the cruciferous vegetables, contain an abundant supply of calcium. In most instances, the anticancer diet described in this book alone should provide you with adequate calcium. In addition, one of the largest studies on the relationship between diet and osteoporosis found that eating a diet high in fruits and vegetables is more protective than taking calcium supplements.[7]

Recent studies have shown a strong link between taking calcium supplements and drinking milk and prostate cancer risk. In the Health Professional Follow-Up Study, in which more than 47,781 men were followed, researchers found that an increased consumption of calcium from any source boosted the risk of advanced prostate cancer 297 percent. The incidence of metastatic disease in the prostate cancer patients with the highest calcium intakes was 457 percent higher.

Chromium

Chromium is a trace metal that is important in the proper metabolism of carbohydrates. Deficiencies in chromium can result in type II diabetes, and many cases of this form of diabetes are improved by supplementing with this mineral. The natural form of chromium is called glucose tolerance factor (GTF) chromium, or polynicotinate chromium. The other acceptable form is chromium picolinate. The recommended dose is 100 to 200 micrograms a day.

Magnesium

Magnesium is one of the most important elements included in nutritional supplements. It plays a critical role in more than 300 biochemical reactions, many of which are a part of the process of energy production. In addition, magnesium is vital for brain protection and for protection against strokes and heart attacks. The cheapest form of magnesium is magnesium oxide. Unfortunately, this form is poorly absorbed, and in some people, it is barely absorbed at all. The best way to gauge your level of absorption of magnesium is by your gastrointestinal response. If you develop stomach cramps or diarrhea, you are absorbing very little. The maximum percentage of magnesium that can be absorbed is about 40 percent.

Other forms of this mineral are magnesium gluconate, magnesium citrate, magnesium glycinate, and magnesium lactate. Of these, the best absorbed is magnesium lactate. But because lactate is a rather large molecule, you have to take a lot of the capsules to get enough of the magnesium. The glycinate form uses the amino acid glycine. The problem with this is that glycine enhances the toxic effect of glutamate. The amount of glycine in the supplement is so low, however, that it probably would not cause a problem.

The form of magnesium that I prefer is called magnesium citramate, which combines the magnesium with citrate and malate, two organic molecules used to make energy in the body. Malate also protects against glutamate toxicity. In addition, it prevents aluminum absorption. The recommended dose is 900 milligrams of magnesium a day.

The only two precautions concerning magnesium involve kidney damage and heart damage. If you have impaired kidney function, you should take magnesium only under medical supervision. This is because your blood levels of magnesium can get very high if you do not have good kidney function. If your kidneys are working well, you have nothing to fear.

Persons with heart conduction defects, such as bundle-branch block, should also take magnesium only under medical supervision. While it is highly unlikely that taking supplemental magnesium would cause any problem, since it is rare for the blood and tissue levels of magnesium to rise above normal, consult your doctor just to be safe. Most problems with magnesium are seen only when the mineral is given in very large doses intravenously.

Manganese

Manganese is a mineral that plays a role in the metabolism of mucopolysacchrides. In addition, it helps to form an antioxidant enzyme complex called manganese-super oxide dismutase (SOD). Very high doses of the mineral are associated with a Parkinson's disease–like syndrome. The maintenance dose of manganese is 2 milligrams a day.

Molybdenum

Molybdenum is an essential mineral that plays a critical role in helping various enzymes to work properly. In particular, it regulates the effectiveness of the enzyme sulfite oxidase, which regulates cysteine, a very important amino acid. When sulfite oxidase works poorly, brain damage and even coma can result. Molybdenum also assists the steroid hormones to work better.

Because molybdenum is needed in only extremely small amounts, it is often referred to as a trace element. Adults require 75 to 100 micrograms a day for good health.

Selenium

Selenium plays a very important role in immune function. Supplementation with selenium greatly enhances cellular immune reactivity, especially of the natural killer cells and T-helper lymphocytes. In addition, numerous studies have highlighted selenium's anticancer effects, especially against prostate cancer. The recommended dose of selenium is 200 micrograms a day. Do not exceed this dose. While the mineral is safe, taken in higher doses it may carry some toxicity. The best source of the mineral is selenium-enhanced garlic. It also comes as selenium citrate, amino acid chelates, and selenomethionine. The last of these should not be taken by cancer patients because of the methionine, even though the amount is very low.

Zinc

Zinc also plays a vital role in numerous reactions in the body. It plays a critical role in brain protection, especially against mercury, lead, and arsenic toxicity. Further, it is important for immune function. Zinc should never be taken at the same time as copper, since the two minerals will compete for absorption by the same mechanism in the gut. Taking zinc in high doses every day will produce a copper deficiency, and vice versa. Instead, take 50 milligrams of zinc twice a week.

Enzymes

Unfortunately, very little hard research has been conducted into the use of digestive enzymes to enhance cancer treatment. However, there are some studies and a lot of theoretical evidence to support their use. I have treated several patients who responded dramatically to supplementation with digestive enzymes, as have other patients.

The idea behind using proteolytic enzymes is based on the observation that cancer cells escape immune destruction by blocking their antigen receptor sites with special covering proteins. The antigen receptor sites are what allow the immune system to identify the cancer cells. In addition, the cancer cells secrete proteins that bind to the antibodies, forming immune-suppressing complexes. The enzymes strip these cancer-protecting proteins away, allowing the immune system to identify and kill the cancer cells.

To be effective, digestive enzymes must be taken on an empty stomach. If they are taken with food, they will be used up digesting the food proteins. Patients with active or recently cured ulcers cannot take these enzymes, since they can erode into the ulcer.

An additional benefit of taking digestive enzymes is that they reduce inflammation in all tissues.

The Flavonoids

The flavonoids, as we have seen, are some of the most powerful components found in edible plants in terms of antioxidant versatility and power, as well as anticancer effects. Approximately 5,000 flavonoids have been identified in plants, several dozen of which have been extensively studied.

Among the phytochemicals having anticancer and antioxidant effects are catechins, epicatechins, anthrocyanins, quercetin, hesperidin, fisetin, apigenin, luteolin, naringenin, ferulic acid, rutin, kaempferol, myricetin, caffeic acid, chlorogenic acid, coumarin, epigallocatechin gallate, hydroxytyrosol, oleuropein, galangin, curcumin, morin, tangeretin, nobiletin, diosmin, and ellagic acid. All of these potent plant chemicals are found in commonly available fruits and vegetables. Some are available as supplements.

Purified flavonoids that are available as supplements include quercetin, herperidin, ferulic acid, curcumin, epigallocatechin gallate, catechin, and epicatechin (as green tea extract). The most versatile as anticancer flavonoids are quercetin and curcumin, both of which have been extensively tested.

Quercetin, in addition, is a powerful antihistamine and can be used to treat allergic reactions and sinusitis. At higher doses, it will lower elevated blood sugar. In addition, it is an anti-inflammatory flavonoid that primarily inhibits the LOX enzyme. The recommended dose is 1,000 milligrams three times a day with meals.

Curcumin is one of the more powerful of the anticancer flavonoids, since it acts at multiple levels of the cancer process to inhibit the growth of cancer cells and to induce apoptosis. In addition, it stimulates the immune system, lowers the blood sugar, thins the blood slightly, and acts as a powerful anti-inflammatory. It is a potent COX-2 enzyme inhibitor, which is very important in preventing the development of prostate, lung, brain, colon, and breast cancers. The recommended dose is 500 milligrams three times a day with food. Curcumin is absorbed best if dissolved in olive oil.

Hesperidin has been shown to inhibit the development of bladder cancer when powerful carcinogens were used in experimental animals.

The other phytochemicals and flavonoids can be obtained as special plant extracts, from blenderized vegetables, and from eating a lot of fruits and vegetables. Luteolin, for example, can be obtained from artichoke extract, while kaempferol, myricetin, and fisetin are found in ginkgo biloba extract. Many of the herbs contain rather high levels of the more powerful flavonoids. For a list of the flavonoids and their food sources, see Table 8.1.

Immune Stimulants

In Chapter 7, I provided a long list of supplements that enhance the immunity. Obviously, you will not want to take all of them. For instance, you should not combine the various immune stimulators that contain beta-glucans, since an excess of the beta-glucans can have the opposite of the desired effect—that is, immune suppression.

However, arabinogalactan and IP-6 can be combined with each other and with any of the beta-glucan-containing immune stimulants, since they have completely different modes of action. Arabinogalactan is especially important when you want to

Table 8.1
Sources of the Cancer-Inhibiting Flavonoids

Flavonoids	*Food Sources*
Anthocyanins	Grapes. Also available as a supplement.
Apigenin	Celery, parsley, ginkgo biloba.
Caffeic acid	Blueberries, apricots, apples, plums, tomatoes.
Catechins	Fruits.
Chlorogenic acid	McIntosh apples, blueberries, eggplant, tomato skin.
Curcumin	Turmeric. Also available as a supplement.
Ellagic acid	Raspberries, muscadine grapes, blackberries, walnut skins, strawberries.
Epicatechins	Teas, hawthorne, fruit.
Epigallocatechins	Green tea, peaches, black and red currants, apples.
Ferulic acid	Fruits. Also available as a supplement.
Hesperidin	Oranges, black currants. Also available as a supplement.
Kaempferol	Kale, turnip greens, broccoli, black tea, strawberries, ginkgo biloba, black currants, green tea.
Lignans (enterodiol)	Flaxseed, asparagus, garlic, soybeans.
Lignans (enterolactone)	Flaxseed, soybeans, sweet potato, carrots, green pepper, broccoli. Also available as a supplement.
Luteolin	Celery, artichoke.
Myricetin	Cranberries, fava beans, red wine, green tea, black tea.

Table 8.1 (cont.)
Sources of the Cancer-Inhibiting Flavonoids

Flavonoids	*Food Sources*
Naringenin	Grapefruit. Also available as a supplement.
Nobeletin	Tangerine oil.
Quercetin	Onions, apples, cranberries, teas, green beans. Also available as a supplement.
Rutin	Sour cherries, tomatoes, asparagus, olives.
Tangeretin	Tangerine oil.

prevent liver metastasis or treat tumors already in the liver. The same is true for the maitake D- and MD-fractions.

You also have to look at the other effects of the immune stimulants. For example, arabinogalactan feeds the good bacteria in the colon in addition to stimulating immunity.

By properly mixing the immune stimulants, you can improve your response to your conventional cancer treatments and boost the ultimate outcome of your disease.

Phytochemicals

Phytochemicals are complex chemicals found in plants. Many phytochemicals have powerful anticancer effects and, in addition, act as very potent antioxidants, immune stimulants, detoxification promoters, and promoters of cellular function. The largest concentrations of these phytochemicals exist in fruits and vegetables, and among the vegetables, within a group called the cruciferous vegetables. The cruciferous vegetables include broccoli, Brussels sprouts, and cauliflower.

Indole-3-Carbinol and DIM

A significant amount of research has been done on indole-3-carbinol (I3C), a compound found in increased concentrations in the cruciferous vegetables. Most of the research has demonstrated a powerful inhibition of certain types of cancer, especially breast cancer. A few of the studies have shown it to increase the cancer rates in experimental animals, but these studies have been criticized as flawed.

In most of the studies, the primary effects of indole-3-carbinol have been in the prevention of cancer, especially breast cancer. A number of the studies have shown it to be effective at suppressing the growth and spread of existing cancers as well. In these last studies, the indole-3-carbinol was shown to cause the arrest of breast cancer cell reproduction, to increase the activity of the cancer cell suicide genes (p53 and p27), and to increase the amount of 2-hydroxyestrone, the cancer-preventing by-product. In fact, one study found that I3C could increase the amount of 2-hydroxy to eighteen times higher than 16-alpha-hydroxy.[8]

Indole-3-carbinol also protects the DNA from oxidation. Like many of the nutrients so far discussed, indole-3 carbinol also enhances the effectiveness of some chemotherapy agents. For example, in one study, indole-3-carbinol combined with tamoxifen caused greater suppression of breast cancer growth than either substance used alone.[9]

This powerful plant extract has also been shown to inhibit the formation in humans of recurrent respiratory papilloma, a benign, virus-caused tumor.[10] I3C inhibits cancer by other mechanisms as well. For example, it has been shown to powerfully stimulate the phase one as well as phase two detoxification enzymes in both the liver and the cells. In one study, it increased cancer cell death by 200 percent. There is also evidence that it can inhibit the formation of liver cancer (hepatocarcinoma) in animals exposed to a powerful carcinogen.[11] Studies have shown that the effective dose of indole-3-carbinol is 300 milligrams a day.

Another product that is gaining popularity is called DIM, which stands for diindolylmethane. DIM is also found in high concentrations in the cruciferous vegetables, particularly in broccoli, Brussels sprouts, and cauliflower. It has no hormone-like properties, but like its cousin I3C, it appears to inhibit the formation and growth of breast cancers.

Modified Citrus Pectin

The search for a drug that blocks metastasis has thus far been futile. However, a natural agent seems to accomplish this purpose and is also very safe to use. Modified citrus pectin is a water-soluble fiber used by plants as cell cement. This fiber consists of a complex of branched sugar molecules that, when modified by treatment with special chemicals, inhibit cancer cell metastasis in experimental animals.

Tests using five different types of human cancers—prostate cancer, two breast cancer types, melanoma, and laryngeal epidermoid carcinoma—have all shown modified citrus pectin to be effective at blocking metastasis. The pectin appears to work by not allowing the cancer cells to adhere to the walls of the blood vessels, a process that has been found to be necessary for a successful metastasis.

HEAVY METALS

Virtually all oncologists ignore the critical step in cancer care of removing the toxic heavy metals from the patient's system. The toxic metals that should be removed include lead, mercury, cadmium, aluminum, and arsenic. Most of these metals not only can cause cancer, but also can promote cancer growth and spread by interfering with the immune function.

For example, mercury has been shown to inhibit cellular immunity and stimulate humoral immunity, just the opposite of what we want. In fact, it is this pattern of immune modulation that leads to the development of the autoimmune diseases, such as lupus and rheumatoid arthritis. There is also evidence that both lead and mercury can cause brain cancers.

I have found many patients with elevated levels of one or more of these toxic metals. Most patients are completely unaware of any exposure to these toxins that they may have had.

Mercury comes from the amalgam fillings in teeth, vaccinations, and seafood. Arsenic can come from drinking water and working with or around treated wood.

In addition to their toxic effects on the immune system, heavy metals also interfere with normal cell metabolism, resulting in impaired detoxification and a weakening of the normal cells in the body.

The diagnosis of heavy metal toxicity depends on proper testing. The most accurate test involves a provocative twenty-four-hour urine collection. By provocative, I mean that it uses a chelating agent, such as dimercaptosuccinic acid (DMSA) combined with alpha-lipoic acid, to remove mercury as well as other toxic metals. By leeching the metals from the tissues and bones, a more accurate measure of toxicity risk is possible.

Several laboratories do heavy metal testing; I prefer the Great Smokies Diagnostic Laboratory. This lab also performs hair analysis and blood erythrocyte levels, which are less accurate but are easier to do on small children. To contact the Great Smokies Diagnostic Laboratory or another lab, see Appendix B.

If elevated levels of heavy metals are found, they will have to be lowered utilizing chelation cycles over a prolonged period of time. For more information on the proper methods of heavy metal removal, see my book *Health and Nutrition Secrets That Can Save Your Life* (Health Press, 2002).

PESTICIDES AND HERBICIDES

As we have seen, pesticides and herbicides can play a major role not only in cancer development, but also in the growth of a cancer once it has developed. Pesticides that have estrogen-like properties, called xenoestrogens, are linked to breast cancer. Recent studies have shown that the flavonoid curcumin can counteract these pesticide estrogens.

Another important way to counteract the effects of pesticides and herbicides is to increase the efficiency of your detoxification systems. As we have already discussed, there are several nutritional ways to do this, including using selected flavonoids, indole-3-carbinol, MSM, glutathione, and the carotenoid vitamins.

By increasing the effectiveness of your detoxification pathways, you can more efficiently eliminate these chemical toxins from your body. This will increase your resistance to the complications of the conventional cancer treatments, since most of the chemotherapy drugs have to be detoxified. In addition, it will improve your immune function by ridding your body of any cancer-related toxins.

It is important to begin the detoxification process early, as your weight loss will release large amounts of these toxins from the fat cells where they were stored. When these toxins are released, they are generally redistributed to other fatty parts of the body, especially to the breasts in women and the brain in both sexes.

A high-fiber diet is also critical to help remove any ingested pesticide and herbicide residues found in foods. The fiber will absorb these residues so that they can be eliminated from the body. It is also important to wash all vegetables thoroughly before eating them.

EXERCISE

Regular moderate exercise has been shown to help prevent cancer as well as reduce the incidence of cancer recurrence. In fact, regular exercise has been shown to reduce the incidence of colon cancer, breast cancer, and lung cancer.[12] The mechanism involves improved immune function, better oxygenation of the tissues (cancer hates oxygen), improved functioning of the antioxidant enzymes, and the release of endorphins from the brain.

Exercise is especially important once we pass our fiftieth birthday. Studies have shown that regular exercise by this age group significantly reduces the complications generally experienced during hospitalization.[13] A study using twins to eliminate the genetic factors found that regular exercise reduced mortality by as much as 66 percent in subjects twenty-five to sixty-four years of age.[14]

Exercise also combats loss of muscle tissue. It has been shown that the loss of muscle tissue in the elderly is due to an excess of TNF-alpha. This immune cytokine is responsible for the muscle loss in cancer patients as well. Supplementation with N-acetyl-L-cysteine has been shown to lower the TNF-alpha levels. As you may recall, this supplement also increases the cellular levels of glutathione, removes mercury from the body, and improves detoxification. The recommended dose of N-acetyl-L-cysteine is 500 milligrams two to three times a day.

The amino acid glutamine plays a major role in muscle building, as well as in the repair of the digestive system. One problem with using this amino acid, however, is that the brain converts it into the excitotoxin glutamic acid. Exercise helps prevent this by removing the glutamine from the blood, allowing it to be used by the muscles instead.

While moderate exercise is very healthy, extreme exercise and aerobics can be very harmful. This is because such extreme exercises greatly increase the metabolism for prolonged periods of time. As we have already discussed, the metabolism is a major source of free radicals. Recent studies have shown that such extremes of exercise can produce significant damage to the cells by this mechanism.[15]

So, what is moderate exercise? Good examples are brisk walking, weight training with cable weights, riding a stationary bicycle in moderation, and other exercises that avoid stressing the body to extreme levels. Marathons, iron man contests, and intense aerobic exercises are not good because they can rapidly deplete the existing antioxidants, suppress immunity, and cause the breakdown of muscle tissue.

An additional advantage of regular moderate exercise is that it has been shown to improve cognitive function in the elderly, especially when combined with improved nutritional intake.

Yeast Infections

When treating cancer, we do not want anything to interfere with the immune system's ability to fight it. This means that the immune system should not be engaged in fighting chronic infections, such as yeast infections. As we have seen, yeast overgrowth is very common in cancer patients exposed to months of chemotherapy, radiation treatments, and/or antibiotic usage.

We are now seeing numerous species of yeast other than *Candida albicans* infecting cancer patients. Once these yeast organisms enter the blood, they can infiltrate numerous organs and tissues. In addition, when they reach the tissues, yeast organisms are very difficult to kill. The result may be months of antiyeast treatments.

Yeast organisms not only tie up the immune system, but also secrete immune-suppressing chemicals that can decrease the ability of the immune cells to attack cancer cells.

For most cancer patients, I recommend a combination stool examination to culture the organisms and blood testing for the yeast antibodies. The Great Smokies Diagnostic Laboratory offers the Yeast Intensive Test, which combines both of these exams. The stool culture also tests the organisms for their sensitivity to specific prescription drugs, as well as to natural products. This helps guide the physician in selecting the most effective treatment to kill the organisms. To contact the Great Smokies Diagnostic Laboratory or another lab, see Appendix B.

FAITH AND THE POWER OF THE WILL

It has been observed many times that people with strong willpower are more likely to have a favorable outcome when facing a serious disease. Newer research, in fact, has shown that these people have better functioning immune systems, especially the cellular immunity, the system that is the most useful in the fight against cancer. Likewise, depression and a sense of hopelessness are more likely to result in a poor outcome and concomitant immune suppression.

A powerful demonstration of this was the observation by Alexander Solzhenitsyn that the inmates in the Gulag system of the Soviet Union were unlikely to survive for very long if they did not possess a strong sense of faith. More modern research has confirmed this, even in the case of some highly fatal diseases.

We know that the nervous system connects to virtually every cell in the body and that even the unconscious mind can influence these cells. This is, in part, how depression suppresses immunity: It acts through the hypothalamus of the brain. It may be that our sense of willpower and strong faith act through this system as well, in ways that go beyond their effects on the immune system.

I firmly believe that God listens to our prayers and answers them. How and when He answers them is up to His discretion. Sometimes, His answer is not the one we may have hoped for, but in the bigger picture, it is the right answer. This is why sometimes our prayers for a miraculous cure seem to go unanswered—God possesses knowledge beyond our understanding. Our failure to conquer our disease is not because we were unworthy of His mercy, but because of a greater purpose that in all His wisdom exceeds our desires.

CONCLUSION

In this book, I have tried to share some of the latest information on the treatment of cancer. For some, cancer can be cured by nutrition alone. For others, a combination of conventional and nutritional treatments may be called for.

As we have seen, numerous studies have now shown that a number of nutritional treatments can offer a great deal in the suppression and elimination of cancer, and that many of the fears expressed by oncologists are completely unfounded.

In fact, not only is there no evidence that nutritional supplements interfere with the traditional cancer treatments, but they have been shown, in well-conducted studies, to enhance the effectiveness of the conventional treatments. In addition, these nutrients can strongly protect the surrounding normal cells from harm by the chemotherapy drugs and radiation treatments. And as we have seen, this is very important in preventing secondary cancers caused by the treatments themselves.

I always emphasize to my patients the critical importance of changing their diet and adhering to their new diet from then on. On many occasions, deviating from the diet in even minor details can mean the difference between success and failure. Reverting to the previous, unhealthful diet becomes a big problem when patients begin to feel really well, full of energy, and relieved of the pain and discomforts of the traditional treatments. The longer patients are free of their tumors, the more likely they are to jump ship and yield to the temptations of their old diet. This can be fatal.

It is vital to understand that, in many cases, the tumors are not eradicated, but only suppressed. As long as your tumors remain suppressed, you will do well. Once activated, however, these cancers may grow and spread with a vengeance. At that stage, they are much more difficult to control. This is also true regarding nutritional supplements. Although many supplements do, in fact, increase the killing of cancers, we have seen the carotenoids, for example, powerfully suppress the growth of a cancer but do not kill it. Once the subjects in one study stopped taking carotenoids, after a long delay, the cancers reappeared.

Even though juicing or blenderizing vegetables can be inconvenient and the resulting drink not very tasty, it is the only way to assure the adequate absorption of the very powerful cancer-suppressing and -destroying nutrients found in produce. This is where the willpower and discipline we just discussed come in.

You will find that, over time, the tasks of preparing your vegetables and other anticancer nutrients will become a part of your routine. Once you arrive at that point, it will seem strange not to do these things. Your greatest problem will come during travel and other situations in which you are forced to eat away from home.

Should you be forced to eat out in a restaurant, choose foods that conform as closely as possible to your new diet, such as salads, lean meats, and steamed vegetables. Avoid gravies and sauces, highly flavored foods, potatoes, fish (especially tuna, swordfish, and salmon), and sweetened desserts.

When traveling, always bring your supplements with you. Purchase only high-quality supplements in the correct forms. When storing your supplements, avoid placing them in heat. This is especially true for probiotics and oils, such as DHA. All of your supplements will last longer and remain more potent if you keep them refrigerated.

While no one can guarantee you success in your battle against this dreaded disease, you can be assured that you will have a much better outcome than if you ignore the importance of nutrition in your treatment. The vast majority of patients treated with nutrition feel better and have far fewer complications than those neglecting this vital addition to their conventional treatment program.

Review the material in this book often. It will not only help to refresh your memory concerning the details of your nutritional treatment, but will remind you of the powerful influence that nutrients can have in controlling your disease.

Notes

CHAPTER 1

1. Steinmetz KA, Potter JD. Vegetables, fruit and cancer prevention: a review. J Am Diet Assoc 96: 1027–1039, 1996.
2. Norell SE, Ahlbom A, et al. Diet and pancreatic cancer: a case-control study. Am J Epidemiol 124: 894–902, 1986.
3. Giovannucci E, Asherio A, et al. Intake of carotenoids and retinol in relation to risk of prostate cancer. J Natl Cancer Inst 87: 1767–1776, 1995.
4. Caltagirone S, Rossi C, et al. Flavonoids apigenin and quercetin inhibit melanoma growth and metastatic potential. In J Cancer 87: 595–600, 2000.
5. Slattery M, Abbott T, et al. Dietary vitamin A, C, and E and selenium as risk factors for cervical cancer. Epidemiol 1: 8–15, 1990.
6. Cole WC, Prasad KN. Heterogeneity of commercial ß-carotene preparations: correlation with biological activities. In: Prasad KN, Cole WC (eds). *Cancer and Nutrition*. Amsterdam: IOS Press, 1998: 99–104.
7. Van den Berg H. Carotenoid interactions. Nutr Reviews 1999: 57: 1–10.
8. Pung A, Rundhaug JE, et al. Beta carotene and canthaxanthin inhibit chemically and physically-induced neoplastic transformation in 10T1/2 cells. Carcinogenesis 9: 1533–1539, 1988.
9. Fahey JW, Zhang Y, Talalay P. Broccoli sprouts: an exceptionally rich source of inducers of enzymes that protect against chemical carcinogens. Proc Natl Acad Sci 94: 10367–10372, 1997.
10. Mason JB, Lavesque T. Folate: effects on carcinogenesis and

the potential for cancer chemoprevention. Oncology 10: 1727–1743, 1996.

11. Folkers K, Brown R, et al. Survival of cancer patients in therapy with coenzyme Q10. Biochem Biophysic Res Comm 192: 241–245, 1993.
12. Layton DW, Bogen KT, et al. Cancer risk of heterocyclic amines in cooked foods: an analysis and implications for research. Carcinogenesis 16: 39–52, 1995.
13. Skog K. Cooking procedures and food mutagens: a literature review. Food Chemical Toxicol 31: 655–675, 1993.
14. Kuijten RR, Bunin GR, et al. Gestational and familial risk factors for childhood astrocytoma: results of a case-controlled study. Cancer Res 50: 2608–2612, 1990.
15. Bunin GR, Kuijten RR, et al. Relation between maternal diet and subsequent primitive neuroectodermal brain tumors in young children. New Eng J Med 329: 536–541, 1993.
16. Shephard SE, Wakabayashi K, Nagao T. Mutagenic activity of peptides and the artificial sweetener aspartame after nitrosation. Chem Tox 31: 323–329, 1993.
17. Tannenbaum SR, Mergens W. Reaction of nitrite with vitamin C and E. Ann NY Acad Sci 355: 267–279, 1980.
18. Blaylock RL. *Excitotoxins: The Taste That Kills*. Health Press, 1997.

Chapter 2

1. Nassani I, Seimiya H, Tsuruo T. Telomerase inhibition, telomere shortening, and senscence of cancer cells by tea catechins. Biochem Biophys Res Comm 249: 391–396, 1998.
2. Trosko JE, Yotti LP, et al. Inhibition of cell-cell communication by tumor promoters. Carcinogenesis 7: 565–585, 1982.
3. Ames BN, Shigenaga MK, Hagen TM. Oxidants, antioxidants and the degenerative diseases of aging. Proc Natl Acad Sci 90: 7915–7922, 1993.
4. Ogle KS, Swanson GM, et al. Cancer and co-morbidity. Redefining chronic diseases. Cancer 88: 653–663, 2000.
5. Dickens BF, Weglicki WB, et al. Magnesium deficiency in vitro enhances free radical–induced intracellular oxidation and cytotoxicity in endothelial cells. Fed Euro Biochem Soc 311: 187–191, 1992.
6. Weijl NI, Hopman GD, et al. Cisplatin combination chemo-

therapy induces a fall in plasma antioxidants of cancer patients. Ann Oncol 9: 1331–1337, 1998.

7. Prasad KN, Cole W, Hovland P. Cancer prevention studies: past, present, and future directions. Nutrition 14: 197–210, 1998.
8. Wei Q, Matanoski GM, et al. DNA repair: a potential marker for cancer susceptibility. Cancer Bull 46: 233–237, 1994.
9. Bishoff FZ, Hansen MF. Genetics of familial breast cancer. Cancer Bull 45: 476–482, 1993.
10. Poulson HE, Prieme H, et al. Role of oxidative DNA damage in cancer initiation and promotion. Eur J Cancer Prevent 7: 9–16, 1998.
11. Ames BN, Gold LS, Willett WC. The causes and prevention of cancer. Proc Natl Acad Sci USA 92: 5258–5265, 1995.
12. Ishioka T, Kuwabara N, et al. Induction of colorectal tumors in rats by sulfinated polysaccharides. CRC Crit Rev Toxicol 17: 215–244, 1987.
13. Reed M. Flavonoids: naturally occurring anti-inflammatory agents. Am J Pathol 147: 235–237, 1995.
14. Raz A, Levine A, Khomiak Y. Acute inflammation potentiates tumor growth in mice. Cancer Lett 148: 115–120, 2000.
15. Hann HL, et al. Antitumor effect of deferoxamine on human hepatocellular carcinoma growing in athymic nude mice. Cancer 70: 2051–2056, 1992.
16. Estrov Z, Tawa A, et al. In vitro and in vivo effect of deferoxamine in neonatal acute leukemia. Blood 69: 757–761, 1987.
17. Weinberg ED. Iron and neoplasia. Biol Trace Elem Res 3: 55–80, 1981.
18. Wyllie S, Liehr JG. Enhancement of estrogen-induced renal tumorigenesis in hamsters by dietary iron. Carcinogenesis 19: 1285–1290, 1998.
19. Sesink ALA, Termont DSML, et al. Red meat and colon cancer: dietary haem-induced colonic cytoxicity and epithelial hyperproliferation are inhibited by calcium. Carcinogenesis 22: 1653–1659, 2001.
20. Fuhr U, Klittich K, Staib AH. Inhibitory effect of grape-fruit juice and its bitter principle, naringenin, on CYP1A2 dependent metabolism of caffeine. Br. J Clin Pharmacol 35: 431–436, 1993.
21. Johnson TM, Nelson BR et al. Matrix metalloproteinases in local tumor invasion in nonmelanoma skin cancer. Cancer Bull 45: 238–244, 1993.
22. Monteagudo C, Merino M, et al. Immunohistological distribu-

tion of type IV collagenase in normal, benign and malignant breast tissue. Am J Pathol. 136: 585, 1990.

23. Talvensaari-Mattila, et al. Matrix metalloproteinase-2 is associated with the risk for relapse in post-menopausal patients with node-positive breast carcinoma, treated with antiestrogen adjuvant therapy. Breast Ca Res Treatment 65: 55–61, 2001.
24. Matrix metalloproteinase-2: a marker for relapse in node positive breast cancer. Cancer Watch 10: 101, 2001.
25. Nicolson GL, Nakajima M, et al. Cancer cell heparanase associated with invasion and metastasis. Adv Enzyme Regulat 38: 19–32, 1998.
26. Nicolson GL. Breast cancer metastasis-associated genes: role in tumor progression to the metastatic state. Biochem Soc Symp 63: 231–243, 1998.
27. Go Y, Chintala SK, et al. Cisplatin but not BCNU inhibits urokinase-type plasminogen activator levels in human glioblastoma cell lines in vitro. Clin Exp Metastasis 15: 447–452, 1997.
28. Rohdewald P. Pycnogenol. In: Rice-Evans CA, Packer L (eds). *Flavonoids in Health and Disease*. New York: Marcel Dekker, Inc., 1998, pp. 405–419.
29. Duthie SJ, Collins AR, et al. Quercetin and myricetin protect against hydrogen peroxide–induced DNA damage (strand breaks and oxidized pyrimidines) in human lymphocytes. Mutat Res 393: 223–231, 1997.
30. Wolff MS, Toniolo PG, et al. Blood levels of organochlorine residues and risk of breast cancer. J Natl Cancer Inst 85: 648–652, 1993.
31. Trocho C, Pardo R, et al. Formaldehyde derived from dietary aspartame binds to tissue components in vivo. Life Sciences 63: 337–349, 1998.
32. Bressler Report, Bureau of Foods, Nov. 8, 1971.
33. Levine AJ. *Viruses*. New York: Scientific American Library, 1992, pp. 87–111.
34. Kovacs E, Almendral A. Reduced DNA repair synthesis in healthy women having first-degree relatives with breast cancer. Eur J Cancer Clin Oncol 23: 1051–1057, 1987.
35. Zhang S, Hunter DJ, et al. A prospective study of folate intake and the risk of breast cancer. JAMA 281: 1632–1637, 1999.
36. Blount BC, Mack MM, et al. Folate deficiency causes uracil misincorporation into human DNA and chromosomal breakage. Proc Natl Acad Sci USA 94: 3290–3295, 1997.

CHAPTER 3

1. Levine EG, Bloomfield CD. Leukemias and myelodysplastic syndromes secondary to drug, radiation, and environmental exposure. Semin Oncol 19: 47–84, 1992.
2. Moss RW. *Questioning Chemotherapy.* Brooklyn, NY: Equinox Press, 1995.
3. Fields KK, et al. Maximum-tolerated doses of ifosfamide, carboplatin and etoposide given over 6 days followed by autologous stem-cell rescue: toxicity profile. J Clinc Oncol 13: 323–332, 1995.
4. Houston SJ, et al. The influence of adjuvant chemotherapy on outcome after relapse in patients with breast cancer. Proc Ann Meet ASCO 11: A108, 1992.
5. McMillian TJ, Hart IR. Can cancer chemotherapy enhance the malignant behavior of tumors? Cancer and Metastasis Rev 6: 503–520, 1987.
6. Skubitz KM, Anderson PM. Oral glutamine to prevent chemotherapy-induced stomatitis: a pilot study. J Lab Clin Med 127: 223–228, 1996.
7. Project ChemoInsight: Quality Performance 1999, Thousand Oaks, CA: Amgen Inc.,
8. Roper Starch Worldwide. "Chemotherapy Experiences" (survey). Jan. 1999.
9. Mizuno Y, Hokamura T, et al. A case of 5-fluorouricil cardiotoxicity simulating acute myocardial infarction. Jpn Circ J 59: 303–307, 1995.
10. Lenzhofer R, Ganzinger U, et al. Acute cardiac toxicity in patients after doxorubicin treatment and the effect of combined tocopherol and nifedipine pretreatment. J Cancer Res Clin Oncol 106: 143–147, 1983.
11. Legha SS, Wang YM, et al. Clinical and pharmacologic investigation of the effects of alpha-tocopherol on adriamycin cardiotoxicity. Ann NY Acad Sci 393: 411–418, 1982.
12. Kurbacher CM, Wagner U, et al. Ascorbic acid (vitamin C) improves the antineoplastic activity of doxorubicin, cisplatin and paclitaxel in human breast carcinoma cells in vitro. Cancer Lett 103: 183–189, 1996.
13. Dimitrov NV, Hay MB. Abrogation of adriamycin-induced cardiotoxicity by selenium in rabbits. Am J Path 126: 376–383, 1987.
14. Meyers C, Borow R, et al. A randomized controlled trial assess-

ing the prevention of doxorubicin cardiomyopathy by N-acetyl-L-cysteine. Semin Oncol 10: Suppl 1; 53–55, 1983.

15. Iarussi D, Auricchio U, et al. Protective effect of coenzyme Q10 on anthacyclines cardiotoxicity: control study in children with acute lymphoblastic leukemia and non-Hodgkins lymphoma. Mol Aspects Med 15: s207–s212, 1994.
16. Chopra S, Pillai KK, et al. Propolis protects against doxorubicin-induced myocardiopathy in rats. Exp Mol Pathol 62: 190–198, 1995.
17. Skubitz KM, Anderson PM. Oral glutamine to prevent chemotherapy-induced stomatitis. J Lab Clin Med 127: 223–228, 1996.
18. Muscaritoli M, Micozzi A, et al. Oral glutamine in the prevention of chemotherapy-induced gastrointestinal toxicity. Eur J Cancer 33: 319–320, 1997.
19. Ueda H, et al. Reduction of cisplatin toxicity and lethality by sodium malate in mice. Bio Pharm Bull 21: 34–43, 1998.
20. Kuhlmann MK, et al. Reduction of cisplatin toxicity in cultured renal tubular cells by the bioflavonoid quercetin. Arch Toxicol 72: 536–540, 1998.
21. Shoskes DA. Effect of bioflavonoids quercetin and curcumin on ischemic renal injury: a new class of renoprotective agents. Transplantation 66: 147–152, 1998.
22. Liu SJ, Zhou SW. Panax notoginseng saponins attenuate cisplatin-induced nephrotoxicity. Acta Pharmacol Sin 21: 257–260, 2000.
23. Zunino F, Tofanetti O, et al. Protective effect of reduced glutathione against cis-dichlorodiammine platinum (II)-induced nephrotoxicity and lethal toxicity. Tumori 69: 105–111, 1983.
24. Zunino F, Pratesti G, et al. Protective effect of reduced glutathione against cisplatin-induced renal and systemic toxicity and its influence on the therapeutic activity of the antitumor drug. Chem Biol Interact 70: 89–101, 1989.
25. Tolley DA. The effect of N-acetyl cysteine on cyclophosphamide cystitis. Br J Urol 49: 659–661, 1977.
26. Kline I, Gang M, et al. Protection with N-acetyl-L-cysteine (NSC–111180) against isophamide (NSC–109724) toxicity and enhancement of therapeutic effect in early murine L1210 leukemia. Cancer Chemother Rep 57: 299–304, 1973.
27. Neglia JP. Cancer survivors: risk of subsequent cancers. Proc Amer Assoc Cancer Res 42: 968, 2001.
28. Cancer Watch 10: 73–74, May 2001.

29. Strumberg D, Brugge S, et al. Evaluation of long-term toxicity in patients after cisplatin-based chemotherapy for non-seminomatous testicular cancer. Ann Oncol 13: 229–236, 2002.
30. Meinardi MT, Gietema JA, et al. Cardiovascular morbidity in long-term survivors of metastatic testicular cancer. J Clin Oncol 18: 1725–1732, 2000.
31. Pedersen-Bjergaard J, Daugaard G, et al. Increased risk of myelodysplasia and leukemia after etoposide, cisplatin, and bleomycin from germ-cell tumors. Lancet 338: 359–363, 1991.
32. Ames BN, Shigenaga MK, Hagen TM. Oxidants, antioxidants and the degenerative diseases of aging. Proc Natl Acad Sci 90: 7915–7922, 1993.
33. Blaylock RL. Phytonutrients and metabolic stimulants as protection against neurodegeneration and excitotoxicity. J Amer Nutr Assoc 2: 30–39, 2000.

Chapter 4

1. Thomlinson RH, Gray LH. The histological structure of some human lung cancers and the possible implication for radiotherapy. Br J Cancer 9: 539–549, 1955.
2. Levenson SM, Rettura G, Seifer E. Effects of supplemental dietary vitamin A and ß-carotene on experimental tumors: local tumor excision, chemotherapy, radiation injury and radiotherapy. In: Butterworth CE, Hutchenson ML (eds). *Nutritional Factors in the Induction and Maintenance of Malignancy*. New York: Academic Press, Inc., 1983, pp. 169–203.
3. Ricoul M, Sabatier L, Dutrillaux B. Increased chromosome radiosensitivity during pregnancy. Mutat Res 374: 73–78, 1997.
4. Patchen ML, MacVittie TJ, et al. Radioprotection by polysaccharides alone and in combination with aminothiols. Adv Space Res 12: 233–248, 1992.
5. Milas L, Nishiguchi I, et al. Radiation protection against early and late effects of ionizing irradiation by prostaglandin inhibitor indomethacin. Adv Space Res 12: 265–271, 1992.
6. Kuttan G. Use of *Withania sominefera Dunal* as an adjuvant during radiation therapy. Indian J Exp Biol 34: 854–856, 1996.
7. Floersheim GL, Racine C. Calcium antagonist radioprotectors do not reduce radiotherapeutic efficacy in three human xenographs. Strahlenther Onkol 171: 403–407, 1995.

8. Salvadori DM, Ribeiro LR, et al. Radioprotection of beta-carotene evaluated on mouse somatic and germ cells. Mutat Res 356: 163–170, 1996.

Chapter 5

1. Popp MB, Kirkemo AK, et al. Tumor and host carcass changes during total parenteral nutrition in an anorectic rat-tumor system. Ann Surg 199: 205–210, 1984.
2. Daly JM, Copeland EM, et al. Relationship of protein nutrition to growth and host immunocompetence. Surg Forum 27: 113–114, 1976.
3. Lasko CM, Good CK, et al. Energy restriction modulates the development of advanced preneoplastic lesions depending on the level of fat in the diet. Nutrition and Cancer 33: 69–75, 1999.
4. Westin T, Stein H, et al. Tumor cytokinetic response to total parenteral nutrition in patients with head and neck cancers. Am J Clin Nutr 53: 764–768, 1991.
5. Durnaton B, Freund JN, et al. Promotion of intestinal carcinogenesis by dietary methionine. Carcinogenesis. 20: 493–497, 1999.
6. American Institute for Cancer Research. *Food, Nutrition and Prevention of Cancer: A Global Perspective*. Washington, DC: American Institute for Cancer Research, 1997.
7. Steinmetz KA, Potter JD. Vegetables, fruit and cancer prevention: a review. J Am Diet Assoc 96: 1027–1039, 1996.
8. Miller NJ. Flavonoids phenylpropanoids as contributors to antioxidant activity of fruit juices. In: Rice-Evans CA, Packer L (eds). *Flavonoids in Health and Disease*. New York: Marcel Dekker, Inc., 1998, 387–403.
9. Raz A, Levine G, Khomiak Y. Acute local inflammation potentiates tumor growth in mice. Cancer Lett 148: 115–120, 2000.
10. Ip C. Controversial issues of dietary fats and experimental mammary carcinogenesis. Prev Med 22: 728–737, 1993.
11. Cohen LA, Thompson DO, et al. Dietary fat and mammary cancer. 1. Promoting effects of differing dietary fats on N-nitromethylurea-induced rat mammary tumorigenesis. JNCI 77: 33–42, 1986.
12. Huang Z, Willett WC, et al. Waist circumference, waist: hip

ratio, and risk of breast cancer in Nurses' Health Study. Am J. Epidemiol 150: 1316–1324, 1999.

13. DeStefani E, Deneo-Pellegrini H, et al. Alpha-linolenic acid and risk of prostate cancer: a case control study in Uruguay. Cancer Epidemiology Biomarkers Prev 9: 335–338, 2000.
14. Qi M, Chen D, et al. Polyunsaturated fatty acids increase skin but not cervical cancer in human papillomavirus–16 transgenic mice. Cancer Res 62: 433–436, 2002.
15. Kelly DA, Branch LB, et al. Dietary alpha-linolenic acid and immunocompetence in humans. Am J Clin Nutr 53: 40–46, 1991.
16. Gogoa CA, Kalfarentzos FE, Zoumbos NC. Effect of different types of total parenteral nutrition on T-lymphocyte subpopulations and NK cells. Am J Clin Nutr 51: 119–122, 1990.
17. Rolland PH, Martin PM, et al. Prostaglandins in human breast cancer: evidence suggesting that an elevated prostaglandin production is a marker of high metastatic potential for neoplastic cells. JNCI 64: 1061–1070, 1980.
18. Kachlap SK, Dange PP, et al. Effect of omega-3 fatty acid (docosahexaenoic acid) on BRACA1 gene expression and growth of MCF-7 cell line. Cancer Biother Radiopharm 16: 257–263, 2001.
19. Mares-Perlman JA, Francis AM, Shrago E. Host and tumor growth and energy substrates in blood of hepatoma-bearing rats receiving high-fat parenteral infusions. Am J Clin Nutr 48: 50–56. 1988.
20. Rijnkels JM, Hollanders VMH, et al. Modulation of dietary fat–enhanced colorectal carcinogenesis in N-methyl-N-Nitrosoguanidine-treated rats by a vegetable-fruit mixture. Nutr Cancer 29: 90–95, 1997.
21. Giovannucci E, Rimm EB, et al. A prospective study of dietary fat and risk of prostate cancer. JNCI 85: 1571–1579, 1993.
22. Attiga FA, Fernandez PM, et al. Inhibitors of prostaglandin synthesis inhibit human prostate tumor cell invasiveness and reduce the release of matrix metalloprotenase. Cancer Res 60: 4629–4637, 2000. Special note: The stimulation of prostate cancer by the N-6 fats is similar to that seen with breast cancers, with most of the effect being due to eicosanoid formation, especially PGE2, 12-HETE and 15-HETE. Blocking the COX-2 enzyme also blocks prostate cancer promotion by these fats. (Rose DP, Connolly JM. Effects of fatty acids and eicosanoid

synthesis inhibitor on the growth of two human prostate cancer cell lines. Prostate 18: 243–254, 1991.) Since omega-3 oils suppress this enzyme, one would expect to see, and sees, significant inhibition of prostate cancer when diets high in these oils or their constituents (EPA and DHA) are eaten.

23. Hamalainen E, Adercreutz C, et al. Diet and serum sex hormones in healthy men. J Steroid Biochem 20: 459–464, 1984.
24. Haven FL. The effect of cod liver oil on tumor growth. Am J Cancer 27: 95–98, 1936.
25. Jenski LJ, Sturdevant LK, et al. Omega-3 fatty acid modification of membrane structure and function. I. Dietary manipulation of tumor susceptibility to cell- and complement-mediated lysis. Nutr Cancer 19: 135–146, 1993.
26. Borgeson CE, Pardini L, et al. Effect of dietary fish oil on human mammary carcinoma and on lipid-metabolizing enzymes. Lipids 24: 290–295, 1989.
27. Morecki S, Yacovlev E, et al. Induction of antitumor immunity by indomethacin. Cancer Immunol Immunother 48: 613–120, 2000.
28. Collett ED, Davidson LA, et al. N-6 and N-3 polyunsaturated fatty acids differentially modulate oncogene RAS activation in colonocytes. Am J Physiol Cell Physiol 280: C1066–C1075, 2001.
29. Chung BH, Mitchell SH, et al. Effects of docosahexaenoic acid and eicosapentaenoic acid on androgen-mediated cell growth and gene expression in LNCaP prostate cancer cells. Carcinogenesis 22: 1201–1206, 2001.
30. Maillard V, Bougnoux P, et al. N-3 and N-6 fatty acids in breast adipose tissue and related risk of breast cancer in a case-control study in Tours, France. In J Cancer 98: 78–83, 2002.
31. Rose DP, Connolly JM. Antiangiogenicity of docosahexaenoic acid and its role in suppression of breast cancer cell growth in nude mice. In J Oncol 15: 1011–1015, 1999.
32. Connolly JM, Gilhooly EM, Rose DP. Effects of reduced dietary linolenic acid intake, alone or combined with an algal source of docosahexaenoic acid, on MDA-MB-231 breast cancer cell growth and apoptosis in nude mice. Nutr Cancer 35: 44–49, 1999.
33. Calviello G, Palozza E, et al. Dietary supplementation with eicosapentaenoic and docosahexaenoic acid inhibits growth of Morris hepatocarcinoma 3924A in rats: effects on proliferation and apoptosis. In J Cancer 75: 699–705, 1998.

34. Thompson LU, Rickard SE, Orcheson LJ, Seidl MM. Flaxseed and its lignan and oil components reduce mammary tumor growth at a late stage of carcinogenesis. Carcinogenesis 17: 1373–1376, 1996.
35. Setchell KD, Lawson AM, et al. Lignans in man and in animal species. Nature 287: 740–742, 1980.
36. Hutchens AM, Martini MC, et al. Flaxseed consumption influences endogenous hormone concentrations in postmenopausal women. Nutr Cancer 39: 58–65, 2001.
37. Pietinen P, Stumpf K, Mannisto S, et al. Serum enterolactone and risk of breast cancer: a case-control study in eastern Finland. Cancer Epidemiol Biomarkers Prev 10: 339–344, 2001.
38. Meilahan EN, DeStavola B, et al. Do urinary oestrogen metabolites predict breast cancer? Guernsey III cohort follow-up. Br J Cancer 78: 1250–1255, 1998.
39. Fishman J, Schneider J, et al. Increased estrogen–16 alpha-hydroxylase activity in women with breast and endometrial cancer. J Steroid Biochem 20: 1077–1081, 1984.
40. Yoo HJ, Sepkovic DW, et al. Estrogen metabolism as a risk factor for head and neck cancer. Otolaryngol Head Neck Surg 124: 241–247, 2001.
41. Bradlow HL, Herschcopf RJ, et al. Estradiol 16 alpha-hydroxylase in the mouse correlates with mammary tumor incidence and presence of murine mammary tumor virus: a possible model for the hormonal etiology of breast cancer in humans. Proc Natl Acad Sci USA 82: 6295–6299, 1985.
42. Wang C, Makela T, et al. Lignans and flavonoids inhibit aromatase in human adiposites. J Steroid Biochem Mol Biol 50: 205–212, 1994.
43. Owen RW, Mier W, et al. Identification of lignans as major components in the phenolic fraction of olive oil. Clin Chem 46: 976–988, 2000.
44. Rickard SE, Yuan YU, et al. Plasma insulin-like growth factor-1 levels in rats are reduced by dietary supplementation of flaxseed or its lignan seoisoloriciresinol diglycoside. Cancer Lett 161: 47–55, 2000.
45. Knekt P, Adercreutz H, et al. Does antibacterial treatment for urinary tract infection contribute to the risk of breast cancer? Br J Cancer 82: 1107–1110, 2000.
46. Mainou-Fowler T, Procter SJ, Dickinson AM. Gamma-linolenic acid induces apoptosis in B-chronic lymphocytic leukemia cells in vitro. Leu Lymphoma 40: 393–403, 2001.

47. Das UN. Tumericidal actions of gamma linolenic acid with particular reference to the therapy of human gliomas. Med Sci Res 23: 507–513, 1995.
48. Lee JH, Sugano M. Effects of linolenic and gamma-linolenic acid on 7,12-dimethyl benzyl(a)anthrecene-induced rat mammary tumors. Nutr Rep Int 34: 1041, 1986.
49. Ip C, Singh M, et al. Conjugated linolenic acid suppressed mammary carcinogenesis and proliferative activity of the mammary gland in the rat. Cancer Res 54: 1212–1215, 1994.
50. Belury MA. Conjugated dienoic linoleate: a polyunsaturated fatty acid with unique chemopreventative properties. Nutr Rev 53: 83–89, 1995.
51. Kohno H, Suzuki R, et al. Dietary conjugated linolenic acid inhibits azoxymethane-induced colonic abberant crypt foci in rats. Jpn J Cancer Res 93: 133–142, 2002.
52. Aro A, Mannistos, et al. Inverse association between dietary and serum conjugated linolenic acid and risk of breast cancer in postmenopausal women. Nutr Cancer 38: 151–157, 2000.
53. Banni S, Anginoni E, et al. Decrease in linolenic acid metabolites as a potential mechanism in cancer risk reduction by conjugated linolenic acid. Carcinogenesis 20: 1019–1024, 1999.
54. Kavanaugh CJ, Liu K-L, Belury MA. Effect of dietary conjugated linolenic acid on phorbol ester-induced PGE2 production and hyperplasia in mouse epidermis. Nutr Cancer 33: 132–138, 1999.
55. Igarashi M, Miyazawa T. Newly recognized cytotoxic effect of conjugated trienoic fatty acids on cultured human tumor cells. Cancer Lett 148: 173–179, 2000.
56. Kimoto Y, Tanji Y, et al. Antitumor effect of medium chain triglyceride and its influence on the self-defense systems of the body. Cancer Detect Trev 22: 219–224, 1998.
57. Kono H, Enomoto N, et al. Medium-chain triglycerides inhibit free radical formation and TNF-alpha production in rats given ethanol. Am J Physiol Gastrointest Liver Physiol 278: G467–G476, 2000.
58. Tsuji H, Kasai M, et al. Dietary medium-chain triacyglycerols suppress accumulation of body fat in a double-blind, controlled trial in healthy men and women. J Nutr 131: 2853–2859, 2001.
59. Shi W, Gould MN. Induction of cytostasis in mammary carcinoma cells treated with the anticancer agent perillyl alcohol. Carcinogenesis 23: 131–142, 2002.

60. Bradley MO, Swindell CS, et al. Tumor targeting by conjugating DHA to paclitaxel. J Control Release 74: 233–236, 2001.
61. Menendez JA, del Mar Barbacid M, et al. Effects of gamma-linolenic acid and oleic acid on paclitaxel cytotoxicity in human breast cancer cells. Eur J Cancer 37: 402–413, 2001.
62. Kenny FS, Gee JM, et al. Effect of dietary GLA/tamoxifen on the growth, ER expression and fatty acid profile of ER positive human breast cancer xenografts. In J Cancer 92: 342–347, 2001.
63. Mainou-Flower T, Procter SJ, Dickenson AM. Gamma-linolenic acid induces apoptosis in B-chronic lymphocytic leukemia cell in vitro. Leu Lymphoma 40: 393–403, 2001.
64. Chen ZY, Istfan NW. Docosahexaenoic acid is a potent inducer of apoptosis in HT-29 colon cancer cells. Prostaglandins Leukot Essent Fatty Acids 63: 301–308, 2000.
65. Cao WX, Cheng QM, et al. A study of preoperative methionine-depleting parenteral nutrition plus chemotherapy in gastric cancer patients. World J Gastroenterol 6: 255–258, 2000.
66. Lu S, Hoestje SM, Choo EM, Epner DE. Methionine restriction induces apoptosis of prostate cancer cells via the c-jun N-terminal kinase-mediated signaling pathway. Cancer Lett 179: 51–58, 2002.
67. Cao WX, Ou JM, Fei XF, et al. Methionine-dependence and combination chemotherapy on human gastric cancer cells in vitro. World J Gastroenterol 8: 230–232, 2002.
68. Paulsen JE, Alexander J. Growth stimulation of intestinal tumors in Apc/Min/+ mice by dietary L-methionine supplementation. Anticancer Res 21: 3281–3284, 2001.
69. Cao WX, Cheng QM, et al. A study of preoperative methionine-depleting parenteral nutrition plus chemotherapy in gastric cancer patients. World J Gastroenterol 6: 255–258, 2000.
70. Xie K, Fidler IJ. Therapy of cancer metastasis by activation of the inducible nitric oxide synthease. Cancer Metastasis 17: 55–75, 1998.
71. Park KG, Heys SD, et al. Stimulation of human breast cancers by dietary L-arginine. Clin Sci (LOND) 82: 413–417, 1992.
72. Blaylock RL. Neurodegeneration and aging of the central nervous system: prevention and treatment by phytochemicals and metabolic nutrients. Integrative Med 1: 117–133, 1998.
73. Takano T, Lin JH, et al. Glutamate release promotes growth of malignant gliomas. Nat Med 7: 994–995, 2001.
74. Ye ZC, Southeimer H. Glioma cells release excitotoxic concentrations of glutamate. Cancer Res 59: 4383–4391, 1999.

75. Yoshida S, Kaibara A, Ishibashi N, Shirouzu K. Glutamine supplementation in cancer patients. Nutrition 17: 766–768, 2001.
76. Neurotransmitter may promote brain tumor growth. Cancer Watch 10: Sept. 2001.
77. Souba WW. Glutamine and cancer. Ann Surg 218: 715–728, 1993.
78. Austgen TR, Dudrick PS, et al. The effects of glutamine-enriched total parenteral nutrition on tumor growth and host tissues. Ann Surg 215: 107–113, 1992.
79. Yoshida S, Kaibara A, et al. Glutamine supplementation in cancer patients. Nutrition 17: 766–768, 2001.
80. Klimmberg VS, Nwodeki E, et al. Glutamine facilitates chemotherapy while reducing toxicity. J Parenter Enteral Nutr 16 (suppl) 83s–87s, 1992.
81. Taudou G, Wiart J, Panijel J. Influence of amino acid deficiency and tRNA aminoacylation on DNA polymerase activity during the secondary immune response in vitro. Mol Immunol 20: 255–262, 1983.
82. Senturker S, Tschirret-Guth R, et al. Induction of apoptosis by chemotherapeutic drugs without generation of reactive oxygen species. Arch Biochem Biophysic 397: 262–272, 2002.
83. The ATBC Cancer Prevention Study Group. The effect of vitamin E and beta-carotene on the incidence of lung cancer and other cancers in male smokers. N Engl J Med 330: 1029–1035, 1994.
84. Hennekens CH, Buring JE, et al. Lack of effect of long-term supplementation with beta-carotene on the incidence of malignant neoplasms and cardiovascular disease. N Engl J Med 334: 1145–1149, 1996.
85. Levin G, Yeshurun M, Mokady S. In vitro antiperoxidative effect of 9-cis beta-carotene compared with that of the all-trans isomer. Nutr Cancer 27: 293–297, 1997.
86. Palozza P, Luberto C, et al. Antioxidant and prooxidant role of beta-carotene in murine normal and tumor thymocytes: effects of oxygen partial pressure. Free Rad Biol Med 22: 1065–1073, 1997.
87. Palozza P, Krinski NI. ß-carotene and alpha-tocopherol are synergistic antioxidants. Arch Biochem Biophys 297: 184–187, 1992.
88. Park CH. Vitamin C in leukemia and preleukemia cell growth, Prog Clin Biol Res 259: 321–330, 1988.

Chapter 6

1. Block JB, Evans MS. A review of recent results addressing the potential interactions of antioxidants with cancer drug therapy. J Amer Nutr Assoc 4: 11–20, 2001.
2. Blaylock RL. A review of conventional cancer prevention and treatment and the adjunctive use of nutraceutical supplements and antioxidant: is there a danger or a significant benefit? J Am Nutr Assoc 3: 17–35, 2000.
3. Wahab MH, Akoul ES, et al. Modulatory effects of melatonin and vitamin E on doxorubicin-induced cardiotoxicity in Ehrlich ascites carcinoma-bearing mice. Tumori 86: 157–162, 2000.
4. Prasad KN, Kumar R. Effect of individual antioxidant vitamins alone and in combination on growth and differentiation of human non-tumorigenic and tumorigenic parotid acinar cells in culture. Nutr Cancer 26: 11–19, 1996.
5. Prasad KN, Hernandez C, et al. Modification of the effect of tamoxifen, cis-platin, DTIC, and interferon-alpha 2b on human melanoma cells in culture by a mixture of vitamins. Nutr Cancer 22: 233–245, 1994.
6. Fukushima S, Imaida K, et al. L-ascorbic acid amplification of second-stage bladder carcinogenesis promotion by NaHCO3. Cancer Res 48: 6317, 1988.
7. Krauhusen U, Blum U, et al. Vitamin B_6 responsive growth of human lung cancers in nude mice. Strahleatherapie und Onkologie 165: 562–563, 1989.
8. Prasad KN, Cole W, Hovland P. Cancer prevention studies: past, present, and future directions. Nutrition 14: 197–210, 1998.
9. Prasad KN, Hernandez C, et al. Modification of the effect of tamoxifen, cis-platin, DTIC, and interferon-alpha 2b on human melanoma cells in culture by a mixture of vitamins. Nutr Cancer 22: 233–245, 1994.
10. Rama BN, Prasad KN. Effect of dl-alpha-tocopheryl succinate in combination with sodium butyrate and cAMP-stimulating agents on neuroblastoma cells in culture. In J Cancer 34: 863–867, 1984.
11. Prasad KN, Edwards-Prasad J. Vitamin E and cancer prevention: recent advances and future potentials. J Am Coll Nutr 11: 487–500, 1992.
12. Block JB, Evans S. A review of recent results addressing the po-

tential interactions of antioxidants with cancer drug therapy. J Am Nutr Assoc 4: 11–20, 2001.
13. Prasad KN, Kumar A, et al. High doses of multiple antioxidant vitamins: essential ingredients in improving the efficacy of standard cancer therapy. J Amer Coll Nutr 18: 13–25, 1999.
14. Bertram JS, Bortkiewicz H. Dietary carotenoids inhibit neoplastic transformation and modulate gene expression in mouse and human cells. Am J Clin Nutr 62 (suppl): 1327S–1336S, 1995.
15. Loft S, Poulsen HE. Cancer risk and oxidative DNA damage in man. J Mol Med 74: 297–312, 1996.
16. Gob SH, Hew NF, et al. Inhibition of tumor promotion by various palm-oil tocotrienols. In J Cancer 57: 529–531, 1994.
17. De Flora S, Bagnasco M, Vainio H. Modulation of genotoxic and related effects by carotenoids and vitamin A in experimental models: mechanistic issues. Mutagenesis 14: 153–172, 1999.
18. Fiala ES, Sodum RS, et al. (-) epigallocatechin gallate, a polyphenolic tea antioxidant, inhibits peroxinitrite-mediated formation of 8-oxodeoxyguanisine and 3-nitrotyrosine. Experimentia 52: 922–926, 1996.
19. Bu-Abbas A, Nunez X, et al. A comparison of the antimutagenic potential of green, black and decaffeinated teas: contribution of flavonols to the antimutagenic effect. Mutagenesis 11: 597–603, 1996.
20. Asano Y, Okamura S, et al. Effect of (-) epigallocatechin gallate on leukemia blast cells from patients with acute myloblastic leukemia. Life Sci 60: 135–142, 1997.
21. Kuo SM. Antiproliferative potency of structurally distinct dietary flavonoids on human colon cancer cells. Cancer Lett 110: 41–48, 1996.
22. Noroozi M, Angerson WJ, Lean ME. Effects of flavonoids and vitamin C on oxidative DNA damage to human lymphocytes. Am J Clin Nutr 67: 1210–1218, 1998.
23. Bhatia N, Zhao J, et al. Inhibition of human carcinoma cell growth and DNA synthesis by silibinin, an active constituent of milk thistle: comparison with silymarin. Cancer Lett 147: 77–84, 1999.
24. Hibasami H, Achiwa Y, et al. Induction of programmed cell death (apoptosis) in human lymphoid leukemia cells by catechin compounds. Anticancer Res 16: 1943–1946, 1996.
25. Huang Y, et al. Br L Pharmacol 128: 999–1010, 1999.

26. Lee SC, et al. Anticancer Res 18: 1117–1121, 1998.
27. Denis L, Morton MS, Griffiths K. Eur Urol 35: 377–387, 1999.
28. Ferriola PC, Cody H. Protein kinase C inhibition by plant flavonoids: kinetic mechanisms and structure-activity relationships. Biochem Pharmacol 38: 1617–1624, 1989.
29. Lin JK, Chen YC, et al. Suppression of protein kinase C and nuclear oncogene expression as possible molecular mechanisms of cancer chemoprevention by apigenin and curcumin. J Cell Biochem (Suppl) 28–29: 39–48, 1997.
30. Mahoney C, Azzi A. Vitamin E inhibits protein kinase C activity. Biochem Biophys Res Commun 154: 694–697, 1988.
31. Gapalakrisgna R, Gudimeda U, Chen Z. Vitamin E succinate inhibits protein kinase C: correlation with its unique inhibitory effects on cell growth and transformation. In: Prasad K, Santamaria L, Williams R (eds). *Nutrients in Cancer Prevention and Treatment*. Totowa, NJ: Humana, 1995, pp. 21–37.
32. Raz A, Levine G, Khomiak Y. Acute local inflammation potentiates tumor growth in mice. Cancer Lett 148: 115–120, 2000.
33. Matasunaga K, Yoshimi N, et al. Inhibitory effects of nebumetone, a cyclooxygenase-2 inhibitor, and esculetin, a lipoxygenase inhibitor, on N-methyl-N-nitrosourea-induced mammary carcinogenesis in rats. Jpn J Cancer Res 89: 496–501, 1998.
34. Liu XH, Rose DP. Differential expression and regulation of cyclooxygenase-1 and -2 in two human breast cancer cell lines. Cancer Res 56: 5125–5127, 1996.
35. Rozic JG, Chakraborty C, Lala PK. Cyclooxygenase inhibitors retard murine mammary tumor progression by reducing tumor cell migration, invasiveness and angiogenesis. In J Cancer 93: 497–506, 2001.
36. Uotila P, Valve E, et al. Increased expression of cyclooxygenase-2 and nitric oxide synthease-2 in human prostate cancer. Urol Res 29: 23–28, 2001.
37. Kirschenbaum A, Liu X, et al. The role of cyclooxygenase-2 in prostate cancer. Urology 58: (2 Suppl 1): 127–131, 2001.
38. Oshima M, Taketo MM. COX selectivity and animal models for colon cancer. Curr Phar Des 8: 1021–1034, 2002.
39. O'Byrne KJ, Daleigsh AG. Chronic immune activation and inflammation as the cause of malignancy. Br J Cancer 85: 473–483, 2001.
40. Denkert C, Kobel M, et al. Expression of cyclooxygenase-2 is an independent prognostic factor in human ovarian carcinoma. Am J Path 160: 893–903, 2002.

41. Sales KJ, Katz AA, et al. Cyclooxygenase-1 is up-regulated in cervical carcinomas: autocrine/paracrine regulation of cyclooxygenase-2. Prostaglandin e receptors, and angiogenic factors by cyclooxygenase-1. Cancer Res 62: 424–432, 2002.
42. Shono T, Tofilon PJ, et al. Cyclooxygynase-2 expression in human gliomas: prognostic significance and molecular correlations. Cancer Res 61: 4375–4381, 2001.
43. Ling JG, Khalili K. Inhibition of human brain tumor cell growth by the anti-inflammatory drug, flurbiprofen. Oncogene 20: 6864–6870, 2001.
44. Kim HP, Mani I, et al. Effects of naturally-occurring flavonoids and biflavonoids on epidermal cyclooxygenase and lipoxygenase from guinea-pigs. Prostagland Leukot Essent Fatty Acids 58: 17–24, 1998.
45. Liang YC, Huang YT, et al. Suppression of inducible cyclooxygenase and inducible nitric oxide synthase by apigenin and related flavonoids in mouse macrophages. Carcinogenesis. 20: 1945–1952, 1999.
46. Connolly JM, Rose DP. Effects of dietary fatty acids on invasion through reconstituted basement membrane (Matrigel) by a human breast cancer cell line. Cancer Lett 75: 137–142, 1993.
47. Lin LI, Ke YF, et al. Curcumin inhibits SK-Hep-1 hepatocellular carcinoma cell invasion in vitro and suppresses matrix metalloproteinase-9 secretion. Oncology 55: 349–353, 1998.
48. Sidhu GS, Singh AK, et al. Enhancement of wound healing by curcumin in animals. Wound Repair Regen 6: 167–177, 1998.
49. Huang Y, et al. Br J Pharmacol 128: 999–1010, 1999.
50. Rohdewald P. Pycnogenol. In: Rice-Evans CA, Packer L (eds). *Flavonoids in Health and Disease*. New York: Marcel Dekker, Inc., 1998, pp. 405–419.
51. Nicotine stimulates angiogenesis and promotes tumor growth and atherosclerosis. Nature Medicine 7: 833–839, 2001.
52. Rose DP, Connally JM. Antiangiogenicity of docosahexaenoic acid and its role in the suppression of breast cancer cell growth in nude mice. In J Oncol 15: 1011–1015, 1999.
53. Fotis T, Pepper MS, et al. Flavonoids, dietary-derived inhibitors of cell proliferation and in vitro angiogenesis. Cancer Res 57: 2916–2921, 1997.
54. Allred CD, Ju YH, et al. Dietary genistin stimulates growth of estrogen-dependent breast cancer tumors similar to that observed with genistein. Carcinogenesis 22: 1667–1673, 2001.
55. Hargreaves DF, Potten CS, et al. Two-week dietary soy supple-

mentation has an estrogenic effect on normal premenopausal breast. J Clin Endocrinol Metab 84: 4017–4024, 1999.
56. Larionov AA, Uporov AV, et al. Correlation between tumor tissue aromatase, histological pattern and reproductive status in patients with breast cancer. Vopr Onkol 44: 37–42, 1998.
57. Santen RJ, Yue W, et al. The potential of aromatase inhibitors in breast cancer prevention. Endoc Relat Cancer 6: 235–243, 1999.
58. Ernster VL, Wrensch MR, et al. Benign and malignant breast disease: initial study results of serum and breast fluid analysis of endogenous estrogens. JNCI 79: 949–960, 1987.
59. Rosenberg RS, Grass L, et al. Modulation of androgen and progesterone receptors by phytochemicals in breast cancer cell lines. Biochem Biophys Res Commun 248: 935–939, 1998.
60. Baker ME, Medlock KL, Sheehan DM. Flavonoids inhibit estrogen binding to rat alpha-fetoprotein. Proc Soc Exp Biol Med 217: 317–321, 1998.
61. Pelissero C, Lenczowski MJ, et al. J Steroid Biochem Mol Biol 57: 215–223, 1996.
62. Spear AT, Sherman AR. Iron deficiency alters DMBA-induced tumor burden and natural killer cell cytotoxicity. J Nutr 122: 46–55, 1992.
63. Van Acker SA, Bast A, Van der Vijgh WJ. Structural aspects of antioxidant activity of flavonoids. In: Rice-Evans CA and Packer L (eds). *Flavonoids in Health and Disease*. New York: Marcel Dekker, Inc., 1998, pp. 221–251.
64. Lautraite S, Musonda AC, et al. Flavonoids inhibit genetic toxicity produced by carcinogens in cells expressing CYP1A2 and CYP1A1. Mutagenesis 17: 45–53, 2002.
65. Blaylock RL. New developments in phytoprevention and treatment of cancer. J Am Nutr Assoc 2: 19–29, 1999.
66. Daly AK, Cholerton S, et al. Metabolic polymorphism. Pharmac Ther 57: 129–160, 1993.
67. Liska DJ. The detoxification enzyme systems. Alter Med Rev 3: 187–198, 1998.
68. Blakely SR, Grundel E, et al. Alterations in ß-carotene and vitamin E status in rats fed ß-carotene and excess vitamin A. Nutr Res 10: 1035–1044, 1990.
69. Prasad KN, Edwards-Prasad J. Effect of tocopherol (vitamin E) acid succinate on morphological alterations and growth inhibition in melanoma cells in culture. Cancer Res 42: 550–555, 1982.

CHAPTER 7

1. Elliott RL, Head JF, McCoy JL. Relationship of serum and tumor levels of iron and iron-binding proteins to lymphocyte immunity against tumor antigen in breast cancer patients. Breast Ca Res Treatment 30: 305–309, 1994.
2. Head JF, Wang F, et al. Assessment of immunological competence and host reactivity against tumor antigens in breast cancer patients. Ann NY Acad Sci 690: 340–342, 1993.
3. Levenson SM, Rettura G, Seifer E. Effects of supplemental dietary vitamin A and ß-carotene on experimental tumors. Local tumor excision, chemotherapy, radiation injury and radiotherapy. In: Butterworth CE and Hutchenson ML (eds). *Nutritional Factors in the Induction and Maintenance of Malignancy*. New York: Academic Press, Inc., 1983 pp. 169–203.
4. Head JF, Elliott RL, McCoy JL. Effect of adjuvant chemotherapy on lymphocyte-mediated immunity in breast cancer patients. Annual Meeting of the Society for Biological Therapy, 1993.
5. DeLaney TF, Afridi N, et al. 13-cis-retinoic acid with alpha-2a-interferon enhances radiation cytotoxicity in head and neck squamous cell carcinoma in vitro. Cancer Res 56: 2277–2280, 1996.
6. Vetvicka V, Terayama K, et al. Pilot study: orally-administered yeast ß1,3-glucan prophylactically protects against anthrax infection and cancer in mice. J Amer Nutr Assoc 5: 1–5, 2002.
7. Kimura Y, Tojima H, et al. Clinical evaluation of sizofilan as assistant immunotherapy in treatment of head and neck cancer. Acta Otolaryngol 511: 192–195, 1994.
8. Mayell M. Maitake extracts and their therapeutic potential—a review. Alternative Medicine Rev 6: 48–60, 2001.
9. Kodama N, Komuta K, Naba H. Can maitake MD-fraction aid cancer patients? Alternative Med Rev 7: 236–239, 2002.
10. Kogan G, Sandula J, et al. Increased efficiency of Lewis lung carcinoma chemotherapy with a macrophage stimulator-yeast carboxymethyl glucan. Int Immunopharmacol 2: 775–781, 2002.
11. Grube BJ, Eng ET, et al. White button mushroom phytochemicals inhibit aromatase activity and breast cancer cell proliferation. J Nutr 131: 3288–3293, 2001.
12. Guo XM, Li JX, Yang XF. Clinical observation on 112 cases

with non-Hodgkin's lymphoma treated by Chinese herbs combined with chemotherapy. Zhongguo Zhong Xi Yi Ie He Za Zhi 17: 325–327, 1997.
13. Kurashiige S, Jin R, et al. Anticarcinogenic effects of shikaron, a preparation of eight Chinese herbs in mice treated with a carcinogen, N-butyl-N-butaolnitrosamine. Cancer Invest 16: 166–169, 1998.
14. Sadava D, Ahn J, et al. Effects of four Chinese herbal extracts on drug-sensitive and multidrug-resistant small-cell lung carcinoma cells. Cancer Chemother Pharmacol 49: 261–266, 2002.
15. Kang LY, Pan XZ, et al. Chinese herbal formula XQ–9302: pilot study of its clinical and in vitro activity against human immunodeficiency virus. Hong Kong Med J 5: 135–139, 1999.
16. Kuhara T, Iigo M, et al. Orally administered lactoferrin exerts an anti-metastatic effect and enhances production of IL–18 in the intestinal epithelium. Nutr Cancer 38: 192–199, 2000.
17. Connely OM. Antiinflammatory activities of lactoferrin. J Amer Coll Nutr 20: (suppl) 389S–395S, 2001.
18. Porterfield H. UsToo PC-SPES surveys: review of studies and update of previous survey results. Mol Urol 4: 289–291, 2000.
19. Pirani JF. The effects of phytotherapeutic agents on prostate cancer: an overview of recent clinical trials of PC-SPES. Urology 58 (2 Suppl 1): 36–38, 2001.
20. Hsieh TC, Wu JM. Mechanism of action of herbal supplement PC-SPES: elucidation of effects of individual herbs of PC-SPES on proliferation and prostate specific gene expression in androgen-dependent LNCaP cells. In J Oncol 20: 583–588, 2002.
21. Hsieh TC, Lu X, et al. Effects of herbal preparation Equiguard™ on hormone-responsive and hormone-refractory prostate carcinoma cells: mechanistic studies. In J Oncol 20: 681–689, 2002.
22. Yun TK, Choi SY. Non-organ specific cancer prevention of ginseng: a prospective study in Korea. In J Epidemiol 27: 359–364, 1998.
23. Kim JY, Germolec DR, Luster MI. Panax ginseng as a potential immunomodulator: studies in mice. Immunopharmacol Immunotoxicol 12: 257–276, 1990.
24. Shinkai K, Akedo H, et al. Inhibition of in vitro tumor cell invasion by ginsenoside Rg3. Jpn J Cancer Res 87: 357–362, 1996.

25. Sato K, Mochoizuki M, et al. Inhibition of tumor angiogenesis and metastasis by a saponin of Panax ginseng, ginsenoside-Rb2. Biol Pharm Bull 17: 635–639, 1994.
26. Oh M, Choi YH, et al. Anti-proliferating effects of ginsenoside Rh2 on MCF-7 human breast cancer cells. In J Oncol 14: 869–875, 1999.
27. Liu WK, Xu SX, Che CT. Anti-proliferative effect of ginseng saponins on human prostate cancer cell line. Life Sci 67: 1297–1306, 2000.
28. Lee YN, Lee HY, et al. In vitro induction of differentiation by ginsenosides in F9 teratocarcinoma cells. Eur J Cancer 32A: 1420–1428, 1996.
29. Mochisuki M, Yoo YC, et al. Inhibitory effect of tumor metastasis in mice by saponins, ginsenoside-Rb2, 20(R)-and 20(S)-ginsenoside-RG3, of red ginseng. Biol Pharm Bull 18: 1197–1202, 1995.
30. Li J, Zhang J. Inhibition of apoptosis by ginsenoside Rg1 in cultured cortical neurons. Chin Med J110: 535–539, 1997.
31. Yun T-K, Choi S-Y, Yun HY. Epidemiological study on cancer prevention by ginseng: are all kinds of cancers preventable by ginseng? J Korean Med Sci 16 (suppl): S19–27, 2001.
32. Harkey MR, Henderson GL, et al. Variability in commercial ginseng products: an analysis of 25 preparations. Am J Clin Nutr 73: 1101–1106, 2001.

Chapter 8

1. Vogelzang N, Breutbart W, et al. Patient, caregiver, and oncologist perceptions of cancer-related fatigue: results of a tripart assessment survey. The Fatigue Coalition. Seminars. Hematology 34 (3 Suppl 2): 4–12, 1997.
2. Lasne C, et al. Transforming activities of sodium fluoride in cultured Syrian hamster embryo and BALB/3T3 cells. Cell Biol Toxicol 4: 311–324, 1988.
3. Taylor A, Taylor NC. Effect of fluoride on tumor growth. Proc Soc Exper Biol Med 65: 252–255, 1965.
4. Yiamouyannis J. *Fluoride: The Aging Factor.* Delaware, Ohio: Health Action Press, 1993, pp. 73–90.
5. Ferrer JF, Kenyon SJ, Gupta P. Milk of dairy cows frequently contains a leukemogenic virus. Science 213: 1014–1016, 1981.
6. Mahmound FA, Rivera N. The role of C-reactive protein as a

prognostic indicator in advanced cancer. Curr Oncol Rep 4: 250–255, 2002.

7. New SA, Robins SP, et al. Dietary influences on bone mass and bone metabolism: further evidence of a positive link between fruit and vegetable consumption and bone health. Am J Clin Nutr 71: 142–151, 2000.
8. Telang NT, Katdare M, et al. Inhibition of proliferation and modulation of estradiol metabolism: novel mechanisms for breast cancer prevention by the phytochemical indole-3-carbinol. Proc Soc Exp Biol Med 216: 246–252, 1997.
9. Cover CM, Hsieh SJ, et al. Indole-3 carbinol inhibits the expression of cyclin-dependent kinase-6 and induces a G1 cell cycle arrest of human breast cancer cells independent of estrogen receptor signaling. J Biol Chem 273: 3838–3847, 1998.
10. Rosen CA, Woodson GE, et al. Preliminary results of the use of indole-3-carbinol for recurrent respiratory papillomatosis. Otolaryngol Head Neck Surg 118: 810–815, 1998.
11. Oganesian A, Hendricks JD, Williams DE. Long-term dietary indole-3-carbinol inhibits diethylnitrosamine-initiated hepatocarcinogenesis in the infant mouse model. Cancer Lett 118: 87–94, 1997.
12. Powell KE, Caspersen CJ, et al. Physical activity and chronic diseases. Am J Clin Nutri 49: 999–1006, 1989.
13. Sullivan DH, Patch GA, et al. Impact of nutrition status on morbidity and mortality in a selected population of geriatric rehabilitation patients. Am J Clin Nutr 51: 749–758, 1990.
14. Kujala UM, Kaprio J, et al. Relationship of lesiure-time physical activity and mortality. The Finnish Twin Cohort. JAMA 279: 440–444, 1998.
15. Packer L. Oxidants, antioxidant nutrients and the athlete. J Sports Sci 15: 353–363, 1997.

Appendix A: Suggested Reading

Altman, Roberta, and Michael J. Sarg. *The Cancer Dictionary.* New York: Checkmark Books, 2000.

Bland, Jeffrey S. *Genetic Nutritioneering: How You Can Modify Inherited Traits and Live a Longer, Healthier Life.* Los Angeles: Keats Publishing, 1999.

Blaylock, Russell L. *Health and Nutrition Secrets That Can Save Your Life.* Albuquerque, NM: Health Press, 2002.

Boik, John C. *Natural Compounds in Cancer Therapy.* Birmingham, AL: American Nutraceutical Association, 2001.

Gordon, James S., and Sharon Curtain. *Comprehensive Cancer Care: Integrating Alternative, Complementary, and Conventional Therapies.* Cambridge, MA: Perseus Publishing, 2000.

Hoffman, Edward Jack. *Cancer and the Search for Selective Biochemical Inhibitors.* Boca Raton, FL: CRC Press, 1999.

Moss, Ralph W. *The Cancer Industry.* New York: Equinox Press, 1999.

Moss, Ralph W. *Cancer Therapy: The Independent Consumer's Guide to Non-Toxic Treatment and Prevention.* New York: Equinox Press, 1996.

Moss, Ralph W. *Questioning Chemotherapy.* New York: Equinox Press, 1995.

Murray, Michael T. *The Healing Power of Foods.* Roseville, CA: Prima Publishing, 1993.

Pizzorno, Joseph. *Total Wellness.* Roseville, CA: Prima Publishing, 1996.

Quillin, Patrick. *Beating Cancer with Nutrition.* Tulsa, OK: Nutrition Times Press, 2001.

Regush, Nicholas. *The Virus Within: A Coming Epidemic.* New York: Dutton, 2000.

Varmus, Harold E., and Robert A. Weinberg. *Genes and the Biology of Cancer.* New York: Scientific American Library, 1993.

World Cancer Research Fund and American Institute for Cancer Research. *Food, Nutrition and the Prevention of Cancer: A Global Perspective.* Washington, DC: American Institute for Cancer Research, 1997.

Appendix B: Diagnostic Laboratories

Great Smokies Diagnostic Laboratory
63 Zillicoa Street
Asheville, NC 28801
Toll-free: 800-522-4762
Fax: 828-252-9303
Website: www.gsdl.com

This lab performs numerous tests, but of special interest to the cancer patient are the tests for Candida infection, disbiosis bowel studies, tests for toxic metals, detoxification tests, extensive estrogen profiles, and lipid profiles that define the balance of the omega-3 and omega-6 fats and their metabolic products. The lab strives for high quality results and uses the newest diagnostic tests.

Great Plains Laboratory
9335 West 75th Street
Overland Park, KS 66204
Phone: 913-341-8949
Toll-free: 888-347-2781
Fax: 913-341-6207
Website: www.greatplainslaboratory.com
E-mail: GPL4U@aol.com

This lab also performs a wide array of tests, overlapping many of the tests described above. It offers tests for toxic metals, tests for Candida infection, detoxification profiles, food allergy tests, and tests for oxidative damage. It offers an immunodeficiency evaluation panel, but unfortunately, it does not include cellular immunity assays. It also offers detailed testing for Candida bowel overgrowth, including systemic infections.

Immunosciences Lab, Inc.
8639 Wilshire Boulevard
Beverly Hills, CA 90211
Toll-free: 800-950-4686
Fax: 310-657-1053
Website: www.immuno-sci-lab.com
E-mail: immunsci@ix.netcom.com

This lab offers a large array of in-depth immune studies, including on the immune complexes, all of the interleukins, natural killer cell cytotoxic activity, and tumor necrosis factor-alpha. It also has a test for the detection of mutated p53. All of these tests are of great interest to doctors treating cancer patients and allow close monitoring of the patients' tumor-fighting immune status.

MetaMetrix Clinical Laboratory
4855 Peachtree Industrial Boulevard
Norcross, GA 30092
Phone: 770-446-5483
Toll-free: 800-221-4640
Fax: 770-441-2237
Website: www.metametrix.com
E-mail: inquiries@metametrix.com

This lab offers a series of high-quality tests, many of which are offered by the other diagnostic laboratories. It has an impressive fatty acid analysis that includes the trans fatty acids and omega-9 fatty acids. In addition, it performs IGF-1 profiles and a test for oxidative damage.

Medical Diagnostics Laboratories
133 Gaither Drive
Suite C
Mt. Laurel, NJ 08054
Toll-free: 877-269-0090
Fax: 856-608-1667
Website: www.mdlab.com
E-mail: Sales@mdlab.com

This lab does extremely accurate testing for numerous viral, mycoplasmal, rickettsial, and bacterial diseases, as well as other highly technical tests.

International Molecular Diagnostics
15162 Triton Lane
Huntington Beach, CA 92649
Phone: 714-799-7177
Website: www.ımmed.org

This lab does a wide variety of testing, including studies for mycoplasma, rickettsia, and other infectious organisms.

Resource List

Compounding Pharmacies

Apothecary Pharmacy
800-889-9159
www.the-apothecary.com

Specialty Pharmacy
877-866-4979
www.specialtyrx.com

Willner Chemists
800-633-1106
www.willner.com

Dental Products

Desert Essence®
800-645-5768
www.desertessence.com

Complete line of antiseptic and cleansing oral care products using tea tree oil for deep cleaning and disinfecting of teeth and gums. All products are animal and eco-friendly and made without artificial colors, sweeteners, or harsh abrasives. They carry a line of Tea Tree Oil Dental Floss, Tea Tree Oil Dental Tape, Tea Tree Oil Dental Pics. They also carry Tea Tree Oil Mouth Wash and Tea Tree Oil Toothpastes that are fluoride free and contain no artificial preservatives, sweeteners, coloring or harsh abrasives. Available in health food stores.

Woodstock Natural Products, Inc.
800-615-6895
The Natural Dentist™

This company has a line of products that include an assortment of toothpaste and mouth rinses. Available in health food stores.

Environmental Products

N.E.E.D.S.
800-634-1380
www.needs.com

This is a total resource for every type of environmental product that is on the market today. They stock air cleaners for house and car and have special air cleaners available for multiple chemical sensitivities. They also stock specific airborne chemical product filters. Filters for airborne mold, toxins and biological problems are also available. They carry the Doulton Water Filter, shower filters and many other environmental products.

Natural Cleaning Products

Allens Naturally
800-352-8971
www.allensnaturally.com

Offers organic dishwasher and washing machine detergents, as well as glass and all-purpose cleansers. Its products are free of perfumes, dyes, and phosphates, and are biodegradable.

Planet
800-858-8449
www.planetinc.com

Products include organic dishwasher and washing machine detergents, and glass and all-purpose cleansers. Its products are free of perfumes, dyes, and phosphates, and are biodegradable.

Nutritional Supplements

The bulk of the supplements recommended in this list are made by the following supplement houses. For further information on any of the supplements, either call the company's toll-free telephone number or check its website. Most of the products listed can be found at your local health food store or obtained through your physician.

Carotec, Inc.
800-522-4279
www.carotec.com

Garden of Life
800-622-8986
www.gardenoflifeusa.com or www.gardenoflife.com

Healthy Origins
888-228-6650
www.healthyorigins.com

Jarrow Formulas®
800-726-0886
www.Jarrow.com

J.R. Carlson Laboratories, Inc.
888-234-5656
www.carlsonlabs.com

Longevity Plus
800-580-PLUS (7587)
www.longevityplus.net

Longevity Science
800-933-9440
www.longevity-science.net

Planetary Formulas
800-606-6226
www.planetaryformulas.com

Source Naturals Inc.
800-815-2333
www.sourcenaturals.com

Thorne Research
800-228-1966
www.thorne.com

Vitamin Research Products
800-877-2447
www.vrp.com

Acetyl-L-Carnitine

J.R. Carlson Laboratories, Inc.
L-Carnitine
Available in either capsule or powder form.

Longevity Science
Acetyl-L-Carnitine
Available in capsule form 500 mg

Source Naturals Inc.
Acetyl L-Carnitine
Each tablet contains Acetyl L-Carnitine 250 mg and 500 mg.

L-Carnitine
Available in capsule form 250 mg

Thorne Research
Carnityl®
Each capsule contains Acetyl-L-Carnitine 500 mg.

Vitamin Research Products
Acetyl-L-Carnitine
Capsule form 500 mg take on empty stomach.

Adaptogens

Gaia Herbs, Inc.
800-831-7780
www.gaiaherbs.com
Rhodiola Rosea
Standardized to full activity. Each liquid filled capsule contains 400 mg.

Alpha Lipoic Acid

Healthy Origins
Alpha Lipoic Acid
Available in 50 mg and 300 mg capsules.

J.R. Carlson Laboratories, Inc.
Alpha Lipoic
Available in tablet form containing 100 mg and 300 mg.

Longevity Science
Alpha Lipoic Acid
Available in capsule form 100 mg.

Source Naturals Inc.
Alpha-Lipoic Acid
Available in tablet form (50 mg, 100 mg, and 200 mg)

Vitamin Research Products
R-Lipoic Acid
Available in capsule form (50 mg). Do not take more than 50 mg a day of this form of Alpha-Lipoic Acid. Higher doses can cause low blood sugar (hypoglycemia).

Antioxidant Combinations

J.R. Carlson Laboratories, Inc.
ACES
Contains Pro-Vitamin A (D. Salina Beta-Carotene) 10,000 I.U., Buffered Vitamin C 1,000 mg., Vitamin E 400 I.U., and Selenium 100 mcg. Provided by two softgels.

Thorne Research
Basic Antioxidant™
Each capsule contains Vitamin A (as Beta Carotene), Vitamin C (as Ascorbic Acid), Vitamin E (d-Alpha Tocopheryl), and Selenium (as selenium Picolinate).

Vitamin Research Products
Extension Antioxidant
A combination including green tea, tumeric, grape seed, vitamin C and other ingredients. Available in capsule form.

Arabinogalactan

Larex, Inc.
800-386-5300
www.larex.com
Cleartrac Ag
Available in powder form (250 gm)

Source Naturals Inc.
Larch Extract™
Standardized to 85% Arabinogalactans in tablet form.

Thorne Research
Arabinex®
Each scoop contains Arabinogalactans (from Larch) 4.7 grams.

Beta-Glucans

ImmuDyne, Inc.
888-246-6839
www.immudyne.com
Macroforce®
Plus C
Contains Beta-1,2 and Beta-1,6 D-Glucan 7.5 mg in vegetable capsules.
Source Naturals Inc.
Beta 1,3/1,6 Glucan
One tablet contains Beta-1,3/1,6-Glucan (250 mg)

Vitamin Research Products
Beta 1,3-D Glucan
Available in capsule form (100 mg).

Beta-Carotene

J.R. Carlson Laboratories, Inc.
Super Beta-Carotene
From *D. salina* algae
Available in softgel containing 16 mg of D. salina beta-carotene.

Jarrow Formulas®
Beta Carotene-Marine
Contains 10,000 I.U. (6 mg) of pro vitamin A activity. Available in softgels.

Thorne Research
Beta Carotene
Each capsule contains Vitamin A (as mixed carotenes) 25,000 I.U.

Bioflavonoids

Source Naturals Inc.
Bioflavonoid Complex
Each tablet contains Vitamin C (magnesium ascorbate) 254 mg, Magnesium (as magnesium ascorbate) 19 mg, Hawthorn Berry Extract 150 mg, Rosemary Leaf Extract 150 mg, Quercetin 100 mg, plus other antioxidants.

Vitamin Research Products
Bioflavonoid Complex with Quercetin
A balanced mix of select bioflavonoids including a standardized extract of quercetin. Available in capsule form.

Biotin

J.R. Carlson Laboratories, Inc.
Biotin
Available in tablet form 1,000 mcg.

Thorne Research
Biotin—8
Available in capsule form (8,000 mcg).

Vitamin Research Products
Biotin
Available in capsule form (10mg).

Blueberry Extract

Herbal Therapeutics, Inc.
800-611-8235
www.herbalist-alchemist.com

Blueberry Solid Extract
Blueberries contain flavonoids, which are potent antioxidants.

Tree of Life
www.treeoflife.com

Blueberry Extract
Derived from wild blueberries and loaded with nutrients.

Borage Seed Oil

Source Naturals Inc.
Mega-GLA 240™ and Mega-GLA 300™
Borage Seed Oil Hexane-Free
GLA (gamma-linolenic acid) is an essential polyunsaturated fatty acid. Each 240 mg softgel contains Gamma Linolenic Acid (GLA).

Boron

Thorne Research
Boron Picolinate
Each capsule contains Boron (as Boron Picolinate) 3mg.

Vitamin Research Products
Boron Caps
Available in capsule form containing 3 mg of boron from boron amino acid chelate.

Broccoli Sprouts Extract

Source Naturals Inc.
Broccoli Sprouts
Standardized Extract
Each tablet contains Broccoli Sprouts Standardized Extract 120 mg yielding 150 mcg Sulforaphane.

Bromelain

Source Naturals Inc.
Bromelain
500 mg, 600 mg, and 2,000 G.D.U./gram
Bromelain is a pineapple enzyme. Each 600 G.D.U./g tablet contains Bromelain 500 mg.

Thorne Research
M.F. Bromelain®
Each capsule contains Bromelain (3,200 m.c.u/gm) 500 mg.

Vitamin Research Products
Bromelain Extract
Helps in digesting protein. Each capsule contains 250 mg and 600 gdu.

Calcium

BioCalth International Inc.
888-275-1717
www.biocalth.com

Calcium L-Threonate
This formulation helps to form new collagen and the calcium is 95% absorbed. Effective for reduction of pain, cramps and weakness in the limbs.

Source Naturals Inc.
Calcium D-Glucarate
Two 500 mg tablets contain Calcium (from 1,000 mg calcium d-glucarate) 123 mg

Thorne Research
Calcium Citramate™
Each capsule contains Calcium (as Calcium Citrate-Malate) 160 mg, Malic Acid (approximately from Calcium Citrate-Malate) 265 mg.

Calcium D-Glucarate
Each capsule contains Calcium D-Glucarate 500 mg.

Vitamin Research Products
Calcium Citrate/Malate Caps
Highly absorbable form of calcium 170 mg in capsule form.

Ca-AEP
Calcium-AEP is essential for neurotransmission, nerve impulse generation, and muscular contractions. Available in capsule form (500 mg)

Celmend™

Contains Calcium glucarate, Ellagic acid and Resveratrol. Available in capsule form.

Carnitine

Vitamin Research Products
L-Carnitine

Available in capsule form (250 mg)

Carotenoids

Vitamin Research Products
CAROTeam™

Contains vitamin E succinate, vitamin C, vitamin A and lutein. Available in capsule form.

Coenzyme Q10

J.R. Carlson Laboratories, Inc.
CoQ10

Softgel form available in 50 mg, 100 mg, 200 mg, and 300 mg.

Carotec, Inc.
CoQ10

Each softgel contains 100 mg co-enzyme Q-10 with 50 mg palm tocotrienols.

Jarrow Formulas®
Q-Absorb™ CoQ10

Available in softgels (100 mg).

Source Naturals Inc.
Coenzyme Q10

Available in 30 mg and 100 mg softgels with Bioperine.

Tishcon Corp
Q-Gel
www.Qgel.com

Comes in 60 and 100 mg doses.

Thorne Research Products
Idebenone 100 mg
May work better than CoQ10 for heart disease.

Lipoquinone-100®
Coenzyme Q10 100 mg (in rice bran oil with Vitamin E as a preservative). Available in gelcaps.

Vitamin Research Products
CoQ10
Available in capsule form 30 mg, 75 mg, 150 mg, and in softgels 100 mg.

Colostrum

Proper Nutrition, Inc.
Colostrum
100% pure Bovine Colostrum in capsule for 500 mg.

Source Naturals Inc.
Colostrum
Available in Powder—650 mg tablets and 500 mg capsules.
Each 500 mg capsule contains Colostrum Powder 500 mg.
Each 650 tablet contains Standardized Colostrum (dried) 650 mg yielding 195 mg of naturally occurring immunoglubulins (proteins).
Each teaspoon of Colostrum powder contains Colostrum (from dried bovine colostrums 2g yielding 600 mg of naturally occurring immunoglobulins (proteins).

Colostrum Transfer Factor™
Supports Immune System Response
One capsule contains: Polyvalent Transfer Factor 5mg (as colostral fraction with minimum 20 potency units).

Vitamin Research Products
Immunesource™
(Liquid Colostrum)
Recommended dosage 1 teaspoon sublingually.

Conjugated Linoleic Acid

Jarrow Formulas®
CLA 750
Conjugated Linoleic Acid
1,000 mg softgel containing a concentrated 750 mg Conjugated Linoleic Acid.

Longevity Science
Tonalin®
Available in softgel 750 mg

Source Naturals Inc.
Tonalin 1000™
Three 1,000 mg sofgels contains Conjugated Linoleic Acid (Tonalin™) 2.22 g

Vitamin Research Products
CLA (Conjugated Linoleic Acid)
Each softgel contains 1,000 mg of CLA.

Cranberry

J.R. Carlson Laboratories, Inc.
Cranberry Concentrate
Available in softgels containing 1,000 mg of cranberry juice concentrate plus 10 mg of Vitamin C.
Vitamin Research Products
Actibotic™
Two capsules contain cranberry berry 400 mg and other ingredients.

Cranberry Concentrate
Capsules containing 600 mg

Curcumin

Jarrow Formulas®
Curcumin-95
Curcuma Longa
500 mg Standardized Turmeric extract. 95% curcuminoids, 18:1 concentrate.

Vitamin Research Products
Turmeric Extract (Curcuma Longa)
Available in capsule form containing 98% curcuminoids.

Dandelion Root Extract

Vitamin Research Products
Dandelion Root Extract (Taraxacum Officinale)
Available in capsule form (500 mg)

Detoxification Products

Thorne Research
Mediclear™
A rice protein-based nutritional supplement useful for allergy relief, bowel and hepatic detoxification and inflammatory control. In powdered form.

Vitamin Research Products
Detox Fiberplex
Fiber rich, Phytonutrient complex promotes detoxification and improves gastrointestinal function. Helps to bind toxic material for elimination.

Digestive Aids

Thorne Research
Betaine HCL and Pepsin
Each capsule contains Betaine Hydrochloride8-grains (520 mg), Pure Lactose Free Pepsin (20 mg).

Diindolylmethane

Source Naturals Inc.
DIM
A metabolite found in cruciferous vegetables. One tablet contains: Viotamin E (as D-alpha tocopheryl) 50 IU, Calcium 53mg, DIM 100 mg, Phosphatidyl Choline 50 mg, and Bioperine 3 mg.

Vitamin Research Products
BioDIM™
Contains DIM, or diindolylmethane, a phytonutrient found in broccoli, cauliflower, cabbage and Brussels sprouts. Available in capsule form 75 mg and 150 mg.

Dimercaptosuccinic Acid

Vitamin Research Products
DMSA

Binds efficiently to mercury, lead, cadmium and zinc. Available in capsule form (100 mg). Take on an empty stomach.

Diosmin–Hesperidin Methyl Chalcone

Thorne Research
Diosmin-HMC

Each capsule contains Diosmin 400 mg and Hesperidin Methyl Chalcone 50 mg.

Docosahexaenoic Acid

Carotec, Inc.
DHA Neuromins®

Each 500 mg softgel of Neuromins® contains 100 mg of DHA from microalgae.

Source Naturals Inc.
DHA Neuromins®

Dietary supplement derived from micro-algae. Available in softgels 100 mg and 200mg. Each softgel contains Docosahexaenoic Acid (DHA).

Thorne Research
DHA
(Omega-3 from algae)

Each gelcap contains DHA (ducosahexaenoic acid from algae oil) 250 mg. Also contains olive oil and Vitamin E.

Vitamin Research Products
DHA

Docosahexaenoic acid is a component of fish oil and is an omega-3 fatty acid. Available in sofgels 135 mg.

Energy Enhancers

Nutritional Therapeutics, Inc.
800-982-9158
www.propax.com

Propax with NT Factor™
Fights fatigue and enhances energy.

Enzymes

Douglas Laboratories
800-245-4440
www.douglaslabs.com

Betaine HCL
Supplement is used to add acid to the stomach.

Garden of Life
Omega Zyme™
Digestive enzyme blend in powdered form.

Longevity Plus
Wobenzym®Med
Used to treat Autoimmune Diseases, Rheumatic Diseases, Vascular Diseases, Inflammations, Injuries, Infections, and Tumors. Also improves the functioning of all body organs/systems. Take on empty stomach.

Pure Encapsulation
800-753-2277
www.PureCaps.com

Pancreatic Vegenzymes L™
Product is derived only from plants. Contains amylase, lipase and protease. Available in capsule form.

Thorne Research
Planti-zyme™
Product derived from plants only. Contains three basic enzymes plus cellulose and lactase in high concentrations.

Tyler Encapsulations
800-869-9705
www.Tyler-inc.com
Has a wide assortment of excellent products for the gastrointestinal tract.

Vitamin Research Products
Digezyme™
For better digestion. Contains Amylase, Neutral Protease, Lactase, Lipase and Cellulase in capsule form.

Evening Primrose Oil

Source Naturals Inc.
Evening Primrose Oil
Hexane-Free 500 mg and 1,350 mg
Softgels contain Oil of Evening Primrose, yielding: Linoleic Acid, GLA (as gamma linolenic acid).

Fiber Sources

Pure Encapsulations, Inc.
Nutra-Flax
Flax seed powder.
Helps maintains ratio of 2-hydroxy and 16-hydroxyestrone.

Prothera™
SpectraFiber™
888-488-2488
www.protheraine.com
Made from glucomannan, prune fiber, apple pectin, celery stalk and leaves, citrus pectin, slippery elm bark, and fennel seed powder.

5-Hydroxytryptophan

Healthy Origins
5-HTP is a naturally occurring standardized extract of Griffonia simplicifolla containing greater than 99% pure 5-hydroxytryptophan (5-HTP).

Vitamin Research Products
5-HTP (5-Hydroxytryptophan)
Available in capsule form (33 mg, 50 mg, 100 mg)

Folic Acid

Thorne Research
Folacal®
Available in capsule form (800 mcg)

Folac Acid Liquid
(.1% dilution w/v)
Provides 50 mcg folate per drop.

Vitamin Research Products
Folic Acid
Available in capsule form (800 mcg)

Gamma Linolenic Acid

Vitamin Research Products
GLA (Gamma Linolenic Acid)
Available in softgels (240 mg)

Garlic

Source Naturals Inc.
Garlic Oil
Tasteless and Odorless
Available in sofgels (0.2 mg)

Vitamin Research Products
Garlic Extract (Allium Sativum)
Immune booster with antimicrobial, antiviral properties. (No less than 10,000 ppm allicin.)

Wakunaga of America
800-421-2998
www.kyolic.com

Kyolic®Aged Garlic Extract (Age)
Highly researched garlic product. Available in capsules as well as in liquid form.

Garlic Products

Kyolic
Aged garlic extract

Contains 700 mg of extract plus enzymes to activate garlic. This is the form of garlic used in most cancer experiments.

Enzymatic Therapy®
Garlinase 4000

Standardized to contain 3.4% alliin. 5000 ug allicin—the active anti-cancer ingredient.

Germanium

Vitamin Research Products
Germanium Sesquioxide
(GE-132)

Germanium is a natural pain killer and nutrient for the immune system. Available in capsules (150 mg).

Ginkgo Biloba Extract

J.R. Carlson Laboratories, Inc.
Ginkgo Biloba

Each standardized softgel contains: Ginkgo Biloba Extract (24% Ginkgoflavone-glycosides) 40 mg and L-Glutamine 200 mg.

Source Naturals Inc.
Ginkgo-24™

Available in 40 mg, 60 mg, and 120 mg tablets.

Vitamin Research Products
Ginko Biloba Extract

Available in 60 mg and 120 mg capsules.

Ginseng

Planetary Formulas
Ginseng Revitalizer

Contains Asian Ginseng root, Licorice root, Astragalus root, plus other ingredients. In tablet form (1000 mg).

Vitamin Research Products
Ginseng Extracts

Two forms of Ginseng, Korean and Siberian, stimulates immune system. 300 mg in capsules.

Glutamine

Source Naturals Inc.
L-Glutamine

Free-form available in 500 mg tablets and powder.

Thorne Research
L-Glutamine

Each capsule contains Glutamine (as L-Glutamine) 500 mg.

Vitamin Research Products
L-Glutamine

Available in capsule form (500 mg)

Glutathione

J.R. Carlson Laboratories, Inc.
Glutathione Booster®

Contains nutrients, which act as a precursor to elevate glutathione in the body in capsule form.

Healthy Origins
L-Glutathione

A naturally derived substance that is a biologically active sulfur amino acid tripeptide compound containing three amino acids: L-Cysteine, L-Glutamic Acid and Glycene produced in Japan through a fermentation process and is pharmaceutical grade. Available in 250 mg capsules.

Source Naturals Inc.
L-Glutathione

Free-form available in tablet form (50 mg and 250 mg)

Grape Seed Extract

J.R. Carlson Laboratories, Inc.
Grape Seed Extract

Cellulose-coated tablets for ease in swallowing. Each tablet contains 130 mg Grape Seed Extract and 50 mg Citrus Bioflavonoids.

Pure Encapsulations
Grape pip 500 mg (grape seed extract)
800-753-2277

Source Naturals Inc.
Grape Seed Extract
Proanthodyn™ 100 mg and 200 mg

Each 100-mg tablet contains Grape Seed Extract (Proanthodyn™) with a proanthocyanidolic value of 95.

Thorne Research
O.P.C.-100™

Each capsule contains Oligomeric proanthocyanidin extract (from Grape Seeds) (95%) 30 mg.

Vitamin Research Products
Grape Seed Extract

Standardized to contain a high concentration of the proanthocyanidins. Available in capsule form (50 mg and 100 mg).

Green Food Complex

Vitamin Research Products
Primary Greens

Contains potent sources of chlorophyll, antioxidant enzymes, essential trace elements, vitamins, polypeptides and pH alkalizers. Available in capsules and powder form.

Green Tea Extract

Carotec, Inc.
Green Tea Phytomicrosphere

Each capsule contains 350 mg of Green Tea Extract and 50 mg of catechins.

Source Naturals Inc.
Green Tea Extract
100 mg tablet

Two 100 mg tablets contain: Green Tea Leaf Standardized Extract (200 mg) yielding 60 mg Epigallocatechin Gallate.

Vitamin Research Products
Green Tea Extract

Contains a potency of 52% polyphenols per capsule with reduced caffeine.

Herbal Supplements

J.R. Carlson Laboratories, Inc.
Bilberry

Standardized each softgel contains Billberry Extract (25% Anthocyanopsides) 25mg, Vitamin A 2,000 IU and Vitamin E 100 IU.

Hawthorn

Nature's long-term assistant. Supports healthy cardiovascular function. Available in 400 mg capsules.

Jarrow Formulas®
Ashwagandha 3%

Standardized 3% with anolides. Available in capsule form (1,000 mg).

Silymarin 80%
Silybum marianum

150 mg. European Mil Thistle 30:1 concentrate yielding 80% or 120 mg Silymarin. Available in capsule form.

Longevity Science
Astragalus Root

Standardized Herbal Extract available in gel capsule 500 mg.

Gaia Herbs, Inc.
800-831-7780
www.gaiaherbs.com

Liquid Phyto-Caps

This company has many herbs in liquid filled vegetarian capsules. They also have a full line of tinctures and other formats.

Planetary Formulas
Astragalus Full Spectrum

Each tablet contains: Astragalus root extract (standardized to 0.4% 4'-hydroxy-3'methoxyisoflavone 7) Astragalyus root. (500 mg)

Cordyceps 450
Full Spectrum

Containing Cordyceps sinensis Mycelia CS-4 standardized extract (0.1% adenosine), Cordyceps sinensis Mycelia. In tablet form. (450 mg)

Ginger Full Spectrum

Contains Ginger Rhizome standardized extract 5% yielding 12.5 mg Gingerols, Ginger Rhizome in tablet form (350 mg).

Silymarin 80

Contains Milk thistle seed extract 80% yielding 168 mg mixed flavanolignans calculated as Silymarin in tablet form.

Source Naturals Inc.
Bilberry Extract

Contains 37% Anthocyanosides 50 mg and 100 mg in tablet form.

Oil of Oregano
Extracted from pure, wildcrafted oregano.

Three drops contain: Wildcrafted Oregano Oil (Origanum vulgare) (22 mg) yielding 70% carvacrol and Extra Virgin Olive Oil (41 mg).

Thorne Research
Asparagus Extract 170MG

Extract has been shown to protect the kidneys. In capsule form.

Berberine
Berbercap®

Each capsule contains Oregon Grape extract (root (Berberis aquifolium) (80% Berberine) 200 mg.

Vitamin Research Products
Artichoke Extract (Cynara Scolymus)

Available in capsule form (500 mg)

Astragalus Extract (Astragalus Membranaceus)

Available in capsule form (500 mg)

Billberry Extract (Vaccinium Myrtillus)

Available in softgels (60 mg)

Boswellia Serrata Extract
Available in capsule form (250 mg)

Bromelain Extract
Available in capsule form (250 mg)

Cat's Claw Extract (Uncaria Tomentosa)
In capsule form (100mg)
Garlic Extract (Allium Sativuim)
In capsule form (500 mg)

Ginger Extract (Zingiber Officinale)
In capsule form (250 mg)

Ginkgo Biloba Extract
Available in capsule form (60 mg) and (120 mg)

Ginseng Extracts
A combination of Korean and Siberian ginsengs. Available in capsule form (300 mg)

Grapefruit Seed Extract (Citrus Grandis)
In capsule form (125 mg)

Gymnema Sylvestre Extract
Contains 24% gymnemic acids. Available in capsule form (200 mg).

Horse Chestnut Extract (Aesculus Hippocastanum)
In capsule form (300 mg)

Immunomax
Effective immune-enhancing botanical extracts. Contains Astragalus 333mg, Cats Claw 33 mg, Echinacea purpurea 25 mg. Available in capsule form.

Propolis Extract
In capsule form (400 mg)

Rosemary Extract (Rosmarinus Officinalis)
In capsule form (300 mg)

Saw Palmetto Berry Extract (Serenoa Repens)
In capsule form (160 mg)

Silymarin Extract (Silybum Marianum)
In capsule form (175 mg)

St. John's Wort Extract (Hypericum Perforatum)
In capsule form (300 mg)

Stinging Nettle Extract (Urtica Dioica)
In capsule form (250 mg)

Uva Ursi (Arctostaphylos Uva-Ursi)
In capsule form (200 mg). A natural diuretic, good for urinary tract infections.

Hesperidin

Thorne Research
HMC Hesperidin™
In capsule form containing Hesperidin methyl chalcone 250 mg.

Immune Enhancers

Longevity Plus
Immuni-T
Dietary Supplement available in capsule form.

Indole-3-Carbinol

Longevity Science
Indole-3-Carbinol
Available in capsule form 400 mg

Thorne Research
Indole-3-Carbinol
In capsule form. Each capsule contains Indole 3-carbinol 200 mg.

Vitamin Research Products
Indole-3-Carbinol
In capsule form 250 mg.

Inositol

Vitamin Research Products
Inositol
Available in capsules (650 mg).

Inositol Phosphate-6

IP-6 International, Inc.
888-276-4ip6
www.ip-6.com

IP6™ with Inositol
Available in capsule and powder form. Contains 3.2g IP-6 per serving, 800 mg Inositol per serving. Formulation of IP-6 and Inositol was developed and patented by Dr. A.K.M. Shamsuddin, MD, PhD, at the University of Maryland.

Source Naturals Inc.
IP-6
Inositol Hexaphosphate 800 mg—Supports Breast, Colon and Prostate Cells
Three 800 mg tablets contain: Calcium (as calcium inositol hexaphosphate), Magnesium (as magnesium inositol hexaphosphate), IP-6 (as calcium and magnesium inositol hexaphosphate.

Vitamin Research Products
IP6 (Inositol Hexaphosphate)
This is a remarkable molecule that can enhance immunity activating natural killer cells. IP6 suppresses the body's production of free radicals. Available in capsule form.

Lactoferrin

Vitamin Research Products
Lactoferrin
The primary component of Colostrum. Available in capsule form (250 mg).

Larch Arabinogalactan

Vitamin Research Products
Larch AG™

The polysaccharide powder derived from the larch tree. Larch AG can be added to water or juice. Research shows it can be beneficial as a cancer protocol.

Liver Protection and Detoxification Aids

Thorne Research
T.A.P.S.™

Contains Milk Thistle extract (seed) (Silybum marianum) (80% Silymarin) 150 mg, Artichoke extract (flower) (Cynara scolymus) 150 mg, Turmeric extract (rhizome) (Curcuma Longa) 150 mg, Picrorhiza Kurroa extract (root) (4% Kutkin) 150 mg. Available in capsule form.

Vitamin Research Products
Hepatogen™

Contains Green Tea, Tumeric, Artichoke, Dandelion and other ingredients in capsule form.

Lutein

J.R. Carlson Laboratories, Inc.
Lutein 15 Mg Plus Kale

Each capsule contains 15 mg Lutein plus 100 mg Kale.

Source Naturals Inc.
Lutein

Antioxidant Carotenoid available in capsule form (6 mg and 20 mg)

Vitamin Research Products
Lutein Caps

Available in softgels (20 mg)

Lycopene

Healthy Origins
Lyc-O-Mato (With Olive Oil)

Contains "Clinical Strength" Lycopene 15 mg per softgel capsule.This non-GMO product, contains no genetically modified organisms. Clinical studies show olive oil when added to Lycopene enhances the absorption of the Lycopene.

Lyc-O-Mato Clinical Trio™

Antioxidant combination. Two capsules contain "Clinical Strength" dosages of Lycopene—30 mg, Selenium—200 mcg, and Natural Vitamin E—400 IU (with 100% mixed tocopherols including l-alpha, beta, gamma and delta tocopherols) in a base of olive oil.

Lyc-O-Mato Plus

Clinically proven Lycopene/Selenium combination for optimal prostate cancer protection. Two capsules contain: Lycopene—30 mg and Selenium—200 mcg. This non-GMO product contains no genetically modified organisms in a base of olive oil.

Vitamin Research Products
Lycopene

An important preventive against diseases of the lungs and prostate. Available in sofgels (10 mg).

Magnesium

Longevity Science
Magna-Calm

Lemon-flavored citrate in powdered form.

Source Naturals Inc.
Magnesium Malate
1,000 mg yielding 825 mg of Malic acid

Three 1,000 mg tablets contain: Magnesium (as magnesium malate) and Malic acid (as magnesium malate)

Thorne Research
Magnesium Citrate

Each capsule contains Magnesium (as Magnesium Citrate) 150 mg.

Vitamin Research Products
Magnesium Ascorbate

Available in capsule form.

Opti-Mag

Contains five different forms of magnesium for excellent absorption. Available in capsule form.

Medium Chain Triglyceride Oil

Vitamin Research Products
MCT Oil

Medium chain Triglycerides, which burn rapidly in the cells and do not contribute to fat storage. Available in sofgels (1000 mg) and also in liquid form.

Melatonin

Source Naturals Inc.
Melatonin Sublinguals

Available in Orange and Peppermint (1mg, 2.5 mg and 5 mg)

Thorne Research
Melatonin-5

Each capsule contains 5 mg Melatonin. Also available in 3 mg and 1 mg.

Vitamin Research Products
Melatonin

Available in capsule form (3mg, 750 mcg, 10mg).

Men's Health Supplements

Dr. Donsbach
888-950-2190
www.donsbach.com

PC Plus
(Replacement for PC SPES) Being used to treat prostate cancer.

This new product formulated by Dr. Donsbach contains virtually the same herbal ingredients that were in PC SPES. The herbs used are Saw Palmetto, Baikal Skullcap, Rabdosia, Licorice, Dyers Wood, Ginseng (Panax), Mum. Also contains sterolins (including 160 mg beta-sitosterol) 400 mg, Quercetin 150 mg. Carried by the following companies:

Thorne Research
Prostate-Guard™

Product designed for individuals having an increased risk of prostate cancer in capsule form.

Vitamin Research Products
PCF (Prostate Care Formula)

Developed by Shari Lieberman, PhD and Friedrich Douwes, M.D., to stimulate immune response. Contains Zinc, Selenium, Quercetin, Beta Sitosterol, Boswellia Serrata, Saw Palmetto, Pygeum, Nettle, and Lycopene. Take three capsules three times per day on an empty stomach.

Methyl-sulfonyl-methane

Vitamin Research Products
MSM

The natural form of organic sulfur. It is also a free radical scavenger. Available in capsule form (500 mg). Also available in powder form.

Minerals

J.R. Carlson Laboratories, Inc.
Chelated Mineral Compleet™

A complete and balanced formulation of major and trace minerals which are chelated and/or complexed by the Albion Patented Process. Available in tablet form.

Selenium

Each capsule contains 200 mcg of Selenium from L-Selenomethionine.

Source Naturals Inc.
Life Minerals™ No Iron

Available in tablet form.

Thorne Research
Chromium Picolinate

Each capsule contains Chromium (as Chromium Picolinate) 500 mcg.

Trace-Minerals

A balanced trace mineral formulation in capsule form.

Vitamin Research Products

Advanced Essential Minerals

A formulation especially designed for seniors. Contains no iron. Available in capsule form.

Modified Citrus Pectin

Longevity Science

Pecta-Sol™

Available in powder and capsule form.

Source Naturals Inc.

Modified Citrus Pectin

Powder

Two teaspoons (5 g) of Modified Citrus Pectin powder contain Modified Citrus Pectin 5g.

Thorne Research

Fractionated Pectin Powder

Water-Soluble

Each scoop contains Fractionated Pectin 6.5 grams.

Vitamin Research Products

Modified Citrus Pectin

Easily absorbed in the gastrointestinal tract and is useful for energy metabolism. Suggested usage two teaspoons daily. Available in powdered form.

Multivitamin-and-Mineral Formulations

J.R. Carlson Laboratories, Inc.

Super 2 Daily™

Easy to swallow softgels. Two softgels supply a super-strength, iron-free, balanced formula rich in EPA & DHA and also contains Lutein.

Jarrow Formulas®

Longevity Multi™

Iron-free vitamin-mineral formula with Methyl B12, Lutein, Lycopene, Silymaarin, and Grape Seed OPCs available in capsule form.

Longevity Science
Revitalize

Multivitamin and mineral complex with botanical detoxifiers and antioxidant. Contains no iron. Available in capsule form.

Source Naturals Inc.
Life Defense™
Multinutrient Program

Fifty-plus nutrients offer a comprehensive, balanced, and potent formula. Available in tablet form.

Life Force™ Multiple
No Iron

Available in tablet form.

Thorne Research
Basic Nutrients I

Without copper and iron. Aspartate Formula in capsule form.

Vitamin Research Products
Extend® Core

Complete vitamin and mineral supplement in capsule form. Three capsules per day formula.

Extend® One

A comprehensive formulation with no iron. Available in capsule form. One capsule per day formula.

Optimum Silver

Formulated for the health needs of mature men and women. It provides a foundation of balanced nutritional ingredients plus extra ingredients like calcium, vitamin K, magnesium, ginkgo biloba and choline. Also contains a digestive system-aiding bacteria. Contains no iron. Six capsules per day formula.

Mushrooms

Carotec, Inc.
Maitakegold404™

The MD fraction contains beta—1,6 glucan with beta 1,3 branched chains—these are special polysaccharides extracted from maitake under a patented process. Available in a vegetarian capsule (15 mgs)

Garden of Life
RM-10™

A proprietary blend of 10 different mushrooms and aloe vera extract. Available in caplet form.

Maitake Products, Inc.
800-747-7418
www.maitake.com
Grifon®-Pro D-Fraction®

Alcohol-Free Extract

One drop of Grifron®-Pro D-fraction® contains approximately 1.1 mg of pure Maitake D-fraction.

Planetary Formulas
Maitake Beta-Factor
Dr. Nanba's

Contains Calcium, Maitake Fruiting body, Maitake Mycelia biomass, Vitamin C, Pure Maitake Beta Glucan fraction in tablet form (163 mg).

Maitake-Pro
Dr. Nanba's

Contains Calcium, Maitake Fruiting body, Maitake Mycelia Biomass, Vitamin C, Pure Maitake Beta Glucan fraction in tablet form double strength (1050 mg).

Thorne Research
Maitakegold™
Liquid

Four drops contain Standardized Extract from Maitake Mushroom (Grifola frondosa) 5.72 mg, Vitamin C 4 mg.

Vitamin Research Products
10 Mushroom Combination

Take between meals in capsule form.

Reishi Mushroom Extract (Ganoderma Lucidum)

Available in capsule form (380 mg)

N-Acetyl Cysteine

Source Naturals Inc.
N-Acetyl Cysteine
Each tablet contains 600 mg and 1000mg N-acetyl cysteine.

Vitamin Research Products
N-Acetyl Cysteine (NAC)
Available in capsule form (600 mg)

Narinase

Thorne Research
Naranise
Available in capsule form containing Naringin 300 mg and Bromelain (2,000 m.c.u./gm) 100 mg.

Nutritional Yeast

Biocodex Laboratories
988-356-7787
www.biocodexUSA.com

Cistrudex™
Flurastor™
Energy supplements containing *Saccharomyces boulardii.*

Olive Leaf Extract

Source Naturals Inc.
Olive Leaf Extract™
Contains 500 mg with 75 mg of oleuropein.

Thorne Research
Olive Leaf Extract
Each capsule contains Olive Leaf extract (20% oleuropein) 500 mg.

Vitamin Research Products
Olive Leaf Extract
Anti-viral, anti-bacterial and anti-fungal benefits. (6% oleuropein) in capsule form (500 mg).

Omega-3 Oils

J.R. Carlson Laboratories, Inc.
GLA

Derived from Black Currant Seed Oil. Available in softgel containing 75 to 85 mg of Gamma-Linolenic Acid and 65 mg of Alpha-Linolenic Acid.

Super DHA™

A softgel containing 500 mg DHA and 200 mg EPA.

Super Omega-3™

Contains special concentrate of fish oil from deep cold-water fish. Available in softgel containing 300 mg EPA and 200 mg DHA.

Oceana™
866-627-4631
www.oceanaproducts.com

Virgin Salmon Oil

Contains Omega-3 fatty acids 250 mg, EPA 80–120 mg, DHA 80–120 mg, and other Omega-3 fatty acids 50 mg. Has a natural lemon flavoring and is available in softgel and liquid form.

Omega-Brite
888-43-OMEGA
www.omegabrite.com

Omega-3 Fish Oil

98% pure Omega-3 fish oil.

Plant Sterols and Sterolins

EPI
877-297-7332
www.moducare.com

Moducare®

Naturally and safely balances, strengthens, and restores the immune system. Formulation of sterols and sterolins in a 100:1 ratio. There are over 4,000 scientific and medical studies on these plant nutrients.

Thorne Research
Moducare®
Each capsule contains 20 mg Sterols and 200 mcg Sterolins

Potassium

Vitamin Research Products
Potassium Caps
Provides two highly bioavailable forms of potassium, potassium chloride (25 mg) and potassium succinate (74 mg). Available in capsule form.

Probiotics

Garden of Life
Primal Defense™
A natural whole food certified organic probiotic blend of homeostatic soil organisms. Contains fourteen different non-dairy probiotic strains including lactobacillus acidophilus, lactobacillus bulgarus, and lactobacillus plantarum in 900 mg caplets.

Longevity Science
Enteropro™
Enteric-coated Probiotic Formula in a vegetarian capsule.

Source Naturals Inc.
Acidophilus
Stabilized Acidophilus Culture in capsule and powder form (300 mg).

Life Flora™
Acidophilus/Bifidus Complex available in capsule and powder form (300 mg and 500 mg).

Vitamin Research Products
Biopro™
Contains over one billion organisms with a long shelf life, even without refrigeration. Available in capsule form.

Culturelle™
High potency—controls overgrowth of harmful bacteria. Contains Lactobacillus GG in capsule form.

Prostate Health

Specialty Pharmacy
Saw Palmetto Pygeum Plus

Contains Nettle and lycopene, important in prostate health. Nettle is a powerful anti-inflammatory.

Longevity Science®
Pecta-sol
Modified citrus pectin. Made to maintain highest standards of purity.

Pycnogenol®

Source Naturals Inc.
Pycnogenol®

Proanthocyanidin Complex available in tablet form at 25 mg, 50 mg, 75 mg, and 100 mg.

Each tablet contains Maritime Pine Bark Extract (Pycnogenol® yielding 90% Proanthocyanidins and Organic Acids).

Quercetin

Jarrow Formulas®
Quercetin 500

500 mg in capsule form. From Eucalyptus.

Source Naturals Inc.
Activated Quercetin™

Three tablets contain Vitamin C (as magnesium ascorbate) 600 mg, Magnesium (as magnesium ascorbate) 47 mg, Quercetin 1,000 mg, Bromelain (2,000 G.D.U. per gram) 300 mg.

Thorne Research
Quercetone®

Each capsule contains Quercetin chalcone 250 mg.

Resveratrol

Source Naturals Inc.
Resveratrol

Antioxidant Protection Available in tablet form (10 mg)

Vitamin Research Products
Resveratrol

Helps to inhibit tumor progression and initiation. Available in capsule form (5 mg)

Selenium

Source Naturals Inc.
Selenomax®

High-Selenium Yeast 100 mcg and 200 mcg Available in tablet form.

Thorne Research
Selenium Citrate

Each capsule contains Selenium (as Selenium Citrate) 200 mcg.

Vitamin Research Products
Selenium Caps

Each capsule supplies 100 mcg of selenium (50% Selenomethionine, 50% Selenium Amino Acid Chelate. In capsule form (100 mg).

Shark Liver Oil

Oceana™
Shark Liver Oil
Extracted from deepwater sharks.

Contains 120 mg Squalene and 120 Alkylglycerols. Available in softgel form.

Vitamin Research Products
Squalene

99.9% pure and extracted from liver oil of sharks. Available in softgels (1,000 mg)

Sleep Aids

Thorne Research
Sedaplus®

Calming botanicals relieve insomnia and promote restful sleep. Contains valerian, kava kava, hops, passion flower extract, and German chamomile extract in capsule form.

Vitamin Research Products
Herbal Sleep

Safe sleep inducing herbs including L-Theanine 150 mg, Hops 133 mg, Valerian 100 mg, and Passion Flower 133 mg in capsule form.

Taurine

Thorne Research
Taurine

In capsule form (500 mg)

Thymus Supplements

Longevity Science
Proboost™

Available in a packet containing 4 mcg freeze-dried purified protein A calf thymus. Also available in a sublingual capsule.

Source Naturals Inc.
Thymic Peptide

A non-animal version of a bovine thymic preparation. One tablet contains: Calcium 60 mg, Thymic Peptide 100mg.

Vitamin Research Products
Proboost Thymic Protein A

Boosts immune function and stamina. Administered sublingually contains 4 mcg. Standard preventive dose is 2–4 mcg's per day. For those with severe ailments take up to 12 mcg per day.

Tocotrienols

Vitamin Research Products
Tocomin Palm Oil (Tocotrienols)

Also contains small amounts of natural carotenoids, phytosterols, and squalene. Available in softgels (572 mg)

Vitamin A

Thorne Research
Vitamin A

Each capsule contains Vitamin A (Palmitate) 25,000 IU. Preservative-free.

Vitamin Research Products
Vitamin A
Available in softgel providing 25,000 IU

Vitamin B

J.R. Carlson Laboratories, Inc.
B-12 SL
Dissolves in mouth. Available in tablet form 1,000 mcg.

B-50-Gel
Available in softgel. 50 mg of each B vitamin except for B_{12}, 50mcg, folate 400 mcg, and Biotin 50 mg.

B Compleet™
B-Compleet provides all the B-Vitamins plus Vitamin C in a balanced formulation. Available in tablet form.

Niacin-Amide
Available in tablet form 100 mg or 500 mg.

Pantothenic Acid
Available in tablet form 250 mg.

Vitamin B_1 (Thiamine Hcl)
Available in tablet form 100 mg.

Vitamin B_2 (Riboflavin)
Available in tablet form 100 mg.

Vitamin B_6 Liquid
Each teaspoon supplies 200 mg of Vitamin B_6.

Carotec, Inc.
Bio B-Complex
Each capsule contains 25 milligrams of each of the "marco" B-vitamins (B_1, B_2, B_6) plus pangthothenic acid; 25 micrograms of B_{12} and D-biotin; 200 micrograms of folic acid; 80 mg of Bioperine®.

Perque LLC
800-525-7372
www.perque.com
B-12 Guard
B-12 Sublingual

Source Naturals Inc.
Coenzymate™ B Complex

This complete B Complex is available in both an orange sublingual and peppermint sublingual. Also available in sublingual form are Vitamins B_1, B_2, B_3, B_5, B_6 and B_{12}.

Thorne Research
Basic B Complex

Contains the entire B Complex in capsule form.

Cobamamide™

Available in capsule form (1,000 mcg).

Vitamin B_2
Riboflavin 5' Phosphate

In capsule form containing 36.5 mg.

Vitamin B_3
Niasafe-600®

In capsule form (510 mg).

Vitamin B_5
Pantethine

Contains 250mg in capsule form.

Vitamin B_6
Pyridoxal 5' Phosphate

Each capsule contains Vitamin B_6 (from 50 mg Pyridoxal 5'-Phosphate) 33.8 mg.

Vitamin Research Products
B_3 (Inositol Hexanicotinate)

Each capsule provides 500 mg niacin and 125 mg of inositol.

B_3 (NADH)

Available in tablet form in either 5 mg or 10 mg.

B_3 (Niacinamide)
Available in capsule form (500 mg).

B_5 (Calcium Pantothenate)
Available in capsule form (545mg).

B_5 (Pantethine)
Available in capsule form (140mg).

P5P (Pyridoxal-5-Phosphate) B6
Available in capsule form (50mg).

B_6 (Pyridoxine HCl)
Available in capsule form (100mg).

B_{12} (Methylcobalamin, Sublingual)
Each ml (one eyedropper) provides 1000 mcg of vitamin B_{12}.

Vitamin B
Extension B-Plex
Provides all the B vitamins. Available in capsule form.

Vitamin C

Pure Encapsulation, Inc
Ascorbyl Palmitate 500 mg.
Buffered Ascorbic Acid capsules 1000 mg.
Buffered Ascorbic Acid powder.

Vitamin Research Products, Inc
Ascorbyl Palmitate (fat soluble vitamin C)
Comes in 400 mg capsules.

Balance (Buffered Vitamin C Drink Mix)
Recommended dose ½ to 1 tsp per day (300 grams). Contains 2,800 mg Vitamin C plus other ingredients.

Mag-C (buffered vitamin C)
Contains 700 mg magnesium ascorbate and 50 mg magnesium.

Vitamin D

Vitamin Research Products
D3 (Cholecalciferol)
One gram supplies 1000 IU of Vitamin D in capsule form.

Vitamin E

J.R. Carlson Laboratories, Inc.
Key E® Powder
Vitamin E Powder
Each level small capful contains approximately 200 IU of Vitamin E (d-alpha-tocopheryl succinate)

Key E® Tablets
E Succinate
Available in chewable tablets l00 IU, 200 IU, and 400 IU.

Tocotrienols
An all-natural source of alpha, beta, gamma and delta tocotrienols with 100 IU of Vitamin E. Available in softgels.

Carotec, Inc.
Vitamin E
Each softgel contains 200 IU alpha tocopherol, 75mg gamma tocopherol, 28 mg delta tocopherol, and 1 mg beta tocopherol.

Healthy Origins
Natural Vitamin E 400IU
Formulated with 100% mixed tocopherols including d-alpha, beta, gamma, and delta tocopherols. No oil fillers. Available in softgels.

Jarrow Formulas®
E-400 (Dry)
Contains 400 IU of 100% Natural d-alpha Tocopheryl succinate. Available in capsule form.

Thorne Research
Ultimate-E (mixed Tocopherols)—500 IU.
Each gelcap contains d-Alpha tocopherol, Beta tocopherol, Gamma tocopherol, and Delta tocopherol.

Vitamin Research Products
D-Alpha Tocopheryl Succinate and Mixed Tocopherols
Vitamin E
Available in capsule form (300 IU)

E-Team
A complete Vitamin E with Tocolpherols and Tocotrienols.

Vitamin K

Vitamin Research Products
Vitamin K (Phytonadione)
Available in capsule form (150 mcg)

Whey Protein

Thorne Research
Hydrolyzed Lactalbumin Protein
Pure Whey Protein
Whey protein boosts level of glutathione in a powder form.

Women's Health Supplements

Thorne Research
Breast-Guard™
Nutritional support for oncology patients in capsule form.

Vitamin Research Products
BCF (Breast Care Formula)
Developed by Dr. Shari Lieberman, PhD. and Friedrich Douwes, M.D.; addresses nutritional needs for women with existing breast care concerns. Available in capsule form. Supports healthy immune functioning.

Zinc

Thorne Research
Zinc Picolinate
Each capsule contains Zinc (as Zinc Picolinate) 15 mg.

Vitamin Research Products
Zinc Monomethionine
This is a 1:1 chelated complex of the antioxidants zinc and methionine. In capsule form (25 mg)

Organic Foods

Culinary Herbs

Natural Lifestyle
800-752-2775
www.natural-lifestyle.com

Certified organic culinary herbs that are nonirradiated, unfumigated, and packed in glass spice jars. Include basil leaves, bay leaves, cayenne pepper, garlic powder, and others.

Eggs

The Country Hen
508-982-5414

Egg contains 170 mg omega-3-FA

EGG-LAND'S Best
1-800-922-3447

Each egg contains 100 mg omega-3-FA. Vegetarian fed hens. Cage free.

Gold Circle Farm Eggs
303-381-8100

Each egg contains 150 mg of omega-3-FA

Flaxseeds

Living Tree Community Foods
800-260-5534
www.livingtreecommunity.com
Organic Golden Flax

Golden flax seeds are larger and softer than the dark brown flax seeds. They have a mild nutty flavor that is really delicious mixed in food. It is also a known source of potassium, magnesium, and boron.

Omega Nutrition
800-661-3529
www.omeganutrition.com

Flax Of Life—Cold-Milled Organic Flax Seeds
Certified organic flax seeds, vacuum packed in a lined, resealable foil bag to retain freshness.

Tree of Life®
www.treeoflife.com
Many health food stores are supplied by a company known as Tree of Life, a distributor of high quality natural foods at moderate prices. Among the many products they carry are frozen organic vegetables, organic fruits, organic extra virgin olive oil, organic tomato sauce products and many others.

Vitamin Research Products
Flax Seed
Dakota Flax Gold. These tiny golden seeds have a rich nutty flavor. Available in seed form.

Mushrooms

Natural Lifestyles
800-752-2775
www.natural-lifestyle.com

Shiitake Mushrooms
High-grade shiitakes in various forms. Shiitakes medicinal capabilities are being used worldwide

Oils

Living Tree Community Foods
800-323-5534
www.livingtreecommunity.com
Living Tree has a raw organic olive oil that is not pressed. It's centrifuged at 75 degrees Fahrenheit, room temperature.

Olive Oil
Made from unrefined, extra-virgin olives that are fresh-pressed and Omegaflo® bottled.

Poultry

Sheltons Poultry, Inc.
800-541-1833
www.sheltons.com

Free-range chickens and turkeys with no added antibiotics. The taste quality of these natural products is far superior to products that are laced with all sorts of additives and hormones. Available in natural food stores.

Sweeteners

Omega Nutrition
800-661-3529
www.omegahealthstore.com

A selection of Stevia products in powdered form and in liquid form and also packet form.

Vitamin Research Products
800-877-2447
www.vrp.com

Unique Sweet®
(Xylitol Crystals)

A unique sweetener in powdered form. Also available in a variety of Xylitol gums.

Wisdom of the Ancients®
800-899-9908
www.wisdomherbs.com

Natural sweetener made from whole leaf Stevia *(Stevia rebaudiana Bertoni)* 6:1 concentrated extract. Available in concentrated tablets, liquid, and as a tea. Hundreds of scientific studies have been conducted on Stevia's effectiveness as a nutritional addition to the diet.

Tea

Maitake Products, Inc.
800-747-7418
www.maitake.com

Maigreen™Tea

Contains organically grown maitake mushroom and premier Japanese green tea (matcha) leaves. Low in caffeine. Available in tea bags.

Rishi Tea
866-747-4483 (866-RISHI TEA)
www.rishi-tea.com

Rishi offers more than two dozen certified organic teas, including ten green tea varietals. While the positive health benefits of regular consumption of green tea are now well documented, this company sells only high quality loose tea including Rooibos Tea, Pu-erh Tea, White Tea, and others.

Triple Leaf Tea, Inc.
800-552-7448
www.tripleleaf-tea.com

Effective authentic, traditional Chinese green, naturally decaffeinated green, medicinal and diet teas, made with authentic Chinese herbs and traditional herbal formulas, packaged in convenient tea bag form. All teas are GMO-free. Triple Leaf's Decaf Green Tea and Decaf Green Tea blends uses a natural solvent-free carbon dioxide decaffeination process. They also carry Decaf Green Tea with Ginseng, Ginko and Decaf Green Tea, American Ginseng Herbal Tea, Ginger Root Tea and Detox Tea.

Water

Mountain Valley Spring Water
800-643-1501
www.mountainvalleyspring.com

This water company has been bottling and distributing their pure spring water since 1871. They are one of the few bottled water companies that still offer some of their products in glass.

Penta™ Purified Drinking Water
800-531-5088
www.hydrateforlife.com

This company uses a system of purifying their water that has less dissolved solvents than either distilled or reverse osmosis purified water.

Index